Your Complete Guide to the
Arizona National Scenic Trail

Matthew J. Nelson
and the Arizona Trail Association

 WILDERNESS PRESS ... *on the trail since 1967*

Your Complete Guide to the Arizona National Scenic Trail

1st EDITION 2014
 3rd printing 2016

Copyright © 2014 by the Arizona Trail Association

Editors: Susan Haynes and Laura Shauger
Project editor: Ritchey Halphen
Overview map: Courtesy of the Arizona Trail Association
Passage maps: Aaron Seifert
Cover design and elevation profiles: Scott McGrew
Text design: Annie Long
Indexer: Galen Schroeder / Dakota Indexing

ISBN: 978-0-89997-747-8; eISBN: 978-0-89997-748-5

Manufactured in the United States of America

Published by: 🐾 **WILDERNESS PRESS**
        An imprint of AdventureKEEN
        2204 First Avenue South, Suite 102
        Birmingham, AL 35233
        800-443-7227
        wildernesspress.com

Distributed by Publishers Group West

FRONT-COVER PHOTOS *Top:* Passage 38, Matthew J. Nelson. *Bottom grid, clockwise from top left:* Passage 20, Robert Luce; Passage 3, Robert Luce; Passage 37, Fred Gaudet; Passage 10, Catherine Peterson; Passage 16, Bill Zimmerman; Passage 15, Scott Morris.

FRONTISPIECE Sunrise over the Rincon Mountains illuminates the Sonoran Desert along Passage 8 of the Arizona National Scenic Trail *(see page 91).* Photo: David Baker.

SAFETY NOTICE Though Wilderness Press and the authors have made every effort to ensure that the information in this book is accurate at press time, they are not responsible for any loss, damage, injury, or inconvenience that may occur while using this book. You are responsible for your own safety and health while in the wilderness. The fact that a trail is described in this book does not mean that it will be safe for you. Be aware that trail conditions can change from day to day. Always check local conditions, know your own limitations, and consult a map.

Overview Map

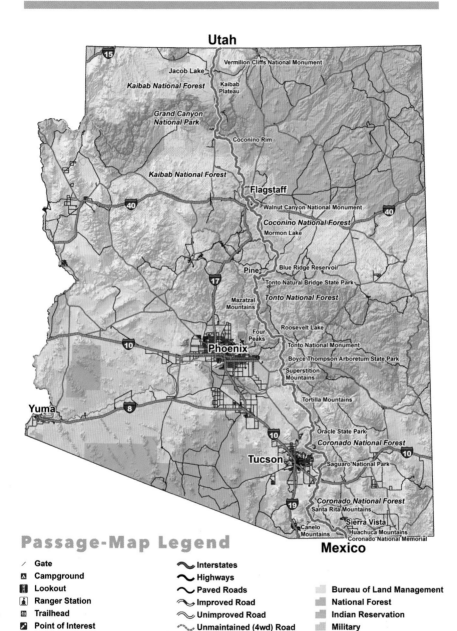

Utah

Vermilion Cliffs National Monument

Jacob Lake

Kaibab National Forest

Kaibab Plateau

Grand Canyon National Park

Coconino Rim

Kaibab National Forest

Flagstaff

Walnut Canyon National Monument

Coconino National Forest

Mormon Lake

Pine

Blue Ridge Reservoir

Tonto Natural Bridge State Park

Tonto National Forest

Mazatzal Mountains

Four Peaks

Roosevelt Lake

Phoenix

Tonto National Monument

Boyce Thompson Arboretum State Park

Superstition Mountains

Tortilla Mountains

Yuma

Oracle State Park

Coronado National Forest

Tucson

Saguaro National Park

Coronado National Forest
Santa Rita Mountains

Sierra Vista

Canelo Mountains

Huachuca Mountains

Coronado National Memorial

Mexico

Passage-Map Legend

⁄ Gate	〜 Interstates	
◭ Campground	〜 Highways	
🏠 Lookout	〜 Paved Roads	▨ Bureau of Land Management
🏠 Ranger Station	〜 Improved Road	▨ National Forest
🅃 Trailhead	〜 Unimproved Road	▨ Indian Reservation
⚑ Point of Interest	〜 Unmaintained (4wd) Road	▨ Military
⛷ Ski Area	🌀 Lake or Pond	▨ National Parks
〜 Other Trails	〜 Perennial Stream	▢ Private
〜 Arizona Trail (Current Passage)	〜 Intermittent Stream	■ Local or State Parks
〜 Arizona Trail (Adjacent Passages)	▢ Wilderness Boundaries	▨ State Trust
⁄ Railroads	▨ BLM National Monuments	▨ Wildlife Refuge

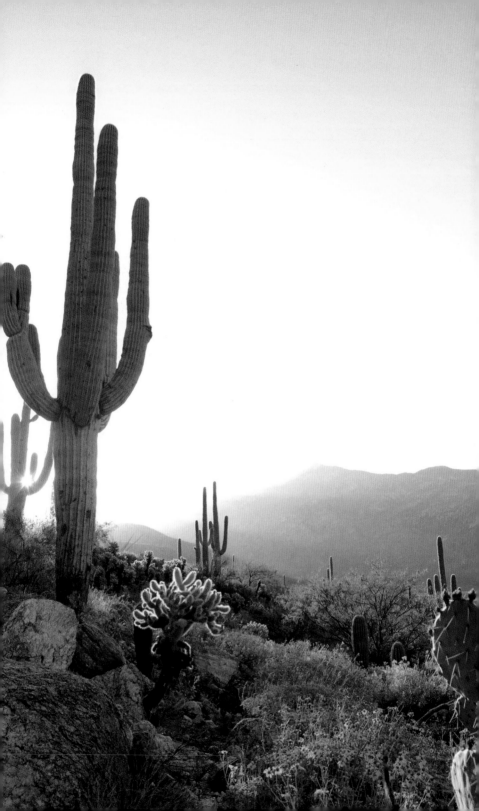

Contents

Dedication

THIS BOOK IS DEDICATED TO DALE R. SHEWALTER (May 16, 1950–January 10, 2010), the author of the following poem. His vision and leadership earned him the title "Father of the Arizona National Scenic Trail."

The Arizona Trail

In the land of Arizona
Through desert heat or snow
Winds a trail for folks to follow
From Utah to Old Mexico.

It's the Arizona Trail
A path through the great Southwest
A diverse track through wood and stone
Your spirit it will test.

Some will push and pedal
And some will hike or run
Others will ride their horse or mule
What else could be more fun?

Oh, sure, you'll sweat and blister
You'll feel the miles each day
You'll shiver at the loneliness
Your feet and seat will pay.

But you'll see moonlight on the borderlands
You'll see stars on the Mogollon
You'll feel the warmth of winter sun
And be thrilled straight through to bone.

The aches and pains will fade away
You'll feel renewed and whole
You'll never be the same again
With Arizona in your soul.

Along the Arizona Trail
A reverence and peace you'll know
Through deserts, canyons and mountains
From Utah to Old Mexico.

Acknowledgments

YOUR COMPLETE GUIDE TO THE ARIZONA NATIONAL SCENIC TRAIL is your ultimate resource for exploring and enjoying the AZT. This magnificent route from Mexico to Utah results from the efforts of thousands of hikers, mountain bikers, equestrians, trail builders, land managers, and donors who participated in building, maintaining, and sustaining the AZT for all. To them and all others who contributed in any way to the development of the trail and this guidebook, we offer our most sincere gratitude.

For that cadre of individuals primarily responsible for the production of this guidebook, we extend additional thanks. Those people include the trail stewards, regional stewards, the trail director, and the board of directors of the Arizona Trail Association (ATA). Seven other contributors deserve to be singled out for their roles in getting this book into your hands:

Sirena Dufault, director of the Arizona Trail Gateway Community Program, has cultivated relationships between trail users and the 32 towns along the trail. She wrote the guide to the AZT's Gateway Communities (see page 297) and authored several passage descriptions throughout the book. Sirena became involved with the Arizona Trail Association in 2007, helping build many miles of trail near Tucson, and she hiked the AZT in 2008–2009. Sirena came to Tucson from Chicago to attend the University of Arizona and has enjoyed exploring the diverse beauty of her adopted state through hiking, backpacking, canyoneering, and rafting.

Fred Gaudet is the ATA's vice president of trail operations, and he manages the association's *Water Source Databook*. For this guidebook, he was instrumental in providing accurate information on water sources (see Appendix 1, "Water Sources Along the AZT," on page 350). Where to locate water is, of course, among the most important items of information for day-trippers and thru-hikers alike. Fred hiked his way into the record books in 2012 when he became one of the few individuals ever to complete the "Triple Crown" of long-distance hiking: the Appalachian Trail, the Pacific Crest Trail, and the Continental Divide Trail. A noted photographer along the AZT, he serves up a panorama at **fredgaudetphotography.com.**

Terri Gay started dreaming of hiking the AZT in 1989, became actively involved with the trail in 2003, and finished section-hiking the route in 2009. She assists the

ATA with projects requiring graphic design, event planning, and promotion. She also compiled photographs and updated descriptions to make this guidebook a success.

Wendy C. Hodgson is coauthor, with Dr. Liz Slauson, of "The Diversity of Botany," starting on page 19. Wendy is the herbarium curator and research botanist at the Desert Botanical Garden in Phoenix, where she has worked since 1974. Her research delves into floristics—rare and endemic plants of the Southwest, particularly the Grand Canyon region; systematics of agaves and yuccas; and Sonoran Desert ethnobotany. She is the author and illustrator of *Food Plants of the Sonoran Desert* (University of Arizona Press), winner of the Mary W. Klinger Book Award presented by the Society for Economic Botany.

Rick Obermiller contributed two key sections to this book: "Welcome to the Geology of Arizona," starting on page 36; and "Geology Features of the AZT," starting on page 338. He has served as a trail steward, board member, and trail builder for more than a decade. Rick has lived in Arizona since 1972, graduated from Arizona State University, and has been hiking and backpacking throughout the state ever since. As an amateur geologist and mineral collector, he finds the Grand Canyon the perfect location for studying and appreciating the forces that have shaped Arizona and the planet.

Aaron Seifert, a certified geographic information systems (GIS) professional, created the passage maps for this book. Aaron has shown his passion for the outdoors by hiking, biking, backpacking, and trail maintenance since his years growing up in Colorado, then living in Phoenix, Sedona, and, currently, Flagstaff. He is a trail steward for Passage 34a. Visit **giseifert.com** for more information about his GIS products and services.

Dr. Liz Slauson is coauthor, with Wendy C. Hodgson, of "The Diversity of Botany." Liz is professor of botany and director of the herbarium at Scottsdale Community College. She holds a BS in urban horticulture and an MS and PhD in botany from Arizona State University. She served as the curator of collections, research botanist, and director of research during her 15-year tenure at the Desert Botanical Garden in Phoenix. As a scientific advisor and committee member, she also has been a key participant with the Center for Plant Conservation, the Texas Rare Plant Task Force and Recovery Team, the International Organization for Succulent Plant Study Congress, the Arizona Native Plant Society, the Boyce Thompson Arboretum, and the Malpai Borderlands.

–Matthew J. Nelson
Executive Director, Arizona Trail Association

(See page 387 for a profile of Matthew J. Nelson.)

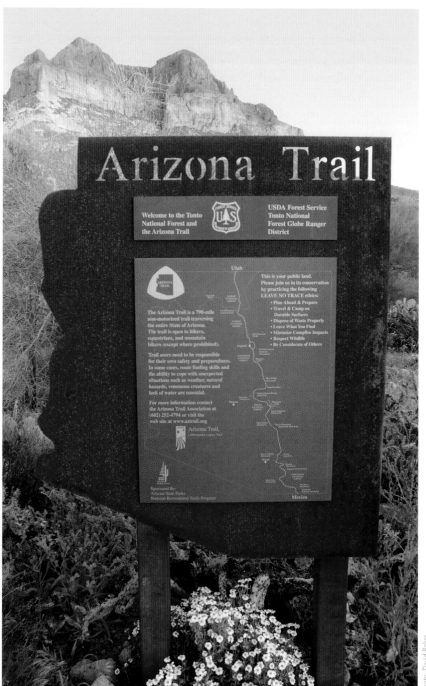

Stretching more than 800 miles through deserts, mountains, and canyons, the Arizona National Scenic Trail features biodiversity unlike that of any other trail.

Introduction

INTRODUCTION to the ARIZONA NATIONAL SCENIC TRAIL

ARIZONA EVOKES IMAGES of breathtaking landscapes, exotic animals, star-filled skies, and dramatic sunsets. Even for those who have never traveled through this wild part of the West, the very concept of the place suggests mystery, beauty, and allure. Glancing at a map of the state reveals an abundance of national forests, national parks, Native American reservations, and huge tracts of land free of roads, cities, or any other semipermanent footprint of modern society. From rolling grasslands and lush Sonoran Desert to alpine peaks and one of the world's deepest canyons, it is a land of biodiversity unlike anywhere else on Earth. This is Arizona.

And through its wild heart runs a single trail—an 800-plus-mile path from Mexico to Utah that links mountains, deserts, forests, canyons, rivers, communities, and people. This is the Arizona National Scenic Trail, or the AZT for short.

One of only 11 National Scenic Trails in the country, and only the third to be completed, the AZT beckons the adventurous at heart to explore the more remote and unknown regions of the state. But it also winds through the Grand Canyon, Saguaro National Park, and other famous natural wonders.

The AZT welcomes all nonmotorized forms of locomotion, and the diversity of trail users is one of the many phenomena that make it unique. On this trail, hikers, runners, and backpackers are just as common as mountain bikers and equestrians, and trail conflicts among these groups are almost unheard of. After all, they worked side-by-side to build the trail. At seasonal trail-maintenance events, you're just as likely to see folks in convertible pants and sun hats as in Lycra and helmets or cowboy hats and Carhartts. Such diversity helps define the trail.

Just because there is a trail through the entire state does not mean it's easily accessible every step of the way. While trailheads and signs exist, the AZT experience is intended to be a personal encounter with nature on its own terms. Unlike other long-distance trails, the AZT offers the possibility of your going for days without seeing humans other than your own companions. Many miles unfold between resupply services on some AZT passages. In fact, you might even forget that "civilization" exists. Yes, you'll see trail signs, but relying on them as a primary means of navigation is foolhardy. And then there's the dry Southwest's lack of water sources other than what you carry in, making a crossing of Arizona a very serious endeavor.

What you will need on this journey in the Grand Canyon State is a reliable guidebook, especially if you want to get to know Arizona a little more intimately. And now you have it—*Your Complete Guide to the Arizona National Scenic Trail*. Whether you plan to attempt the entire AZT in one crossing or, like most trail enthusiasts, will spend the next decade section-hiking (or section-biking or section-horseback-riding) the trail one passage at a time, this book will help you plan and navigate appropriately. We created it to inform, entertain, and inspire you.

Directions in these pages will lead you to trailheads, water sources, and the twists and turns you'll need to stay on the trail and keep from getting lost. You'll also find profiles on Gateway Communities—the small towns near the trail where you can make segues to basic supplies (such as Advil and peanut butter) and sustenance and services (Mexican food and massage therapy, for instance). Gateway Communities, by the way, make great weekend destinations for your one-day and overnight AZT adventures.

We've also included information about Arizona's geology and botany. The more you learn about the forces that shaped this wild landscape and the organisms that have adapted to live here, the more you'll become enamored of Arizona.

Most of all, we hope you enjoy the AZT. And in the words of the late, great Edward Abbey (as he wrote in *Desert Solitaire*), "May your trails be crooked, winding, lonesome, dangerous, leading to the most amazing view . . . where storms come and go as lightning clangs upon the high crags, where something strange and more beautiful and more full of wonder than your deepest dreams waits for you. . . ."

■ History

Dale Shewalter, a fifth-grade schoolteacher, had a dream, and that dream became the AZT. After attending college in Illinois, Dale wanted to hike the Appalachian Trail (AT), but he couldn't afford to do it right away. As a geophysicist, he felt Tucson would be a promising area for finding work and putting some money into the bank before striking out on the AT. But when he moved to Arizona, in 1974, his priorities soon changed: "I saw the Sonoran Desert, and I was instantly converted," he said.

Dale busied himself with work, volunteering at local schools, and getting his teaching certificate. He moved to Flagstaff in 1978 to teach full-time. His thirst for exploration was strong, and in 1982 he walked the length of the Mogollon Rim, the fantastic easterly–westerly escarpment that divides the lower-elevation deserts in southern Arizona from the pine-clad plateaus of the north. After completing this route, he started to look for a south–north hike. "I saw all the forests along the way, and I thought I could link them in one continuous hike," he recalled.

Thus, in 1985, Dale started near Nogales, along the Mexico–U.S. border, and made it to Flagstaff in just a couple of weeks. He continued on to Fredonia, a short distance from the Utah border, proving that a continuous trail linking the wildest parts of Arizona might be possible.

Immediately thereafter, he began traveling around the state giving presentations on his vision of a trail connecting communities, mountains, canyons, deserts, forests, public lands, historic sites, various trail systems, wilderness areas, and other points of interest. The idea was embraced by all types of trails users throughout Arizona and by official bodies that included Arizona State Parks; four national forests—Coconino, Coronado, Kaibab, and Tonto; the U.S. Bureau of Land Management (BLM); and the National Park Service (NPS). (Arizona's Prescott and Apache National Forests are not on the route, so they were not involved.)

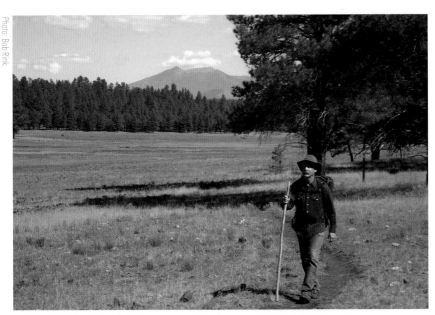

Photo: Bob Rink

Dale Shewalter, the "Father of the Arizona National Scenic Trail," walks a sinuous ribbon of trail he helped develop near the mountain town of Flagstaff.

Dale's presentation to the Arizona Hiking and Equestrian Trails Committee, an advocacy group for nonmotorized trails, was pivotal to the development of the AZT. Members' instant enthusiasm evolved into strong public and governmental support. Then–Governor Bruce Babbitt created a coalition focused on recreation and public lands, and Shewalter's dream gained momentum.

In the late 1980s Kaibab National Forest management hired Dale as the first paid coordinator for the AZT, and all the agencies noted above began establishing segments of the envisioned route. In 1988 the U.S. Forest Service (USFS) dedicated the first segment of the trail: it ran 54 miles, from Grand Canyon National Park's boundary, north toward Utah.

By 1990 two needs became apparent: a formal partnership among all pertinent governmental agencies to better coordinate efforts, coupled with communication and a nonprofit organization to lead the effort and sustain the trail into the future. Arizona State Parks assumed the lead role and employed coordinators for the AZT throughout the 1990s. To accomplish this work, and along with its own financial contributions, Arizona State Parks used funds from the four proximate national forests cited above, and from the BLM and NPS.

■ *Arizona Trail Association*

In 1994, the Arizona Trail Association (ATA) incorporated as a 501(c)(3) nonprofit organization and became an organized advocate for the trail that unites people from throughout the state: day-hikers, backpackers, equestrians, mountain bicyclists, runners, trail builders, nature enthusiasts, cross-country skiers, and packers (folks who use horses, mules, llamas, and other animals to haul gear). These committed individuals provided route identification to close the information gaps along the unfinished route. They became the volunteers necessary for building and maintaining the trail; created maps and provided GPS coordinates; identified water sources and resupply points; and raised money and awareness for the ATA. Individuals, families, and businesses purchasing memberships through the ATA have been a tremendous source of financial support since 1994, and they've been as important to building the trail as those physically charting the route.

Organized trail crews spent extended periods of time maintaining and repairing the trail. Those groups included various youth corps crews, Sierra Club service trips, American Hiking Society volunteer vacationers, scouting and college groups, Volunteers for Outdoor Arizona, REI service trips, Backcountry Horsemen of America,

International Mountain Bicycling Association trail-care crews, and many others. Much of the work took these trail crews deep into the backcountry, where logistics for a typical weekend volunteer work project are challenging.

Many large donors—from outdoor stores and clubs, to large corporations, to small businesses—have provided valuable funding for the AZT. Because of their generous donations, the trail was completed in record time. Additionally, many Land Managers have aggressively pursued Arizona Heritage Fund grants for the trail.

Since the new century began, the once seemingly impossible milestones include:

≈ seeking and gaining National Scenic Trail status;

≈ establishing easements and building the trail on Arizona State Lands in Pima and Pinal Counties;

≈ working to reestablish the trail in areas severely affected by major wildfires;

≈ traversing the challenging topography north of the Gila River;

≈ negotiating through private-land-owner opposition;

≈ developing outstanding maps and GPS data to better guide trail users through remote AZT areas;

≈ building the ATA to its current level of membership and community involvement;

≈ organizing events and trail work parties;

≈ creating AZT products.

Altogether, the above efforts have supported the ATA's mission to build, maintain, promote, protect, and sustain the AZT as a unique encounter with the land. It is a place for the adventure of a lifetime through some of the most incredible landscapes on Earth.

In sharing the more than 800 miles of the AZT, hikers, backpackers, equestrians, mountain bikers, cross-country skiers, nature photographers, and wildlife enthusiasts also take responsibility for its construction, maintenance, and preservation. The best way to support this spectacular long-distance trail is by becoming a member of the Arizona Trail Association (ATA). A 501(c)(3) nonprofit organization, the ATA welcomes contributions, whether in the form of membership dues or donations designated expressly for trail development. All contributions are tax-deductible.

To help ensure the legacy of the AZT and its important role in Arizona's history and its future, please contact the ATA:

Arizona Trail Association
P.O. Box 36736
Phoenix, AZ 85067
602-252-4794
aztrail.org

The ATA website provides up-to-date narrative information about the trail, GPS and map data, and a comprehensive databook. The latter is an online spreadsheet giving a play-by-play of the entire trail's water sources, intersections, and other vital information. The ATA relies on your membership dollars to support such endeavors.

Additionally, as a member, you can communicate with other long-distance trail users, land-management personnel, the 5 regional stewards, and some 100 trail stewards. The ATA website offers a complete, up-to-date list of the trail stewards, who are excellent resources regarding specific AZT passages. These committed individuals help keep the entire trail corridor healthy—physically maintaining the tread. They do this individually, with friends, and, when the need arises, with organized, major work events.

■ *Use at Your Own Risk*

Within nature are the great unknowns, that which attracts the adventurous among us to explore, attempt, and risk, with the hope of gaining an experience that will enrich our lives. Risk is always a factor in backcountry travel. Many of the activities described in this book can be dangerous, especially when weather is adverse or unpredictable or when unforeseen events or conditions create a hazardous situation.

The ATA has done its best to provide the reader with accurate information about backcountry travel, as well as point out some of its potential hazards. It is the responsibility of the users of this guide to learn the necessary skills for safe backcountry travel and to exercise caution in potentially hazardous areas. The ATA disclaims any liability for injury or other damage caused by backcountry traveling or performing any other activity described in this book. Use it at your own risk, accept responsibility for yourself and those around you, and be prepared for anything you may encounter along the way.

■ *Planning Your Trip*

Careful planning can eliminate many problems on the trail. For a long hike, you need to prepare an itinerary, arrange food drops and water caches, acquire and break in the gear you'll need, and get in shape—not necessarily in that order. Make a detailed checklist and review it carefully. No matter how much you prepare, however, you must remain flexible once you hit the trail because bad weather, illness, and other problems may upset the best-laid plans. In the words of AZT hiker and former Executive Director Dave Hicks, "Fail to plan—plan to fail."

When to Go

Avoid low deserts in the summer months and higher alpine areas in late fall, winter, and early spring. South–north travelers usually start sometime in late winter or early spring, while north–south travelers will need to start in late summer or early autumn. To maximize the experience and take advantage of the seasons, travel from Mexico's border to the Mogollon Rim in the springtime to catch the wildflowers, and from Utah to the Mogollon Rim in autumn to see the changing colors.

Permits

The NPS tightly regulates camping and travel in Saguaro National Park (Passage 9) and Grand Canyon National Park (Passages 37–39). Backpackers wishing to stay in these areas must reserve campsites well in advance. Permits are not required on most of the AZT as long as you're passing through, but you must get a permit to camp along the trail in certain areas.

The USFS and the BLM allow camping anywhere along the trail on most of the land they manage. Camping in Saguaro National Park and Grand Canyon National Park, both of which are managed by the NPS, requires a permit and is restricted to designated campgrounds. Colossal Cave Mountain Park charges a fee, and you must stay within the designated campground.

All areas of Arizona State Land require a permit if you camp or travel outside the 15-foot trail corridor. Approximately 95 miles of the AZT cross State Land. Though a permit is not required to use this part of the trail, trail users are encouraged to purchase one. That permit allows users to lawfully camp and wander outside the trail corridor, and funds collected from permits benefit state schools and other nonprofit organizations.

For a complete list of Land Managers and the contact information to obtain permits, consult Appendix 2, "Land-Management Agencies," on page 366.

Fences and Gates

Arizona has a long history of cattle ranching, mining, and homesteading. These brave families attempt to carve out a living in an inhospitable environment, and many of them have been in operation for generations. The AZT corridor was established with support from many of these families, with the understanding that trail users would have minimal impact upon the land and no adverse effect on their operations. Every trail user is an ambassador, and maintaining positive relationships with ranching families is necessary to keep this 800-plus-mile path from Mexico to Utah open and available to all.

You will encounter many gates and fences along the way, and because every one of them has pedestrian access, you'll never have to hop over a fence. The standard rule is this: close the gate unless it's been intentionally wired open. Even if you find the gate open, please close it. Gates that are accidentally left open, blown open by storms, or by cattle rubbing against them can separate animals from their water sources—a death sentence for the animal and a loss of precious resources for the family.

Backcountry Safety

The AZT was intentionally routed through wild, remote parts of the state to provide the backcountry traveler a primitive experience. In some places help will be far away, so preparing for hazards is essential. Anyone considering a hike along the AZT should carefully evaluate his or her ability to cope with potential dangers. Remember that self-rescue is always the primary means of dealing with an emergency, and is often the fastest. Search-and-rescue missions to assist lost or injured trail users can take a very long time, depending on how far from the nearest road they are.

Mobile-phone coverage is intermittent and unreliable along much of the AZT. Carrying a satellite telephone or personal rescue transponder is a better option, but neither of these pieces of equipment is a substitute for good trail sense and on-the-ground experience.

It's always smart to leave a detailed itinerary with a reliable friend or family member and check in regularly to acknowledge that you're OK and on-track. Knowing when a person was last seen or heard from is a vital piece of information for rescue personnel.

■ Water

The single biggest challenge of the AZT is finding, carrying—and consuming—enough water. Because water does not occur naturally throughout most of the state, you must carry enough for yourself or cache it ahead of time along the trail. Bringing enough of it can mean carrying an additional 25–30 pounds of liquid on your back for some passages. Consult Appendix 1, "Water Sources, Along the AZT" on page 350, to determine which passages may require caches of water.

The ATA has been building and installing bear boxes and metal storage containers at key locations along the trail to provide designated locations, reduce trash along the trail, minimize plastic bottles' sun exposure, and give trail angels specific places to leave fresh bottles for the next thirsty trail user. Community water caches are typically visible to the public, while private caches are usually hidden or marked with dates of anticipated use. Passages 1, 4, 5, 7, 13, 14, 18, 19, 20, 22, 23, 27, 31, 32, 33, and 40 list alternate access points in addition to the main southern and northern access points. Keep those passages in mind for expanding your proximity to water sources or for starting a hike or ride with ample water.

Rancher-developed water on leased federal land or State Land is the rancher's private property and cannot be used without first getting permission from the rancher, unless it's a life-or-death situation. Please respect the property rights of others.

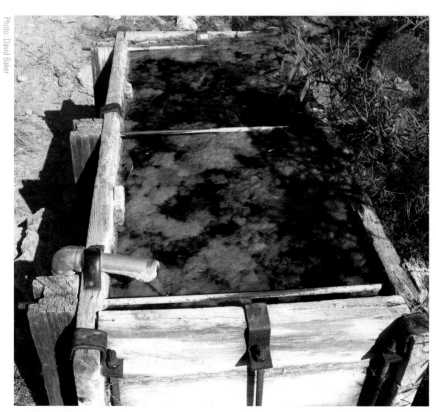

Photo: David Baker

You're more likely to encounter algae-filled cattle tanks than sparkling mountain streams on the AZT, but each water source is precious and should not be overlooked.

A GPS unit may be useful for making and finding water caches, but remember that the GPS is not foolproof and is subject to failure or operator error. Be confident that you can find your water caches without it.

▪ Contaminated Water

The greatest peril of drinking natural water is contamination, especially from *Giardia lamblia* and *Cryptosporidium,* small parasites that cause severe intestinal distress in humans. A lightweight water-filtration system is the best defense against such impurities. Always carry two means to treat water (chemical, mechanical, or ultraviolet, for example), in case one system fails or your supply dwindles. Drinking contaminated water is a better option than not drinking at all; you can survive a bout with giardia, but dehydration kills quickly.

▪ Dehydration

Arizona's low humidity, combined with the increased breathing rate you will likely experience when hiking strenuously, can result in potentially dangerous dehydration. Hikers may need a gallon of water per day, which they must carry or cache ahead of time along the route unless there are guaranteed natural sources. Consult "Appendix 1: Water Sources," as well as the ATA's website (**aztrail.org;** see the drop-down "Trail Resources" menu). On the website, you can easily connect with stewards, land managers, and many recent trail users to confirm water availability. (Also see "Conserve Water," on page 16.)

▪ Heat Exhaustion

The intense sun and heat along much of the AZT can pose a serious health threat during at least half the year. Heat exhaustion can overtake a person rapidly, and because disorientation and confusion are common symptoms, victims may never realize they are in trouble. Keep an eye on yourself and your companions, and take seriously such warning signs as chills, clammy skin, stumbling, muscle weakness, or nausea.

If heat exhaustion advances, it may turn into heatstroke, which is even more serious than heat exhaustion—and often deadly. Signs include the skin going from clammy to hot and dry, and unconsciousness may follow. Rapid and immediate cooling of the entire body is the only backcountry response, and emergency medical personnel should be contacted immediately.

■ *Hypothermia*

Arizona's weather is extreme and can change at any time. Even in the low-elevation deserts, snow and cold rain are possible. An emergency Mylar blanket, which is easy to fit into your first-aid kit, can help retain body heat in emergency situations.

■ *Flash Floods*

Floods kill several people each year, and often with just a few seconds' warning. Survivors have described flash floods as sudden, raging walls of water—not gradually increasing flows. To avoid these calamities, stay aware of the weather and the terrain. Flash floods occur when thunderstorms drop a large amount of rain and the ground cannot quickly absorb all of the water. Obviously, dark skies and the sound of distant thunder are warning signs, but floods can develop many miles away, and the storm may not be evident downstream.

As for terrain, floods follow established waterways and seek the lowest ground. Thus it is important not to camp or linger in dry washes or near streams or rivers, especially during the rainy season or thunderstorms. Low-lying areas that are not obvious waterways can also be inundated. Err on the side of caution and always camp on high ground. Never enter an enclosed canyon when thunderstorms are present or likely.

■ *Lightning*

This danger can strike anywhere, but it is most threatening at exposed high elevations, such as Arizona's sky islands, isolated mountain ranges rising from valleys or flat lands. Other examples the AZT user will encounter include the high ridges of such wilderness areas as the Superstitions, Mazatzals, and San Francisco Peaks. Lightning is most likely during Arizona's monsoon rainstorms of June, July, and August, and it usually occurs in the afternoon. If you become caught in a storm, look for a low, treeless spot, and squat there until the weather passes. A low-elevation stand of trees of uniform height can also make for a suitable shelter. Hiding in caves is dangerous as they provide an ideal conduit for ground currents.

■ *Animals, Reptiles, and Insects*

Most animals you encounter in the backcountry will be more frightened of you than you are of them. However, a large animal occasionally may exhibit protective or aggressive behavior. Animals and their prey, may be attracted by the smell of food. Maintain a clean camp and keep food in one place (such as a stuff sack) 100 yards from your tent to minimize the chance of confronting a hungry visitor. When there are trees near your campsite, hang food high off the ground from a slender branch.

Mountain lions and black bears inhabit Arizona but, for the most part, they are shy of humans. Black bears, which can be black or brown, have poor eyesight and will often stand up on their hind legs simply to get a better look at you. In the unlikely event that you have a threatening encounter with either creature, experts suggest standing up tall, waving your arms, making noise, and slowly backing up. Throwing rocks or a walking stick at a persistent mountain lion may also be effective. If a mountain lion attacks you, fight back.

The best defense against snakes, scorpions, and spiders is to avoid putting your hands and feet in places you can't see into, such as deep grass, rock crevices, and holes. The majority of snakebites occur on the hands and faces of victims because they are harassing the snake. If you see a rattlesnake, back away and leave the snake an escape route. This beautiful creature uses camouflage as its primary defense, its rattle as a secondary defense, and ots fangs as a last resort.

In spite of their reputation, rattlesnake bites are rarely fatal, although they are extremely painful and victims who are envenomated can lose muscle and tissue to

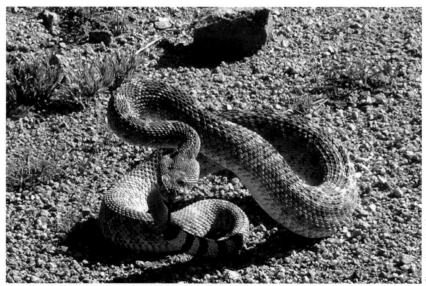

Arizona is home to 13 species of rattlesnakes, and during the warmer months you're likely to share the trail with a few of them.

necrosis. If you are bitten, remain as calm as you can and get professional medical attention as soon as possible. Keeping your heart rate down slows the spread of venom through your body. Do not apply a tourniquet, pack the bit with ice or ice water, cut the wound, or suck out the venom by mouth.

The Gila monster is a rare creature, one of only two venomous lizards in the world, with the ability to lock its jaw on a victim and pump venom into the wounds from ridges in its teeth. It has a flat snout, a thick, stubby tail, and black and orange (sometimes pink) dots. Watch it from a distance without harassing it, and you'll enjoy an exciting and rare sighting.

Africanized honeybees, also called killer bees, are hybrids of African bees and European honeybees, the most common bees in North America. Africanized bees are more aggressive and persistent, attack in larger numbers, and may pursue intruders farther from their hives than European bees do. Their venom is the same as that of the European bee. Because it is difficult to distinguish between the two kinds of bees, it is best to treat all bees with respect. Wear light-colored clothing and avoid shiny jewelry. If you enter an area with a lot of bees, move away calmly. Never swat or kill a bee, because sudden movements and the odor of an injured bee stimulate the attack instinct in Africanized bees.

If you are attacked by Africanized bees, run away and keep running. Cover your head and face with clothing, because these are the first places bees will sting. Seek shelter. Unleash pets so they can escape too. If you are stung, scrape away the stinger; squeezing it releases more venom.

Children are more vulnerable to all wild creatures than adults are, so keep an eye on them. Avoid direct physical contact with any wild animal, regardless of its size, and never feed them.

■ Mine Shafts

Thousands of abandoned mine shafts dot the hillsides of Arizona. They are unmaintained and are extremely dangerous. Not only are they subject to collapsing rock, but they also may contain toxic fumes that could overcome a careless explorer. And there is very little to see; they have been picked clean of any interesting artifacts. Give them a wide berth, and avoid the temptation to use them as shelter from rainstorms.

■ Snags

Snags are dead trees whose root structures may be decayed to the point that the tree is ready to topple over. They are particularly prevalent in burned areas that, unfortunately, are common along the AZT. Although the danger of being hit by a falling tree is slight, snags have killed people. Don't camp under snags (or large dead branches on live trees), and remember that even live trees are susceptible to blowing over in a strong storm.

Leave No Trace

As the popularity of backcountry adventures grows, it's the responsibility of each one of us who visits the American wilderness to preserve it in its natural state. Toward this end, the USFS and various partners developed the principles of **Leave No Trace,** which should govern the behavior of every visitor along the Arizona National Scenic Trail.

For more information on low-impact hiking and camping in various environments, contact the Leave No Trace organization at 800-332-4100 or **lnt.org.**

■ *Plan Ahead and Prepare*

By equipping yourself with the right equipment, maps, and information, you can reduce your impact on the land. If you know your route, for example, you're less likely to get lost and trample the vegetation. If you have an adequate sleeping bag, you won't need to build fires in sensitive resource areas to keep warm. Gathering knowledge of the terrain before your trip will help you pick appropriate campsites, plan your use of water, and prepare for the adventure ahead.

■ *Backcountry Etiquette*

Respect other visitors' desire for a remote backcountry experience by keeping a low profile and picking campsites screened from the trail by trees or terrain features— always following permit requirements (see "Permits," on page 7). When you meet other trail users, be courteous and give them room to pass. The standard rule is that mountain bikers and hikers yield to horses, and bikers yield to hikers—but the prudent hiker always makes room for a mountain biker. When encountering a horse or other livestock, move off the trail on the lowest side and talk to the rider and animal until everyone has passed. Don't make sudden movements or loud noises that might spook the horse or livestock.

■ *Travel and Camp on Durable Surfaces*

Most of the AZT follows established trails and roads. Hiking single-file and staying on the trail keeps you from trampling fragile plants and soft ground, which can take years to recover from boots, hooves, and tires. Be especially careful to avoid cryptobiotic soil

(soil with primitive organisms), which is essential to the ecology of arid lands. Please avoid disturbing these very sensitive soils.

In places where there is no trail or where it is necessary to leave the trail, walk on the most durable surfaces: rocks, dry ground, or a carpet of pine needles. Groups should fan out to disperse their impact. Equestrians should avoid stepping off the trail and traveling cross-country whenever possible. Mountain bikers should be cautious to avoid riding after storms, when tire tracks will create channels in muddy soils.

When camping, try to select an established campsite that has already seen a lot of use; camping in an established site helps preserve the surrounding area. For a tent site, choose hard, dry ground with the least amount of vegetation. Make sure your camp is at least 200 feet from streams, lakes, and trails. While moving about camp, be aware that each step is potentially harmful. If you are in a heavily used area, choose existing trails instead of tromping down new ones. In less-visited areas, try not to take the same route each time you travel around camp; this practice preserves any single area from becoming worn. Switch from hard-soled hiking boots to lightweight shoes once you arrive at camp.

■ Equestrians

Horses and mules are welcomed on the AZT, but please be sure they are in good condition. Several sections of the trail are unsafe for equines; plan your ride accordingly, and check the ATA website for current conditions. Forest fires, flash floods, and other uncontrollable events can impact the suitability of any one section of the trail.

If you plan to use pack animals on the trail, please learn to minimize the impact of large creatures. Bring collapsible buckets to carry water to the animals so they do not drink directly from streams and thereby damage stream banks. At camp, hitch horses to a highline. Avoid tethering them in a small area, which will concentrate their impact. Bring your own feed, and make sure it is certified weed-free to avoid introducing invasive plant species.

Locating adequate water for equines is a challenge on many passages. Often, you will need to haul water in for horses. You may want to carry a list of veterinarians willing to make "trail calls" from nearby communities, but be as self-sufficient in this regard as possible.

■ Leave What You Find

Leave the natural wonders along the trail for other visitors to enjoy. Don't break boughs off trees, hammer nails into trees, or pick flowers. It is unethical and illegal to remove cultural artifacts, such as potsherds and flaked stone. If you encounter ruins, consider viewing them from a distance.

■ *Use Fire Responsibly*

Travelers in the natural world have long regarded campfires as a source of warmth and comfort, providing a sense of security in the vast darkness of the outdoors. But fires have an unnatural impact on the environment, leaving scars, gobbling up nutrients, and sterilizing the soil. Mismanaged campfires have burned hundreds of thousands of acres throughout the Southwest, including portions of the AZT. A small backpacking stove provides a quick, efficient way to cook.

The AZT hiker is encouraged to experience the darkness of the forest or the desert on its own terms, without the glaring interruption of a fire. You'll see things you would have missed when blinded by flames, and you will hear sounds otherwise drowned out. If you must build a fire, make sure it's far from water sources or wetlands, in an area where there is an abundant supply of dead and downed wood. Never cut firewood from a standing tree, even if the tree is dead. Never build a new fire ring, though it's okay to use an existing ring. Or learn how to build a low-impact mound fire if you don't already know how. You can find how-to videos online.

■ *Conserve Water*

In the deserts and arid forests of Arizona, water is precious. Use it sparingly and avoid polluting it. On many stretches of the AZT, you'll have to carry your own water or cache it along the way. When you do encounter a water source, camp at least 200 yards away from it whenever possible. Use containers to carry water far from its source to bathe or cook. Don't let your animals trample stream banks or relieve themselves in water sources.

Arizona's rare riparian corridors—green strips of life cutting a line through the surrounding dry land—are inviting places for campers and hikers. But avoid the temptation to linger in these places. The vegetation is easily trampled, and the animals that rely on the water are frightened away by human presence.

Water is life, but it may be here today and can be gone tomorrow. If we treat it with care and respect, it's likely to be around a little bit longer.

■ *Pack It In, Pack It Out*

Please do not leave anything in the forest or the desert that wasn't there before you arrived, with the exception of human waste. Everything else, including toilet paper,

Photo: David Baker

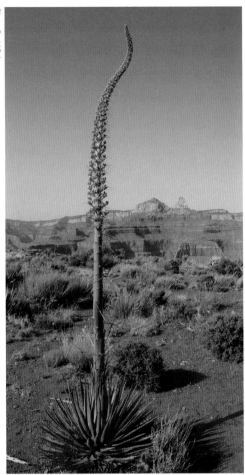

Fragile ecosystems, such as those along the Tonto Platform of the Grand Canyon, should be traversed with care. Here, plants grow by the inch and die by the foot.

personal hygiene items, and uneaten food, should be packed out. Most trash, even paper, will not burn completely in a campfire. Also, never feed animals. Leaving food for animals or feeding them directly habituates them to humans, alters their diet, and makes them less self-sufficient.

Waste Disposal

The best way to dispose of solid human waste is with the cathole method, which entails digging a hole 6–8 inches deep and filling it in with dirt after you use it. Catholes should be at least 200 feet from water or potential waterways, such as dry washes. Toilet paper should be packed out; a double plastic bag works well for this.

Use soap sparingly; even so-called biodegradable soap is an unnatural chemical in an outdoor environment. Never use soap near a water source. Use a small strainer to remove food particles when rinsing plates and pans, and pack out the solids. Spread the remaining wastewater over a large, dry area to disperse its concentration.

■ Wilderness Areas

The AZT passes through many designated wilderness areas. Within national forests are specially protected areas where, as the Wilderness Act of 1964 defines them, "the earth and its community of life are untrammeled by man, where man himself is a visitor who does not remain." Please follow these guidelines while traveling through the wilderness:

≈ Camp out of sight, at least 200 feet from lakes and streams, on dry, durable surfaces.

≈ Use a campstove. If you must have a fire, use existing fire rings, or build mound fires.

≈ Keep water sources clean by washing at least 200 feet from them.

≈ Bury human waste 6–8 inches deep and 200 feet from lakes and streams.

≈ Pack out toilet paper and other used toiletry items.

≈ Hobble or picket livestock at least 200 feet from lakes and streams, and use only treated, weed-free feed and grain.

≈ Keep all dogs on a leash.

≈ Do not ride a mountain bike in the wilderness.

≈ Pack out all trash; don't burn it.

The Botany of Diversity

By Wendy C. Hodgson and Dr. Liz Slauson

ARIZONA NOT ONLY OFFERS, but also *is,* beauty in all shapes, sizes, forms, and colors. Within this state's borders, myriad national parks, monuments, and other public lands reflect the great biological, geological, and cultural diversity that is its heritage. Arizona's geographical position and range of altitude and climates contribute greatly to its more than 4,000 vascular plant species (ferns, fern allies, and flowering plants) and to its overall plant variation. Here you'll find vegetation from tall columnars to tiny, almost invisible cacti, from succulent and nonsucculent trees and shrubs to alpine ground-huggers. In fact, according to NatureServe's 2002 report to The Nature Conservancy, only California and Texas outrank Arizona for diversity.

Additionally, no fewer than 13 natural biotic communities occur in Arizona, and the Arizona National Scenic Trail (AZT) travels through all of them except two: the Lower Colorado Desert subdivision of the Sonoran Desert and the Alpine Tundra. Characteristics of the latter two include the most extremes in elevation, temperature, and rainfall. Thus, the AZT is the most scenic route for viewing plant communities in Arizona.

But more than scenery unfolds within this botanical kingdom. Traveling along the AZT, trail users cross through cultural landscapes where past cultures—as far back as hundreds (if not thousands) of years—have altered plants and their habitats. This legacy remains apparent to those who look closely. For example, along the Saddle Mountain Passage in the Mazatzal Mountains grows the rare Tonto Basin agave (*Agave delamateri*), believed to be a living relict of plants once grown by pre-Columbian farmers.

In order of encounter along the trail's three regions, from South to Central to North, the botanical communities and the pertinent regions are as follows:

Arizona Upland (South and Central Regions)

Semidesert Grassland (South and Central Regions)

Interior Chaparral (South and Central Regions)

For further reading, the authors recommend *Biotic Communities: Southwestern United States and Northwestern Mexico,* edited by David Brown (University of Utah Press, 1994).

Madrean Evergreen Forest Woodland (South Region)

Plains Grassland (South Region)

Rocky Mountain Montane Conifer Forest (South, Central, and North Regions)

Great Basin Conifer Woodland (Central and North Regions)

Relict Conifer Woodland (Central Region)

Great Basin Desert Scrub (North Region)

Mohave Desert Scrub (North Region)

Subalpine Community (North Region)

The region-by-region lists below offer highlights of these diverse plant communities along the AZT. Within the three regions, all vegetation is listed in alphabetical order.

South Region (Passages 1–15)

From the Plains Grassland of Mexico's northern state of Sonora, at the southern beginning of the AZT, Madrean Evergreen Forest Woodland appears in the Huachuca Mountains before culminating in the Rocky Mountain Montane Conifer Forest at the mountain's top. **Proceeding north, AZT users descend into the oak- and grassland-dominated Canelo Hills area, where they can look for the following:**

Alkali sacaton (*Sporobolus airoides*)

Cane bluestem (*Bothriochloa barbinodis*)

Emory and Mexican blue oaks (*Quercus emoryi* and *Q. oblongifolia*)

Grama grasses (including *Bouteloua curtipendula, B. eriopoda, B. gracilis,* and *B. hirsuta*)

Indian rice-grass (*Achnatherum hymenoides*)

James galleta (*Hilaria jamesii*)

Plains lovegrass (*Eragrostis intermedia*)

Shrubs here include:

Arizona madrone (*Arbutus arizonica*)

Ashy silktassel (*Garrya flavescens*)

Coralbean (*Erythrina flabelliformis*)

Evergreen sumac (*Rhus virens* variety *choriophylla*)

Firecracker bush (*Bouvardia ternifolia*)

Hairy mountain mahogany (*Cercocarpus montanus* variety *paucidentatus*)

Manzanita (*Arctostaphylos pringlei* and *A. pungens*)

Ocotillo (*Fouquieria splendens*)

Tahitian kidneywood (*Eysenhardtia orthocarpa*)

Velvetpod mimosa (*Mimosa dysocarpa*)

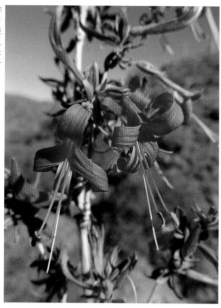

Photo: Wendy Hodgson

Hummingbird bush (*Anisacanthus thurberi*), commonly found within the Arizona Upland and Interior Chaparral ecosystems, provides ample nectar for pollinators.

Among the riparian trees visible along the Southern Region are:

Arizona sycamore (*Platanus wrightii*)

Frémont cottonwood (*Populus fremontii*)

Netleaf hackberry (*Celtis reticulata*)

New Mexican locust (*Robinia neomexicana*)

Seep-willow (*Baccharis salicifolia*)

Velvet ash (*Fraxinus velutina*)

Here are the noted leaf and stem succulent plants that will catch your eye:

Beargrass (*Nolina microcarpa*)

Cane cholla (*Cylindropuntia spinosior*)

Fendler hedgehog cactus (*Echinocereus fendleri* variety *fendleri*)

Hoary yucca (*Yucca madrensis* [synonym, *Y. schottii*])

Rainbow hedgehog cactus (*Echinocereus rigidissimus*)

Sotol (*Dasylirion wheeleri*)

Significant among the region's numerous herbaceous plants are:

Dwarf morning-glories (*Evolvulus alsinoides, E. arizonicus,* and *E. sericeus*)

Fameflower (*Phemeranthus aurantiacus* [synonym, *Talinum aurantiacum*])

Jewel-of-opal (*Talinum paniculatum*)

Mexican star (*Milla biflora*)

Morning-glories (including *Ipomoea costellata, I. cristulata,* and *I. longifolia*)

Purslanes (*Portulaca pilosa, P. suffrutescens,* and *P. umbraticola*)

Saiya (*Amoreuxia palmatifida*)

Southwestern cosmos (*Cosmos parviflorus*)

Still in the Southern Region, in the foothills of the Santa Rita Mountains, you transition from Semidesert Grassland to the Madrean Evergreen Forest Woodland, then descend through Arizona Upland and Interior Chaparral, and then back to Semidesert Grassland near the Empire Mountains. **At the very top of the Santa Catalina Mountains, you can encounter a relatively small area of Rocky Mountain Montane Conifer Forest embracing:**

Ponderosa pine (*Pinus ponderosa*)

Southwestern white pine (*Pinus strobiformis*)

Subalpine fir (*Abies lasiocarpa*)

White fir (*Abies concolor*)

The diverse understory in the Santa Rita Mountains includes:

Apache plant (*Guardiola platyphylla*)

Brickellbush (*Brickellia amplexicaulis, B. coulteri, B. eupatorioides* variety *chlorolepis, B. floribunda, B. grandiflora,* and *B. venosa*)

Buckwheats (including *Eriogonum abertianum, E. jamesii,* and *E. wrightii*)

Grama grasses (including *Bouteloua curtipendula, B. eriopoda, B. gracilis,* and *B. hirsuta*)

Lupines (including *Lupinus concinnus* and *L. sparsiflorus*)

Morning-glories (*Ipomoea* several species)

Muhly grasses (*Muhlenbergia* several species)

Ocotillo (*Fouquieria splendens*)

Penstemons (*Penstemon* several species)

Turpentine bush (*Isocoma tenuisecta*)

Wild beans (*Macroptilium gibbosifolium, Phaseolus acutifolius, P. maculatus* subspecies *ritensis,* and *P. parvulus*)

Among myriad displays of succulents, AZT users can see:

Banana and hoary yucca (*Yucca baccata* and *Y. madrensis* [synonym, *Y. schottii*])

Barrel cactus (*Ferocactus wislizeni*)

Beargrass (*Nolina microcarpa*)

Beehive cactus (*Coryphantha vivipara* variety *vivipara*)

Cane cholla (*Cylindropuntia spinosior*)

Fendler's and rainbow hedgehog cactus (*Echinocereus fendleri* variety *fendleri* and *E. rigidissimus*)

Macdougal's pincushion cactus (*Mammillaria macdougalii*)

Palmer, Parry, and Schott's agave (*Agave palmeri, A. parryi,* and *A. schottii*)

Prickly-pears (*Opuntia engelmannii* variety *engelmannii, O. macrorhiza,* and *O. santa-rita*)

Leaving the high Santa Catalina Mountains and heading north, AZT travelers pass through Madrean Evergreen Forest Woodland and Interior Chaparral, which is characterized by mild winters and wet summers. **The vegetation here consists mainly of:**

Alligator juniper (*Juniperus deppeana*)

Arizona cypress (*Cupressus arizonicus*) on north-facing slopes

Arizona madrone (*Arbutus arizonica*)

Oaks (*Quercus arizonica, Q. emoryi, Q. gambelii, Q. grisea, Q. hypoleucoides, Q. oblongifolia,* and *Q. turbinella*)

Pines (including *Pinus arizonica, P. cembroides, P. leiophylla* variety *chihuahuana,* and *P. ponderosa*)

Walnut (*Juglans major*)

Other shrubs include:

Arizona rosewood (*Vauquelinia californica*)

Evergreen sumac (*Rhus virens* variety *choriophylla*)

Pointleaf manzanita (*Arctostaphylos pungens*)

Wright's silktassel (*Garrya wrightii*)

Finally arriving back in the Semidesert Grassland near Oracle, AZT users can observe:

Grassland species, such as brome (*Bromus* several species), cane bluestem (*Bothriochloa barbinodis*), dropseed (*Sporobolus* several species), lovegrass (*Eragrostis* several species), muhly (*Muhlenbergia* several species), three awn (*Aristida* several species), and grama (*Bouteloua* several species)

Kearney's snakewood (*Condalia warnockii* variety *kearneyana*)

Central Region (Passages 16–27)

Along the Black Hills and Tortilla Mountains Passages, trail users continue through Arizona Upland, which is characterized by a typical plant community of palo verde (*Parkinsonia florida, P. microphylla* [synonyms, *Cercidium floridum, C. microphyllum*])

and saguaro (*Carnegiea gigantea*). **In addition, common in this particular area you will see:**

Kelvin's cholla (*Cylindropuntia ×kelvinensis*), a hybrid of cane cholla
(*C. spinosior*) and chainfruit cholla (*C. fulgida*)

Along certain stretches, trail users might find it difficult to determine the plant community because what appears to be Semidesert Grassland mingles with Arizona Upland throughout the hilly topography. **Occasional riparian areas also intersect these passages, which shelter such species as:**

Arizona sycamore (*Platanus wrightii*)

Frémont cottonwood (*Populus fremontii*)

Seep-willow (*Baccharis salicifolia*)

Traveling west from Kearny along the Gila River, trail users alternately travel along an extensive riparian corridor and beautiful Arizona Upland Sonoran Desert before heading due north through immense canyons along the Gila River Canyons Passage. **Characteristic species of the riparian corridor include:**

Frémont cottonwood (*Populus fremontii*)

Goodding's willow (*Salix gooddingii*)

Salt-cedar (*Tamarix ramosissima*)

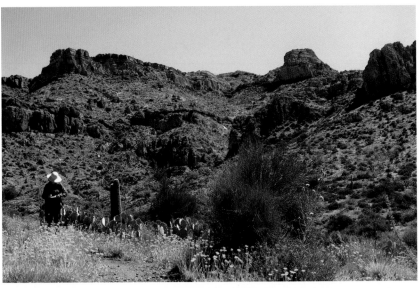

Photo: Liz Slauson

The Arizona Upland ecosystem, south of Picketpost Mountain along Passage 17, is surprisingly diverse and colorful.

As trail users approach Picketpost Mountain along the Alamo Canyon Passage, the vegetation is characteristic of the Arizona Upland biotic community. Fires in 2011 and 2012 have transformed this non-fire-adapted plant community to one dominated by red brome (*Bromus rubens*), a nonnative grass.

Approaching the Superstition Mountains along the Reavis Canyon and Superstition Wilderness Passages, AZT users continue to travel through mostly Arizona Upland. **Characteristic plants of the Arizona Upland along these stretches include numerous succulents, such as:**

Arizona pencil cholla (*Cylindropuntia arbuscula*)

Banana and soaptree yuccas (*Yucca baccata* and *Y. elata*)

Barrel cactus (*Ferocactus cylindraceus* and *F. wislizenii*)

Buckhorn cholla (*Cylindropuntia acanthocarpa*)

Cane cholla (*Cylindropuntia spinosior*)

Chainfruit (*Cylindropuntia fulgida*)

Hedgehog cactus (*Echinocereus engelmannii* variety *engelmannii*)

Pencil cholla (*Cylindropuntia leptocaulis*)

Pincushion cacti (*Mammillaria grahamii* and *M. viridiflora*)

Prickly-pears (*Opuntia engelmannii* variety *engelmannii, O. phaeacantha,* and their hybrids)

Saguaro (*Carnegiea gigantea*)

Teddybear cholla (*Cylindropuntia bigelovii*)

While creosote (*Larrea tridentata*) is occasionally observed, common trees and shrubs include:

Blue and littleleaf palo verde (*Parkinsonia florida* and *P. microphylla* [synonyms, *Cercidium floridum* and *C. microphyllum*])

Fairy duster (*Calliandra eriophylla*)

Frémont wolfberry (*Lycium fremontii*)

Graythorn (*Ziziphus obtusifolius* variety *canescens*)

Ocotillo (*Fouquieria splendens*)

Red barberry (*Berberis haematocarpa*)

Scrub-live oak (*Quercus turbinella*)

Snapdragon-penstemon (*Keckiella antirrhinoides* subspecies *microphylla*)

Turpentine bush (*Ericameria laricifolia*)

Velvet mesquite (*Prosopis velutina*)

Whitethorn acacia (*Vachellia constricta* [synonym, *Acacia constricta*])

Among the shrubs, California flannelbush (*Fremontodendron californicum*) is an attractive yellow-flowered species that occurs only in a few places in Arizona, including in the Superstition Mountains of the AZT's Central Region.

Common herbaceous perennials and annuals in this area include:

Bluedicks (*Dichelostemma capitatum* subspecies *pauciflorum*)

Brittlebush (*Encelia farinosa*)

California poppies (*Eschscholzia californica* subspecies *mexicana*)

Creamcups (*Platystemon californica*)

Desert chicory (*Rafinesquia neomexicana*)

Desert rock pea (*Lotus rigidus*)

Desert windflower (*Emmenanthe penduliflora*)

Fringed red maids (*Calandrinia ciliata*)

Globemallows (*Sphaeralcea ambigua, S. coccinea,* and *S. rusbyi*)

Lupines (*Lupinus arizonicus, L. concinnus,* and *L. sparsiflorus*)

Sego-lily (*Calochortus kennedyi*)

Continuing north, AZT users traverse through Arizona Upland until this biocommunity gives way to the Interior Chaparral on the eastern foothills of the Mazatzal Mountains and finally trail users also encounter Great Basin Conifer Woodland and Relict Conifer Woodland. **Within the Great Basin Conifer Woodland, trail users can expect to see:**

Arizona alder (*Alnus oblongifolia*)

Holly-leaf buckthorn (*Rhamnus crocea*)

Junipers (*Juniperus coahuilensis* and *J. deppeana*)

Oaks, including Arizona oak, canyon live oak, Emory oak, Gambel oak, and scrub-live oak (*Quercus arizonica, Q. chrysolepis, Q. emoryi, Q. gambelii,* and *Q. turbinella*)

Piñon pine (*Pinus edulis*)

Red barberry (*Berberis haematocarpa*)

Serviceberry (*Amelanchier utahensis*)

Silktassels (*Garrya flavescens* and *G. wrightii*)

Skunkbush (*Rhus aromatica* variety *trilobata* [synonym, *Rhus trilobata* variety *anisophylla*])

Sugar sumac (*Rhus ovata*)

Herbaceous plants in this area include:

Buckwheats (including *Eriogonum abertianum* and *E. wrightii*)

Globemallows (*Sphaeralcea ambigua, S. coulteri,* and *S. rusbyi*)

Lupines (including *Lupinus argenteus, L. concinnus, L. palmeri,* and *L. sparsiflorus*)

Penstemons (including *Penstemon barbatus, P. eatonii,* and *P. pseudospectabilis*)

Sego-lily (*Calochortus flexuosus*)

Wormwood (*Artemisia ludoviciana*)

Succulents are frequent here and include:

Beehive cactus (*Coryphantha vivipara* variety *vivipara*)

Claret cup hedgehog cacti (*Echinocereus coccineus* and *E. mojavensis*)

Golden-flowered agave (*Agave chrysantha*)

Parry's agave (*Agave parryi*)

Prickly-pears (*Opuntia chlorotica, O. engelmannii* variety *engelmannii,* and *O. phaeacantha*)

Whipple cholla (*Cylindropuntia whipplei*)

You will find the Relict Conifer Woodland in localized areas within Interior Chaparral, where Arizona cypress (*Cupressus arizonica*) occurs on north slopes and in canyons below the Mogollon Rim.

Along the Four Peaks and Pine Mountain Passages, trail users continue their travel through Interior Chaparral and Semidesert Grassland communities, the latter characterized by:

Barberry (*Berberis haematocarpa*)

Catclaw acacia (*Senegalia greggii* [synonym, *Acacia greggii*])

Desert hackberry (*Celtis pallida*)

Graythorn (*Ziziphus obtusifolia* variety *canescens*)

Ocotillo (*Fouquieria splendens*)

One-seeded juniper (*Juniperus monosperma*)

Velvet mesquite (*Prosopis velutina*)

Grasses are numerous and include, among others:

Curly-mesquite (*Hilaria belangeri*)

Fluff grass (*Dasyochloa pulchella*)

Grama grasses (*Bouteloua* several species)

Slim tridens (*Tridens muticus*)

Tanglehead (*Heteropogon contortus*)

Three awn (*Aristida* several species)

Succulents include:

Banana yucca (*Yucca baccata*)

Barrel cactus (*Ferocactus cylindraceus*)

Beargrass (*Nolina microcarpa*)

Beehive cactus (*Coryphantha vivipara* variety *vivipara*)

Brown-spined prickly-pear cactus (*Opuntia phaeacantha*)

Cane cholla (*Cylindropuntia spinosior*)

Engelmann prickly-pear (*Opuntia engelmannii* variety *engelmannii*)

Golden-flowered agave (*Agave chrysantha*)

Hedgehog cacti (*Echinocereus coccineus, E. engelmannii* variety *engelmannii*, and variety *fasciculatus, E. fendleri* variety *bonkerae*, and *E. mojavensis*)

Pancake prickly-pear (*Opuntia chlorotica*)

Parry's agaves (*Agave parryi*)

Soaptree yucca (*Yucca elata* variety *elata*)

Sotol (*Dasylirion wheeleri*)

As trail users travel from the Mazatzal Mountains toward Pine, the AZT continues through Rocky Mountain Montane Conifer Forest, Great Basin Conifer Woodland, riparian areas, and Interior Chaparral. Fire-adapted woody shrubs with deep roots and leathery leaves make up much of the vegetation in the Interior Chaparral.

Common trees or shrubs you can view here include:

Birchleaf mahogany (*Cercocarpus montanus*)

Ceanothus (*Ceanothus greggii, C. fendleri*, and *C. integerrimus*)

Holly-leaf buckthorn (*Rhamnus crocea*)

Manzanita (*Arctostaphylos pringlei* and *A. pungens*)

Shrub live oak (*Quercus turbinella*)

Silktassels (*Garrya flavescens* and *G. wrightii*)

Skunkbush (*Rhus aromatic* variety *trilobata* [synonym, *Rhus trilobata* variety *anisophylla*])

Stansbury cliffrose (*Purshia stansburyana* [synonym, *Cowania mexicana* variety *stansburiana*])

Common succulents include:

Agaves–golden flowered, Parry's, and Toumey's (*Agave chrysantha, A. parryi*, and *A. toumeyana* variety *bella* and variety *toumeyana*)

Banana and soaptree yuccas (*Yucca baccata* and *Y. elata* variety *elata*)

Barrel cactus (*Ferocactus cylindraceus*)

Beargrass (*Nolina microcarpa*)

Beehive cactus (*Coryphantha vivipara* variety *vivipara*)

Buckhorn cholla (*Cylindropuntia acanthocarpa* variety *coloradensis* and variety *thornberi*)

Cane cholla (*Cylindropuntia spinosior*)

Hedgehog cacti (*Echinocereus coccineus, E. engelmannii* variety *engelmannii* and variety *fasciculatus* and *E. fendleri* variety *bonkerae*)

Prickly-pears (*Opuntia chlorotica, O. engelmannii* variety *engelmannii, O. phaeacantha*, and *O. macrorhiza*)

Rock echeveria (*Dudleya saxosa* subspecies *collomiae*)

Sotol (*Dasylirion wheeleri*)

Whipple's cholla (*Cylindropuntia whipplei*)

Traveling north toward the Grand Canyon, AZT users continue to encounter mainly Great Basin Conifer Woodland and Rocky Mountain Montane Conifer Forest.

North Region (Passages 28–43)

The Grand Canyon is known not only for its jaw-dropping views, geological wonders, and immensity but also, to botanists, for its diverse flora. Nearly *half* of Arizona's flora occurs in the Grand Canyon, owing to all the factors that contribute to the state's diversity: elevation, geographic position, climate variation, and variety of niches. The canyon's diversity also can be attributed to the presence of five of the seven life zones and three of the four desert types in North America.

At the canyon's edge, the plants that grow on the Kaibab Limestone are more characteristic of lower and warmer elevations. **Commonly found near and at the edges—due to the "edge effect," when warm air from the canyon bottom rises and increases the temperature and aridity at the canyon's edge—are these plants:**

Banana yucca (*Yucca baccata*)

Claret cup hedgehog cacti (*Echinocereus coccineus* and *E. mohavensis*)

Rabbitbrush (including *Chrysothamnus depressus, C. greenei, Ericameria arizonica, E. nauseosa* [synonym, *Chrysothamnus nauseosa*], and *E. parryi*)

Stansbury cliffrose (*Purshia stansburyana* [synonym, *Cowania mexicana* variety *stansburiana*])

Traveling from the South Rim to the North Rim of Grand Canyon, hikers and other AZT users pass from Rocky Mountain Montane Conifer Forest and Great Basin Conifer Woodland through Great Basin Desert Scrub and, finally, Mohave Desert Scrub near the Colorado River. **Vegetation near the river is adapted to arid environments and includes:**

Alkaline goldenbush (*Isocoma acradenia*)

Apache plume (*Fallugia paradoxa*)

Chuckwalla's delight (*Bebbia juncea*)

Longleaf brickellbush (*Brickellia longifolia*)

Mohave brittlebush (*Encelia resinifera*)

Rabbitfoot (*Acourtia wrightii*)

Sacred datura (*Datura wrightii*)

Spearleaf brickellbush (*Brickellia atractyloides*)

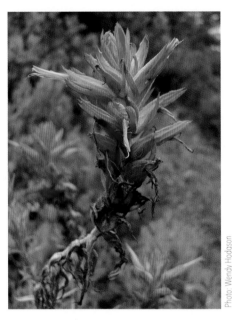

Wyoming paintbrush
(*Castilleja linariifolia*)
is a common wildflower in the
Great Basin Conifer Woodland and
Rocky Mountain Montane Conifer Forest.

Watson's dutchman-pipe (*Aristolochia watsonii*)

Western bernardia (*Bernardia incana*)

Succulents include:

Engelmann hedgehog cactus (*Echinocereus engelmannii* variety *engelmannii*)

Pincushion cacti (*Mammillaria grahamii* and *M. tetrancistra*)

Prickly-pears (*Opuntia engelmannii* variety *engelmannii, O. phaeacantha, O. chlorotica, O. polyacantha,* and several hybrids)

Soaptree yucca (*Yucca elata* variety *elata*)

Many of the Sonoran Desert species occur within the canyon bottom. They include:

Brittlebush (*Encelia farinosa*)

Desert-chicory (*Rafinesquia neomexicana*)

Odora (*Porophyllum gracile*), a fragrant species

Slender janusia (*Cottsia gracilis* [synonym, *Janusia gracilis*])

Among the Grand Canyon-endemic species that AZT trail users might see as they pass through are:

Arizona prickle-poppy (*Argemone arizonica*)

Arizona turpentine bush (*Ericameria arizonica*)

Glow willowweed (*Lorandersonia salicina*)

Kaibab agave (*Agave utahensis* subspecies *kaibabensis*)

Near-endemic plants–species that are found only in and just outside the Grand Canyon region–include:

Barrel cactus (*Echinocactus xeranthemoides*)

Giant hellebore orchid (*Epipactis gigantea*)

Grand Canyon beavertail cactus (*Opuntia basilaris* variety *longiareolata*)

Riparian areas abound along Garden and Pipe Creeks (west of the AZT), characterized by such plants as maidenhair fern (*Adiantum capillus-veneris*), redbud (*Cercis orbiculata*), and red monkeyflower (*Mimulus verbenaceus*).

Leaving the Colorado River, trail users traverse the same Grand Canyon communities in reverse order; however, the North Rim of the canyon averages altitudes that are approximately 1,200 feet higher than the South Rim. The Great Basin Subalpine Conifer Forest begins abruptly at the North Rim—literally, at the edge of the canyon. In addition, heading up toward the North Rim, AZT users encounter riparian areas that are found along various creeks including Bright Angel, Phantom, Wall, and Manzanita.

Across the Kaibab Plateau, the vegetation slowly transitions from Great Basin Subalpine Conifer Forest to Rocky Mountain Montane Conifer Forest, characterized by ponderosa pine. **In addition, four dominant trees occur here:**

Corkbark fir (*Abies lasiocarpa* variety *arizonica*)

Gambel oak (*Quercus gambelii*)

Quaking aspen (*Populus tremuloides*)

White fir (*Abies concolor*)

Other trees include:

Blue spruce (*Picea pungens*)

Engelmann spruce (*Picea engelmannii*)

Common shrubs include:

Buckwheats (*Eriogonum arcuatum* variety *arcuatum*, *E. heermannii*, *E. microthecum,* and *E. umbellatum*)

Currants (*Ribes* several species)

Dwarf juniper (*Juniperus communis*)

Elderberry (*Sambucus nigra* and *S. racemosa*)

Fendler's ceanothus (*Ceanothus fendleri*)

Gambel oak (*Quercus gambelii*)

Greenleaf manzanita (*Arctostaphylos patula*)

New Mexican locust (*Robinia neomexicana*)

Parry's rabbitbrush (*Ericameria parryi*)

Raspberry (*Rubus* several species)

Smooth sumac (*Rhus glabra*)

Snowberry (*Symphoricarpos oreophilus* and *S. rotundifolius*)

Herbaceous plants are common in more open areas, especially following the summer monsoons. They include, in addition to numerous grasses:

Bracken fern (*Pteridium aquilinum*), especially common

Buckwheats (*Eriogonum inflatum* and *E. racemosum*)

Cinquefoils (*Potentilla crinita, P. hippiana,* and *P. norvegica*)

Columbines (*Aquilegia chrysantha, A. desertorum,* and hybrids)

Fleabane daisies (including *Erigeron divergens, E. flagellaris, E. formosissimus, E. pumilus,* and *E. speciosus*)

Geraniums (*Geranium caespitosum, G. eremophilum,* and *G. richardsonii*)

Golden-eye (*Heliomeris multiflora*)

Goldenrods (*Oreochrysum parryi* [synonym, *Solidago parryi*], *Solidago altissima, S. multiradiata, S. nana,* and *S. velutina*)

Groundsels (*Packera multilobata* and *P. werneriifolia* [synonyms, *Senicio multilobatus, S. werneriifolius*])

Hairy golden aster (*Heterotheca villosa*)

Indian paintbrush (*Castilleja chromosa, C. kaibabensis, C. linariifolia,* and *C. miniata*)

Lotus (*Lotus utahensis* and *L. wrightii*)

Lupines (including *Lupinus argenteus* and *L. hillii*)

Meadow-rue (*Thalictrum fendleri*)

Parry's bellflower (*Campanula parryi*)

Peavine (*Lathyrus lanszwertii*)

Penstemons (including *Penstemon barbatus, P. eatonii, P. linarioides, P. pachyphyllus,* and *P. rydbergii*)

Puccoon (*Lithospermum incisum* and *L. multiflora*)

Pussytoes (*Antennaria parvifolia, A. marginata,* and *A. rosea*)

Thistles (*Cirsium arizonicum, C. pulchellum, C. undulatum,* and *C. wheeleri*)

Western and white prairie asters (*Symphyotrichum ascendens* [synonym, *Aster ascendens*] and *S. falcatum* variety *commutatus* [synonym, *Aster commutatus*])

Wild strawberry (*Fragaria* several species)

Wormwood (including *Artemisia bigelovii, A. campestris, A. ludoviciana,* and *A. tridentata*)

Yarrow *(Achillea millefolium)*

Yellow hawkweed (*Hieracium fendleri*)

Succulents are few on the Kaibab Plateau, but a watchful eye might find the small, fragile prickly-pear (*Opuntia fragilis*) hiding among the pine-needle litter.

Open areas or parks are interspersed with ponds, which are home to numerous aquatic species, such as:

Bulrush (*Schoenoplectus* several species)

Buttercups (including *Ranunculus flammula, R. cymbalaria,* and the invasive *R. testiculatus*)

Rushes (*Juncus* several species)

Sedges (*Carex* several species)

Water plantain (*Alisma plantago-aquatica*)

As the elevation gradually declines from the high Kaibab Plateau toward the Arizona–Utah border, trail users enter the Great Basin Conifer Woodland plant community. **One of the most extensive vegetative types in the Southwest, it is dominated by:**

Big sagebrush (*Artemisia tridentata*)

Juniper (*Juniperus monosperma, J. osteosperma,* and *J. scopulorum*)

Piñon pine (*Pinus edulis*)

Other trees and shrubs encountered in this community include:

Fern-bush (*Chamaebatiaria millefolia*)

Frémont barberry (*Berberis fremontii*)

Gambel oak (*Quercus gambelii*)

Hop-bush (*Ptelea trifoliata*)

Mormon-tea (*Ephedra viridis*)

Rabbitbrush (*Ericameria nauseosa* [synonym, *Chrysothamnus nauseosus*])

Serviceberry (*Amelanchier utahensis*)

Stansbury cliffrose (*Purshia stansburyana* [synonym, *Cowania mexicana* variety *stansburiana*])

Succulent plants include:

Banana and Bailey's yucca (*Yucca baccata* and *Y. baileyi*)

Beehive cactus (*Coryphantha vivipara* variety *vivipara*)

Claret cup hedgehog cacti (*Echinocereus mohavensis* and *E. coccineus*)

Prickly-pears (including *Opuntia macrorhiza, O. phaeacantha,* and *O. polyacantha*)

Whipple cholla (*Cylindropuntia whipplei*)

Herbaceous plants include:

Cutleaf (*Hymenopappus filifolius*)

Penstemons (*Penstemon barbatus, P. eatoni, P. linarioides, P. pachyphyllus,* and *P. thompsoniae*)

Phacelia (*Phacelia crenulata* and *P. heterophylla*)

Sego-lilies (*Calochortus flexuosus* and *C. nuttallii*)

Wild onions (*Allium acuminatum, A. bisceptrum,* and *A. nevadense*)

Additional herbaceous plants in this community are:

Bladderpods (including *Physaria arizonica, P. intermedia,* and *P. rectipes*)

Buckwheats (*Eriogonum alatum, E. arcuatum* variety *arcuatum, E. microthecum,* and *E. racemosum*)

Evening-primrose (*Oenothera caespitosa*)

Grasses such as muttongrass (*Poa fendleriana*) and squirreltail (*Elymus elymoides*)

Groundsel (*Packera multilobata* [synonym, *Senicio multilobatus*])

Indian paintbrush (*Castilleja linariifolia*)

Locoweed (including *Astragalus amphioxys, A. calycosus, A. lentiginosus,* and *A. preussii*)

Phlox (*Phlox austromontana* and *P. longifolia*)

Pinque rubberweed (*Hymenoxys richardsonii*)

Sedges, such as clustered field sedge (*Carex praegracilis*) and western sedge (*C. occidentalis*)

Wild cabbage (*Caulanthus crassicaulis*)–unusual and thick-stemmed

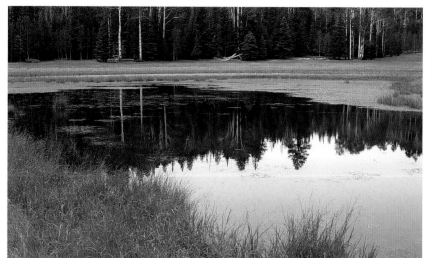

Duck Lake, north of the Grand Canyon along Passage 40, is one of many pockets of water that support an abundance of plant and animal life.

Ongoing Observations

Along the AZT, a number of rare species and their documentation—through photographs and herbarium specimens—provide additional information regarding their distribution and morphology. For example, we know that satintail grass (*Imperata brevifolia*), which is found along streams and seeps, was once known from Texas to California prior to the mid-1900s. The water-loving plant is now found only in Arizona and northern Sonora. The largest populations exist in the Grand Canyon, representing recent relict populations safe from groundwater pumping that destroys their habitat. Hiking up the AZT along Bright Angel Creek (Passage 38: Grand Canyon: Inner Gorge and Passage 39: North Rim), trail users can find numerous populations of this beautiful grass.

Additionally, although most people probably do not think of ferns as especially common in Arizona and along the AZT, they actually are, and they occupy every biotic community in the state. It is not yet known how many species of vascular plants will be documented or observed along the trail, and without a doubt, any such number will continually increase. Thus far, for the Central Region alone, we have documented approximately 650 species—all along a narrow trail corridor only 15 feet wide.

Arizona is a special place, and the Arizona National Scenic Trail provides an extraordinary venue that showcases our state's beauty, geology, wildlife, history, and culture, and of course, its plants. The trail provides unlimited opportunities, not only to enjoy Arizona, but also to learn about its many wonders. Through education comes appreciation and understanding, and through appreciation and understanding comes better stewardship and care of Arizona's treasures.

An important tool to help everyone learn about the plants of Arizona and the AZT is SEINet (swbiodiversity.org)—the Southwestern Environmental Information Network. The network operates under the umbrella of the Southwest Biodiversity Consortium. SEINet provides a tremendous amount of information on plant characteristics and distribution, as well as images, interactive keys, and more, thereby making it an important educational tool for everybody at all expertise levels.

As this book goes to press, Wendy Hodgson and Dr. Liz Slauson (see profiles on page xi) continue to conduct in-depth research to document the myriad species and extensive botanical habitats along the AZT. The information and photographs gleaned from their ongoing work will be uploaded to **aztrail.org.** *The coauthors also plan AZT-botany field guides with detailed descriptions and photographs to be published in the future.*

Welcome to the Geology of Arizona

By Rick Obermiller

SOME GEOLOGISTS CLAIM THAT GEOLOGY is the father of all sciences. Indeed, life on earth could not have begun or continue to exist without geological forces. The atmosphere, oceans, nutrients, and minerals that enrich the soil and power our technology; the magnetic field that protects us from solar radiation; the awe-inspiring scenery, including the magnificent mountains, canyons, valleys, and river systems, all owe their existence to the geological forces that began with the formation of the solar system and continue with the dynamic geology that shapes our planet today.

In Arizona, we have the unique privilege of viewing, studying, and experiencing many geologic processes that are more evident here than in other parts of the country, in large part to Arizona's wide open spaces, absence of dense forest canopy, and the lack of human development over most of the state. Arizona has been volcanically active and subject to the tectonic forces that built mountains and basins, canyons and mesas, and plateaus and escarpments. Much of the state has been under water as sea levels have risen and fallen over time. Arizona is a geologist's dream.

Anyone hiking, biking, or riding on the Arizona National Scenic Trail (AZT) will experience Arizona geology intimately. Thus, this guidebook provides geological descriptions for some of the major points of interest along the trail. However, our focus on these major points does not mean that there isn't interesting geology to be found all along the trail.

To understand what geology means to the state, consider the four fundamental areas of geology, particularly within the context of Arizona's three physiographic zones that are described in the last part of this section:

≈ geological time scale

≈ plate tectonics

≈ rock classifications

≈ rock cycle

Geological Time Scale

Earth's geological history began about 4.5 billion years ago. The appearance of dinosaurs in the fossil record begins in the Triassic Period around 230 million years ago. Early hominids date back 4.4 million years, according to a recent fossil find in Ethiopia, and the Egyptian civilization dates back only 5,000 years. By comparison, our tenure on the planet is a very small fraction of the earth's age. It's very hard to comprehend such a vast expanse of time.

One way to help absorb this concept is to transfer the time scale to something we can relate to. At the Grand Canyon's South Rim you'll find an impressive treatment of geological time in an outdoor interpretive exhibit called *The Trail of Time*. Grand Canyon National Park offers the following description: "The exhibit follows the existing paved rim trail on the South Rim of Grand Canyon between Yavapai Observation Station and Grand Canyon Village and is marked by brass markers every meter, representing one million years of time. Viewing tubes and other interpretive materials help visitors connect the rocks visible in Grand Canyon to their place along the geologic timeline."

Using this technique we can visualize the oldest exposed rocks in Grand Canyon and the state, the Elves Chasm Granodiorite: 1.8 billion years old as 1.8 kilometers in length

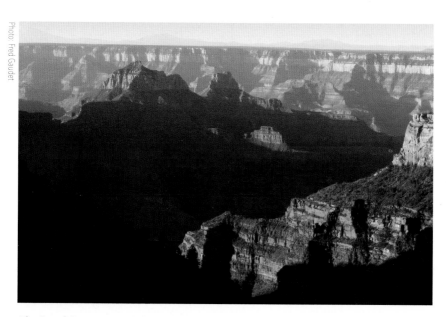

Photo: Fred Gaudet

The Grand Canyon presents a rare opportunity to view layers of geological history unlike those found anywhere else on the planet.

DIVISIONS OF GEOLOGIC TIME

EON	ERA	PERIOD	EPOCH	MILLION YEARS AGO
PHANEROZOIC	CENOZOIC	QUATERNARY	HOLOCENE PLEISTOCENE	1.8
		TERTIARY	PLIOCENE MIOCENE OLIGIOCENE EOCENE PALEOCENE	65
	MESOZOIC	CRETACEOUS	LATE EARLY	144
		JURASSIC	LATE MIDDLE EARLY	206
		TRIASSIC	LATE EARLY	248
	PALEOZOIC	PERMIAN	LATE EARLY	290
		PENNSYLVANIAN	LATE MIDDLE EARLY	323
		MISSISSIPPIAN	LATE EARLY	354
		DEVONIAN	LATE MIDDLE EARLY	417
		SILURIAN	LATE MIDDLE EARLY	443
		ORDOVICIAN	LATE MIDDLE EARLY	490
		CAMBRIAN	LATE MIDDLE EARLY	540
PROTEROZOIC	LATE PROTEROZOIC MIDDLE PROTEROZOIC EARLY PROTEROZOIC			2,500
ARCHEAN	LATE ARCHEAN MIDDLE ARCHEAN EARLY ARCHEAN			3,800
PRE-ARCHEAN				4,500

Illustration: Terri Gay (content courtesy of the U.S. Geological Survey)

from the present; the appearance of dinosaurs: 230 million years ago as 230 meters; the caldera eruption in the Superstitions: 30 million years ago as 30 meters; the appearance of hominids: 4.4 million years ago as 4.4 meters; and the age of the Egyptian civilization: 5,000 years as 0.5 millimeters (the thickness of a human hair!) from the present.

Geologists use a standard chart that delineates vertically from the largest-to-smallest span of time—and horizontally from the oldest-to-newest by Eon, Era, Period, and Epoch. (See "Divisions of Geologic Time," above.)

View the chart to grasp that we are currently in the Phanerozoic Eon, the Cenozoic Era, the Quaternary Period, and the Holocene Epoch, which began 10,000 years ago, roughly the end of the last ice age. There are no exposed rocks on the planet from the Archean Eon. However, Arizona does have exposed rock dating back to the Proterozoic Eon.

Plate Tectonics

The generally accepted concept of plate tectonics was proposed as a theory in the late 1970s. Since that time, scientific evidence has well supported the theory, citing plate tectonics as the driving force of crustal movements that build mountains, create volcanic eruptions, cause earthquakes, and separate continents.

The top layer of the earth is called the *lithosphere,* which reaches a depth of about 75 miles. The upper part of the lithosphere is called the *crust.* Except for isolated bodies of molten magma (melted rock), the lithosphere is solid rock. The continental crust averages 21 miles in depth, and the oceanic crust averages only 5 miles in depth. Beneath the lithosphere is the *asthenosphere,* composed of plastic, semimolten rock; it extends to a depth of 155 miles. That's just the outer skin of the earth. As with geological time, we humans find it hard to imagine the size of the earth. It is 3,976 miles from the surface to the inner solid-iron core!

The lithosphere is made up of nine discrete areas of crust called *tectonic plates* and various minor ones that raft on top of the semimolten asthenosphere and move in relation to each other ever so slowly, up to 13 centimeters (about 5 inches) per year. The mechanisms that allow the plates to move relative to one another are not well understood. However, it appears that midocean ridges cause magma to upwell, which in turn causes the seafloor to spread; this process creates a conveyor-belt action that moves the ocean crust in opposite directions from the ocean ridge as it creates new crust. The ocean plates then move and influence the movement of other plates in various directions. There is one place on earth where a midocean ridge can be observed at the surface: the island nation of Iceland, which is constantly growing new crust with intense volcanism.

When ocean crust meets continental crust, the ocean crust dives, or *subducts,* below the continental crust. The diving action over time produces melting because of intense heat and pressure as the crust returns to the mantle. The subduction also results in a gravity-assisted pulling action that may work in tandem with seafloor spreading to facilitate plate movements. It also produces volcanic activity and mountain ranges on the continental crust by exerting pressure on the crust, resulting in folding and faulting of rock.

The oceanic Pacific Plate is subducting under the Continental Plates around the Pacific Ocean. Subduction by the Pacific Plate around the Pacific Rim (called the Rim of Fire) encourages much volcanic activity. The islands of Japan and the Andes Mountains in South America are the result of subduction tectonics, as are the Rocky Mountains in the United States. Between subduction, where crust is returned to the mantle, and seafloor spreading, where crust is created, the net result is a static amount of crust on the surface.

When continental crusts meet at plate boundaries, the result is a collision that can build huge mountain ranges; for example, the collision of the Indian Plate and Eurasian Plate is what formed the Himalaya Range. As this collision continues, the mountains are pushed up by a few centimeters per year. The Appalachian Mountains are remnants of a plate collision that created a mountain range as high as the Himalayas are now, but the former have been subject to erosion over a very long period of time.

Another type of plate action, *transform,* occurs when one plate slides by another instead of colliding. Along the San Andreas Fault system in California, for instance, part of California and Baja California west of the San Andreas sits on the Pacific Plate and is moving north relative to the rest of California, which sits on the North American Plate and is moving relatively south. This grinding of two plates creates regular earthquake activity. Sometimes one plate will drag the other and couple it, which can cause crustal extension in the plate being dragged. This action is believed to have caused the Basin and Range Disturbance, which created the northwest-to-southeast-trending mountains and basins in the Basin and Range Province in Arizona.

Rock Classifications

There are three basic rock types: *igneous, sedimentary,* and *metamorphic.* Igneous rocks are the rocks from which the other two types are formed.

Igneous rocks are formed from the crystallization of *magma,* which is molten rock formed in the mantle or lithosphere as a result of melting of other rock. Because magma is less dense than solid rock, it finds its way upward through cracks, faults, and ruptures in overlying rocks in a variety of volcanic eruptions. Igneous rocks that solidify on the surface are called *extrusive.* However, much magma, called *intrusive,* never reaches the surface and cools slowly beneath the surface. A common extrusive igneous rock is basalt. Granite is an example of a common intrusive igneous rock.

Sedimentary rocks are the erosional and weathered remains of other rocks such as sandstone, the remains of sea creatures that settle to the bottoms of oceans (limestone), or rocks, such as gypsum, that form out of chemical solution. Sedimentary rocks are usually deposited in flat layers. Grand Canyon has 4,000 feet of flat-lying sedimentary rocks. Much of the Basin and Range Province is composed of tilted sedimentary block mountains.

Metamorphic rocks are igneous and sedimentary rocks that have been changed and deformed by extreme temperature and pressure by burial deep within the crust or by proximity to volcanic heat sources. If rocks are subjected to enough pressure and temperature, they will melt and create new igneous rocks. Melting occurs either by the deep subduction of oceanic crust or by continuous layering and burial of sediments and igneous rocks over time. Examples of metamorphic rocks are the schists and gneisses of the Inner Gorge of the Grand Canyon (see the text and "Grand Canyon's Three Sets of Rocks" in "The Grand Canyon: A Geological Masterpiece," on page 346).

The Rock Cycle

Igneous rocks that become sedimentary rocks or metamorphic rocks and once again become igneous rocks are said to have completed the rock cycle. If we compare it with a law of physics known as The Conservation of Energy, the rock cycle (see the illustration on the next page) could be called The Conservation of Rock.

You can see an example of the rock cycle in Arizona's Superstition Mountains. There, volcanic rock is eroded by wind and water and ends up as deposits of sand in the Phoenix Basin. The Phoenix Basin contains about 4,000 feet of accumulated sediments of sand, gravel, and mud eroded from the surrounding mountains. The tremendous weight of these sediments is already transforming the sediments into sandstones and mudstones. Looking ahead in geologic time as the basins continue to fill, extreme pressures and temperatures of burial will turn the sedimentary rock into metamorphic rocks. As burial continues, the metamorphic rocks will ultimately melt and become magma and erupt again as igneous rocks.

Physiographic Provinces

Above in this section, you've been reading about the four fundamental areas of geology—all described within the context of Arizona's three physiographic provinces. They are the state's distinct divisions, according to physical geography and geology. From

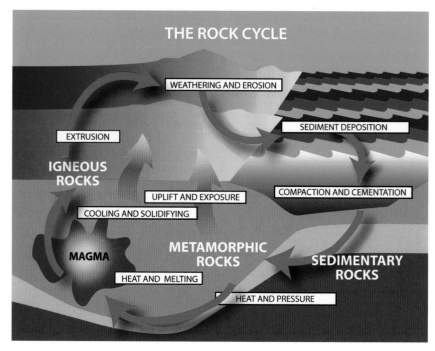

Illustration: Terri Gay (content courtesy of the Arizona Trail Association)

south to north, they are the Basin and Range Province, the Transition Zone Province (also known as the Central Highlands), and the Colorado Plateau Province. (See the illustration on page 44.)

■ Basin and Range Province (Passages 1-18)

This zone extends from the Mexico–U.S. border to the mountains of the Central Highlands. Geographically, the Sonoran Desert dominates this province, which covers virtually all the Basin and Range Province and the Transition Zone Province. The Sonoran Desert is one of the largest and hottest deserts in North America, covering 120,000 square miles. Besides its breadth in Arizona, it extends into California and northwestern Mexico.

The Sonoran Desert exists because of the rain shadow effect of California's Sierra Nevada and ancillary southern mountains. The rain shadow creates a desert because Pacific moisture traveling east with the prevailing wind drops most of its moisture on the western flanks of the Sierra and across its range, except for major storms. Consequently, little moisture remains when air reaches Arizona and Mexico.

Geologically, the Basin and Range Province is characterized by low elevation, parallel mountain ranges, and broad valleys that trend from northwest to southeast and that also extend into southern Nevada, California, and Mexico. These mountains and basins were formed during a period called the Basin and Range Orogeny (an *orogeny* is a mountain-building episode), sometimes called the Basin and Range Disturbance.

The disturbing orogeny occurred between 15 and 8 MYA (million years ago) and was caused by a pull action on the earth's crust to the northwest from tectonic plate movements. Pull action is known as *crustal extension* and causes faulting, which results in crustal blocks being uplifted (mountain formation) and other blocks being down-dropped—thus forming basins.

During this period, much volcanic activity occurred in Arizona. Some of the rocks that make up this area are very old marine limestone, shale, and sandstones that date to the Paleozoic Era, 570–240 MYA; volcanic rocks, marine sandstones, shales, and carbonates dating to the Mesozoic Era, 63–240 MYA; and primarily volcanic rocks during the Cenozoic Era, 63–2 MYA. The Phoenix Mountains and the Hualapai Mountains in Kingman are good examples of Basin and Range Mountains.

■ Transition Zone Province (Passages 19-27)

The Transition Zone separates and transitions the major zone to the north, the Colorado Plateau, and the major zone to the south, the Basin and Range. Its northern border is the escarpment known as the Mogollon Rim. Rugged and severely faulted mountains of Proterozoic age characterize the Transition Zone. Proterozoic, shown as Precambrian in the illustration on page 348, represents rocks that are very old—at least 500 million years or more. The zone lacks the sedimentary rocks found in the other zones and also has an absence of Mesozoic and Cenozoic rocks. If they were present at one time, they have since eroded away. All the important copper-mining districts from Jerome to Morenci are located in the Transition Zone. Rocks found in this zone are igneous (volcanic) and metamorphic rocks—those formed by extreme heat and pressure. The Mazatzal Mountains are a good example of Transition Zone geology.

■ Colorado Plateau Province (Passages 28-43)

In Arizona, this zone extends from the Mogollon Rim to the Utah border. Geographically, the Colorado Plateau continues into southern Utah, western Colorado all the way to the Rockies, and northwestern New Mexico—with Arizona's Four Corners area as its center. It also contains the highest concentration of national parks in the nation,

ARIZONA'S
PHYSIOGRAPHIC PROVINCES

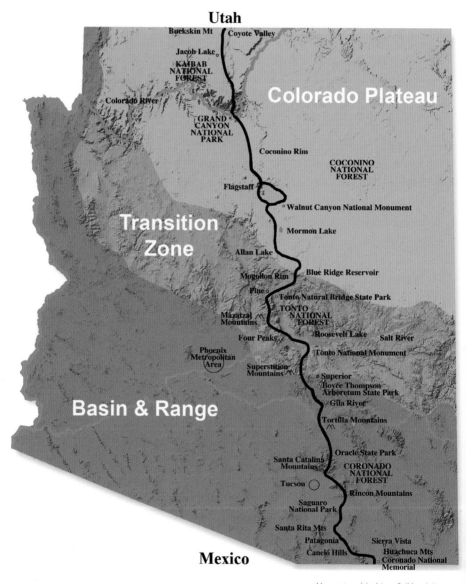

Map courtesy of the Arizona Trail Association

including Zion, Bryce Canyon, Canyonlands, Grand Canyon, and Petrified Forest, to name just a few. Most of the Colorado Plateau is drained by the Colorado River and its tributaries. It also has the highest average elevation of the three physiographic provinces.

Geologically, the Colorado Plateau was uplifted as a block and, except for volcanics, does not seem to have been affected by the faulting and deformation that occurred in the other two zones in the past 600 million years. The Plateau Province also exhibits much more layering of sedimentary rock than do the Transition Zone and the Basin and Range, although erosion may have eliminated the layers in those zones. The flat-lying stability of the zone is evidenced in the Grand Canyon. Most of the rocks in this province are Paleozoic sedimentary rocks, with some Mesozoic sedimentary rocks to the north. In the Mesozoic Moenkopi formation (a mudstone), many dinosaur fossils have been found.

Despite its stability, much erosion has occurred on the plateau that has created some of the great scenic wonders of the state, such as the Grand Canyon and Monument Valley. Most of the mountains found on the Plateau are Cenozoic volcanics that have erupted on top of the Mesozoic sediments, such as those found on the southern margin of the plateau in the San Francisco Volcanic Field near Flagstaff.

(See page xi for a profile of Rick Obermiller, author of the preceding section.)

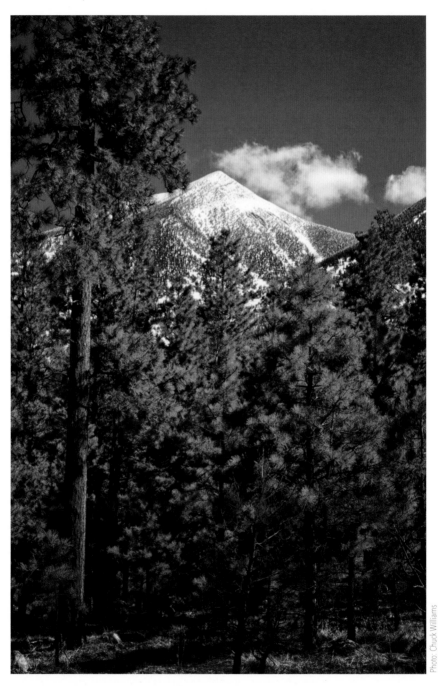

Photo: Chuck Williams

Despite a massive eruption that significantly reduced the height of the mountain, the mighty San Francisco Peaks still dominate the skyline of the Colorado Plateau.

The Arizona National Scenic Trail:
SOUTH, CENTRAL, and NORTH

LONG BEFORE THE ARIZONA NATIONAL SCENIC TRAIL (AZT) was created, Dale Shewalter was determined to cross the Grand Canyon State on foot, linking mountains, deserts, canyons, forests, and communities along a single path. Dale started this visionary adventure at the Mexico–U.S. border and walked north toward his home in Flagstaff, and eventually to the invisible line that separates Arizona and Utah. Thus, when the AZT was built, it was oriented from south to north to honor Dale's journey and his vision.

As you will see in this guidebook, Passage 1 begins at the southern boundary, between Mexico and the United States, at the Arizona line; and the trail's final link, Passage 43, terminates at the northern boundary, the Arizona–Utah border.

Within that geographic order, the passages are divided into three segments: South (Passages 1–15, pages 49–138), Central (Passages 16–27, pages 139–210), and North (Passages 28–43, pages 211–296).

Likewise, the 32 Gateway Communities (pages 297–337) and the Geology Sites (pages 338–349) unfold from south to north.

Each passage's length in miles—and its often-challenging terrain—can present a full day's hike, and sometimes more, if you want to complete the entire passage. But all trail users should feel welcome to enjoy partial distances along each passage, according to their available time and energy. Therefore, you will note that the narrative description for each passage includes a southern access point and a northern access point—and often yet an additional alternate access. This gives hikers, backpackers, mountain bikers, and equestrians more options for hitting the trail. It also invites opportunities to set up shuttle transportation for each passage. For example, in Passage 1, you could arrange for a car to be parked near that passage's northern access, at the Parker Canyon

Lake Trailhead, or near the Sunnyside Canyon Trailhead. Meanwhile, you could begin the hike at the southern access, at Montezuma Pass.

Another aspect for trail users to consider is each passage's terrain. Thus, the difficulty rating in the key info section at the top of each entry indicates the level of energy, stamina, and hiking prowess needed for that stretch of the AZT. Following are this guidebook's difficulty criteria:

STRENUOUS: Extreme elevation challenges, rough terrain, harsh environmental concerns, and expert route-finding skills are often required. Appropriate for well-seasoned outdoor adventurers.

DIFFICULT: Steep grades, long distances between water sources, rough terrain, and good route-finding skills required. Appropriate for skilled hikers, mountain bikers, and equestrians familiar with Arizona's unique challenges.

MODERATE: Rolling terrain, well-maintained tread, and ample water. Appropriate for hikers, runners, and other trail users who are prepared for remote outings.

EASY: Level terrain that presents few environmental challenges. Appropriate for most ability levels.

AZT South Section

Passages 1 through 15

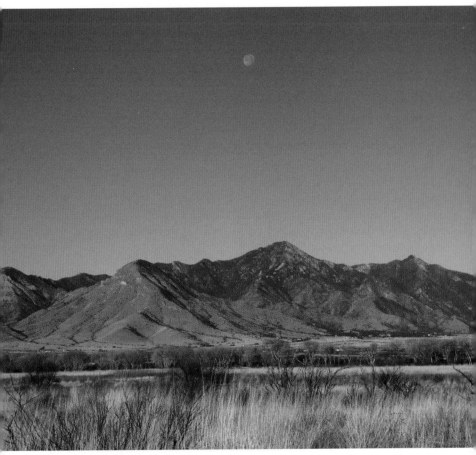

The AZT begins by climbing from the Mexico–U.S. border into the Huachuca Mountains, a formidable range that rises to a height of 9,466 feet.

Photo: Matthew J. Nelson

Huachuca Mountains

KEY INFO

LOCATION Mexico–United States Border to Parker Canyon Lake Trailhead

DISTANCE 21.7 miles one-way (22.7 miles if you summit Miller Peak)

DAY-TRIP OPTION See turnaround note in the trail description.

SHUTTLE RECOMMENDATION Sunnyside Canyon Trailhead (Passage 1, mile 16.6)

DIFFICULTY Strenuous

LAND MANAGERS Coronado National Forest, Sierra Vista Ranger District, **www.fs.usda.gov/coronado,** 520-378-0311; Coronado National Memorial, **nps.gov/coro,** 520-366-5515

RECOMMENDED MONTHS March–November

GATEWAY COMMUNITY See Sierra Vista (page 303).

GEOLOGY HIGHLIGHTS Not applicable

OVERVIEW

A historic obelisk and simple barbed-wire fence at the Mexico–U.S. border mark the official start of the Arizona National Scenic Trail (AZT) from its southernmost point. Here, before your eyes unfolds the expansive San Rafael Valley—a unique Sonoran grassland environment that is beautiful during all seasons. Passage 1 is unique, however, because you must already be *on* it in order to access this true beginning! But that's easier than it sounds, as described later (see Southern Access, page 56).

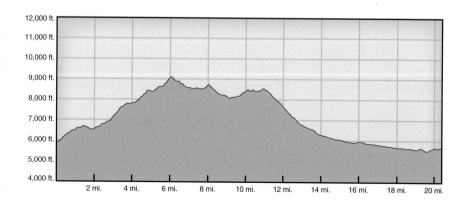

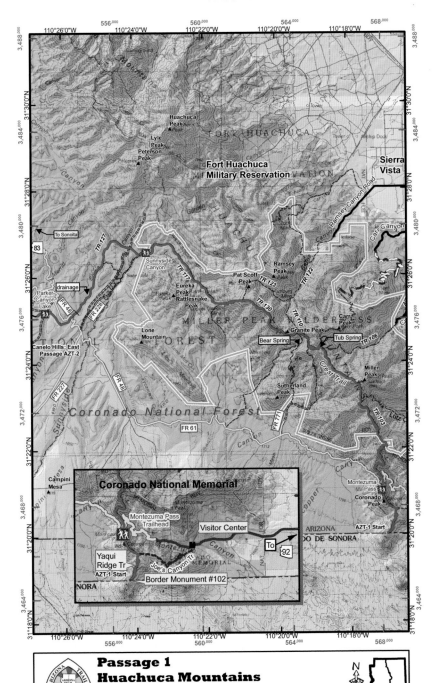

Passage 1
Huachuca Mountains

A. Seifert v1.0
10/30/2013

Lat/Long WGS 84
UTM NAD 83 12N
Scale: 1:160,000

0   0.5   1   2
Miles

N

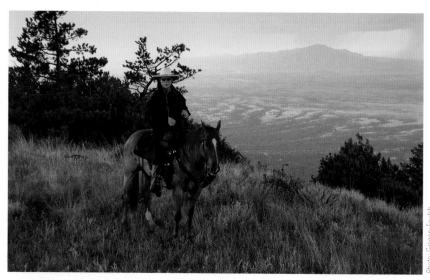

Photo: Gregory Foutch

The Huachuca Mountains are rich with cultural history, biodiversity, and expansive views into Mexico's northern state of Sonora.

After touching the monument and traveling north for almost 2 miles, you arrive at a trailhead at Montezuma Pass. Getting there is worth the effort, as you will no doubt agree when the passage climbs onto the first of several landforms called sky islands, which are unique to Arizona. These isolated mountain ranges rise several thousand feet above the surrounding desert, resulting in dramatically different life zones from those found at lower elevations only a few miles away. These elevated biotic communities are evidence of what the Sonoran Desert climate was like 10,000-plus years ago, and as the climate has warmed, the plants and animals have retreated higher into the hills. Thus, these sky islands are surrounded by a sea—of desert.

On the Passage 1 map (see previous page), you will see the Huachuca Mountains represented at the top. As the AZT follows the spine of the Huachucas, flat ground becomes a precious commodity, and campsites are rare. Level places occur along the trail at mile 3.9 (not recommended for camping), mile 5.8 (no water), mile 8.5 (water usually found at mile 8.3), mile 9.7 (no water), miles 10.4 to 11.1 (no water), and from mile 13.8 to the end of the passage.

For thru-hikers, Passage 1 may present other difficulties. Because of its high elevation, it holds snow later than nearby sections of the AZT. If you plan to hike here in late winter or spring, call the Sierra Vista Ranger District (see page 50) or check local hiking blogs for reports on current conditions.

The Monument Fire of 2011 affected the southern portion of the AZT in the Huachuca Mountains. Trail crews addressed major trail issues during the autumn of 2011; you may, however, encounter some tread erosion, missing or downed signs, blowdowns, and other adverse conditions.

Extensive immigration traffic flows through the Huachuca Mountains, and as on any wilderness route, you must always be alert to your surroundings. At press time for this book, however, AZT users have reported no negative encounters with immigrants illegally entering the country via this passage. For current information—and before setting out on Passage 1—contact the Coronado National Forest's Sierra Vista Ranger District (see page 50 and also Appendix 2, page 366). District agents can provide updates about immigration use, level of risk along this passage, and what to do if you encounter suspicious individuals or groups. Note that such trail users sometimes create what are called wildcat trails that can be confused easily with the AZT route. And while it's always wise to hike with companions, this is especially true when traveling through remote wilderness areas in the international borderlands.

ON THE TRAIL

At the Passage 1 starting point, the corner of two fences near the obelisk indicates the beginning of the AZT at the Mexico border. After pausing for a moment to take in the view, turn back, north-northeast, to essentially retrace your steps and follow the winding trail as it climbs to a saddle and returns to the intersection with Joe's Canyon Trail at mile 1.1.

Turn left (west) and climb a short distance, and then drop through several switchbacks to meet the Coronado Peak Trail at mile 1.8. Turn right and descend 0.1 mile to the parking lot at 6,570-foot Montezuma Pass. If you were to make a left turn at mile 1.8, it would lead a short distance off the AZT to the top of Coronado Peak, where Flagstaff schoolteacher Dale Shewalter sat with friends on a clear, cool evening and presented the question of whether it would be possible to link a series of trails across the entire state.

Walk to the road (FR 61) at the north end of the parking lot, turn right (northeast), and continue 25 yards to the Crest Trail, a clear singletrack that takes off on the left (north). The trail climbs through many switchbacks along the east side of the ridge. You reach the ridgecrest at mile 2.5. This portion of the AZT is within the Coronado National Memorial, a historically significant region of Arizona that commemorates the first organized expedition into the Southwest by conquistador Francisco Vásquez de Coronado.

At mile 3.9 the trail crests the main ridge, with great views to the east. In another 50 yards, the trail enters the Miller Peak Wilderness. Avoid side trails to Lutz Canyon and Bond Spring as you continue straight ahead to mile 6.5, where the trail crests the ridge at an intersection with the trail to the top of Miller Peak (9,050 feet). To climb Miller Peak, turn right and continue 0.5 mile to the 9,466-foot summit. The views from the summit of this sky island make the side trip worth every step.

TURNAROUND NOTE: If you're day-hiking and you haven't arranged for a car shuttle at Sunnyside Canyon or Parker Canyon Lake Trailheads, this is a great spot to reverse and retrace your steps back toward Montezuma Pass. The views to the south are incredible, and if your timing is right, you'll enjoy the sunset across the seemingly endless grasslands of the San Rafael Valley.

To continue on the trail, the AZT follows the ridge to the northwest for about a mile before dropping off to the east side and passing Tub Spring at mile 8.3 (8,550 feet). This water source, which flows into an old bathtub, is reliable in springtime and year-round if

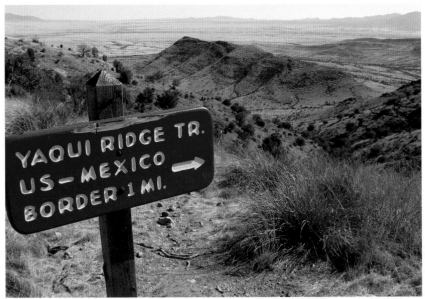

Photo: David Baker

For its first mile, the AZT follows the Yaqui Ridge Trail from the international boundary to Montezuma Pass.

conditions are favorable. Camping is prohibited within 200 feet of the spring—and there are better sites at mile 8.5 anyway. Thirty yards past the spring, reach an intersection with the Miller Canyon Trail (Trail 106), which descends to the right. Turn sharply left (due north) and follow a sign for the Crest Trail.

Climb briefly to mile 8.5 where you should avoid the Carr Peak Trail by staying on the Crest Trail to the left (west). There are a few flat spots here for camping.

Negotiate the steep descent to an intersection with the Oversite Canyon Trail at mile 9.8. Stay on the Crest Trail, and walk due north, crossing a streambed in 0.1 mile. Cross through Bear Saddle, where there is one flat spot to pitch a tent about 2 feet off the trail. *Be aware that this area, especially Bear Spring, is heavily used by immigrants crossing into the United States illegally.*

If you turn left (south) at Bear Saddle onto the Bear Canyon Trail, you can descend 0.5 mile (with an elevation loss of 500 feet) to reliable Bear Spring and some nice campsites. Note that this detour takes you off the AZT.

If you have not made that detour—or once you've returned to the AZT if you did take the detour—climb steeply west through pines until the trail crosses the ridge.

At mile 11.6, the AZT reaches the crest again and then becomes fainter as it descends to an intersection at mile 11.8. Leave the Crest Trail here by turning left (west-northwest) onto the signed Sunnyside Canyon Trail (Trail 117, at 8,500 feet). Stay on the Sunnyside Canyon Trail as it intersects the Eureka Canyon Trail at mile 12.8 and the Copper Glance Trail at mile 13.5.

The bottom of Sunnyside Canyon often contains flowing water during snowmelt. Continue to the wilderness boundary at mile 16.6. There is a small parking area here (see Alternate Access, page 57), and a good camping area is less than 0.1 mile down the road.

To continue on the AZT, follow the rough road through a turn to the left in 0.1 mile. Look for a somewhat obscure AZT sign on the right (north) side of the road. Turn onto the singletrack, cross a drainage, turn left to follow this drainage, and then veer right (west) in 0.1 mile.

At mile 17.2, cross a dirt road at a right angle and enter a confusing series of dirt roads. From the sign on the far side of the road, walk due west about 50 yards, and look for more signs indicating the singletrack to the northwest. Cross a wash for the first of several times at mile 17.3.

At mile 18.9, join an old road and turn right to descend along a wash to the south-southwest. At mile 19.5, go straight through a gate and continue to follow the road down lower Scotia Canyon. As you approach FR 48, leave the drainage, and follow cairns and signs as you hike through a flat parking area on the east side of FR 48. Cross the road where the AZT sign directs you to a trail on the west side of FR 48 at about mile 20.4.

To continue on the AZT, follow the singletrack through a pleasant, forested bench going south-southwest. Descend to and cross a major wash following cairns and signs. Continue through a vehicle-accessible camping area, and then pick up a clear singletrack that climbs a short but steep hill.

Cross an old jeep road (at about mile 21.2), a wash, a corral and gate, and another road. On the other side of this road is a parking area and a kiosk identifying the AZT. It marks the end of Passage 1.

Mountain Bike Notes

Bikes are not permitted on trails in Coronado National Memorial or Miller Peak Wilderness. Cyclists wishing to start at the international border will have to improvise by using roads outside the memorial boundary. An easier alternative is to start at Montezuma Pass and ride west on FR 61 to FR 48 and the beginning of Passage 2, near Parker Canyon Lake. Mountain bikers also can ride the AZT in Passage 1 outside of the Miller Peak Wilderness, from Parker Canyon Lake Trailhead to the wilderness boundary in Sunnyside Canyon. Starting and finishing at Parker Canyon Lake and connecting Scotia and Sunnyside Canyons makes for an excellent loop. *For detailed information about scenic mountain biking routes around wilderness areas, vi*sit aztrail.org. *Note:* Passage 2 (see page 58) provides good mountain biking for advanced riders.

SOUTHERN ACCESS: Mexico-U.S. Border

As referenced in the overview, above, to access the true beginning of Passage 1, at the international border, you must walk southbound on the trail itself, starting at mile 1.9 atop Montezuma Pass.

To reach Montezuma Pass from the town of Sonoita, follow AZ 83 south 30 miles to its intersection with FR 48. Turn left (south) onto FR 48 and continue 5.4 miles to FR 61. Continue east 8.8 miles on a rough dirt road to a large parking area at the summit of the pass.

To reach Montezuma Pass from Sierra Vista, travel 14 miles south on AZ 92 and turn right (south) on South Coronado Memorial Road. Continue 8.3 miles, generally south and west, to the large parking area at the summit of the pass. Shortly after you pass the Coronado Memorial Visitor Center, the road turns to dirt and climbs to the pass via switchbacks. This road is unsafe for vehicles hauling horse trailers (use the approach from FR 61 instead).

From your car, at Montezuma Pass, hike toward the Passage 1 start at the Mexico border by heading to the kiosk in the southeast end of the Coronado National Memorial Visitor Center parking lot. Climb a short distance on a clear tread, and follow a sign for the Coronado Peak Trail. After 0.1 mile, turn left onto Joe's Canyon Trail, which follows the ridgeline to the southeast. Descend to a saddle and an intersection at mile 0.8, turn right (south) on the combined AZT and Yaqui Ridge Trail, and follow switchbacks down Yaqui Ridge. At 1.9 miles from the parking lot, reach the fence that separates Mexico from the United States and another fence that runs up the ridge to the north. An obelisk here notes that the Treaty of 1853 established the international boundary and marks the true beginning of the AZT.

You could also access the combined AZT and Yaqui Ridge Trail to the border by hiking Joe's Canyon Trail from where it starts near the Coronado National Memorial Visitor Center, but that option is longer and more strenuous.

Note: It is illegal to cross the fence line into the Mexican state of Sonora.

ALTERNATE ACCESS: Sunnyside Canyon Trailhead

As noted in the Key Info on page 50, this trailhead, at AZT mile 16.6, is a good place to leave a vehicle for a shuttle hike in order to shorten the distance you must cover in a single push. From the town of Sonoita, drive AZ 83 south 30 miles to its intersection with FR 48. Turn left (south) onto FR 48, continue 2.2 miles, and turn left (east) onto FR 228. Drive 0.9 mile to a fork and stay left. Continue 1.6 miles to a T-intersection and turn right on FR 204. Drive 0.3 mile to a Y-intersection and bear left on FR 204. Over the next 0.2 mile, ignore three left turns, following the road as it winds back to the right to intersect another road at a sharp angle. Turn left here and drive 0.5 mile to meet the AZT, which leaves the road on the left. Continue 0.1 mile to a small parking area at the wilderness boundary.

NORTHERN ACCESS: Parker Canyon Lake Trailhead

If you want to hit the trail from here, please follow the trail description in reverse order. From the town of Sonoita, follow AZ 83 south 30 miles to its intersection with FR 48. Turn left (south) onto FR 48, continue 0.5 mile, and turn right onto South Lake Drive. Proceed 0.5 mile to a parking area near an AZT kiosk.

Canelo Hills: East

KEY INFO

LOCATION Parker Canyon Lake Trailhead to Canelo Pass

DISTANCE 14.5 miles one-way

DAY-TRIP OPTION See turnaround note in the trail description.

SHUTTLE RECOMMENDATION Canelo Road (passage mile 9.0)

DIFFICULTY Moderate

LAND MANAGERS Coronado National Forest, Sierra Vista Ranger District, **www.fs.usda.gov/coronado,** 520-378-0311

RECOMMENDED MONTHS September–May

GATEWAY COMMUNITY Not applicable

GEOLOGY HIGHLIGHTS Not applicable

OVERVIEW

Very few outdoor enthusiasts explore the hills north of Parker Canyon Lake. Because they don't command the respect of higher mountain ranges nearby, the Canelo Hills go relatively unnoticed. But as with many of Arizona's natural wonders, careful examination reveals incredible beauty. The trail follows a rolling path up and down hills and crosses many arroyos. Although this is not a designated wilderness area, there is little evidence of humans along the trail.

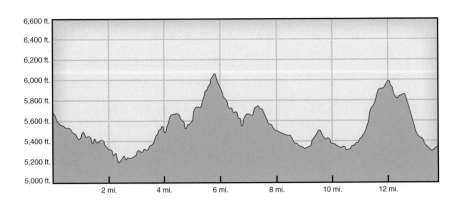

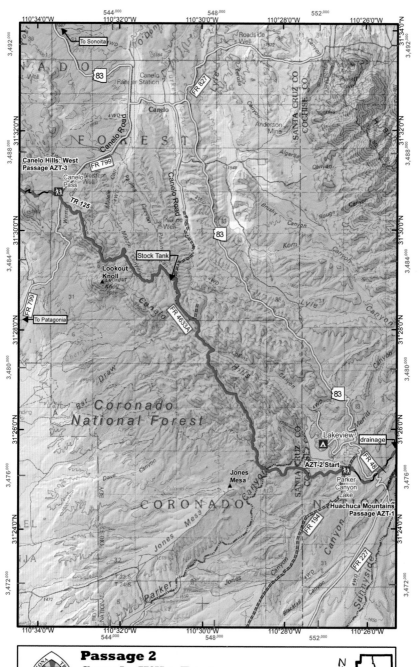

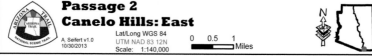

Campsites are plentiful, but water is scarce. It's a good idea to stock up at the beginning of the passage and leave a cache at Canelo Pass. In springtime, after a wet winter, water may trickle down the network of small canyons crossed by the trail, nurturing lush growth. Grasslands, oak savannahs, and groves of gnarled mesquite provide cover for healthy populations of wildlife, including the Mexican opossum. The trail is easy to follow except in the frequent drainage crossings, where cairns mark the way. Camping is permitted unless signs indicate otherwise.

ON THE TRAIL

From the southern access point, northbound travelers should head for the kiosk at the trailhead (at 5,680 feet) and follow an old, rocky road that descends to the west and reaches a CLOSED TO ALL VEHICLES sign. A side trail to Parker Canyon Lake leaves the Arizona National Scenic Trail (AZT) here. The AZT heads to the right of the road-closed sign and gradually climbs a ridge where you soon have a view of Parker Canyon Lake, a popular destination for anglers, swimmers, and campers.

Descending for the next 0.1 mile, pass through a gate and continue another 0.1 mile to cross the drainage at the bottom of Parker Canyon. Clear water flows here throughout much of the year.

The AZT goes through another gate and contours above a side canyon, and then crosses it several times over the next 0.5 mile. After passing through another gate, join a drainage heading north for about 100 yards. Head out of the drainage to the left (west) and make a substantial climb to the top of a small ridge.

TURNAROUND NOTE: Ups and downs ensue until a sustained climb begins, lasting until the AZT reaches a saddle—an ideal turnaround spot for day-hikers who haven't arranged a car shuttle.

The trail descends along steep switchbacks, bottoms out, bends right (north), and starts to climb again. Pass through a gate and top out in a saddle, then bear left (north-northwest) to cross a ridge. To continue on the trail, turn left (west) onto an old road, and climb 0.1 mile to an AZT trail marker (a four-by-four wooden post). From the marker, the road curves to the right (north) and descends gradually to reveal impressive views to the northeast. Follow trail makers through a gate to the left (south). Stay on this new road (FR 4633A) as it bends to the right (west) in about 25 yards.

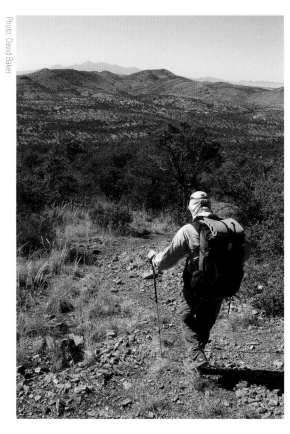

Photo: David Baker

The AZT follows a rugged, rocky path through the seldom-traveled Canelo Hills.

Near mile 9, you pass a stock tank that sometimes has murky water, then bend to the right (northwest). Stands of sturdy ponderosa pines adorn the trail here. As you descend, a deep forest of pine, juniper, and oak envelops you. In the heart of these woods, turn left (south) onto an intersecting jeep road.

The AZT climbs over a ridge before descending to cross an arroyo. From here, *don't* follow the road as it climbs a steep hill to the southwest. Instead, turn right (north-northwest) onto singletrack that dances in and out of a small wash for the next 0.5 mile. The trail starts a committing climb, bends right (north) near the top of a ridge, and continues a gentler climb along a fence to a high point (5,980 feet). From this stretch, the sharp peak of Mount Wrightson, monarch of Passage 5, dominates the horizon to the west-northwest.

As Canelo Pass Road (FR 799) comes into view, pass through a gate in the fence, and begin a switchbacking descent to the west. The trail comes within 20 feet of the road, and then it turns right (north) and climbs to cross the road at mile 14.5, the end of Passage 2. If you are desperate for water, walk onto the road here, turn left, and follow it to the first road sign on your right. Follow the faint jeep track on your right to a dirt tank that may have water.

Mountain Bike Notes

Although this passage is not particularly technical, it has countless climbs, loose rock, steep grades, and sandy wash crossings. Pedaling with a full load makes it harder still. It's also a lot of fun, and a rare opportunity for a long bike ride into remote grassland and oak woodland ecosystems. Grazing over the past century has dispersed a mountain biker's nemesis, catclaw acacia, widely across the landscape. Use a liquid sealant or tubeless system, or plan on patching dozens of punctures along this passage. *For more information about mountain biking along the Arizona National Scenic Trail, visit* **aztrail.org.**

SOUTHERN ACCESS: Parker Canyon Lake Trailhead

From the town of Sonoita, follow AZ 83 south 30 miles to its intersection with FR 48. Turn left (south) onto FR 48, continue 0.5 mile, and turn right onto South Lake Drive. Proceed 0.5 mile to a parking area near an AZT kiosk.

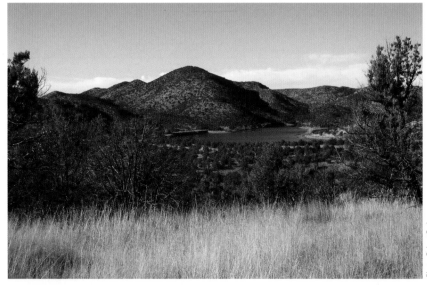

Photo: Robert Garber

Parker Canyon Lake, marking the beginning of Passage 2, is a pleasant oasis nestled among the oaks.

NORTHERN ACCESS: Canelo Pass Trailhead

If you want to hit the trail from here, please follow the trail description in reverse order.
From the town of Patagonia, follow Harshaw Road (FR 58) east 14 miles to an intersection where FR 58 makes a 90-degree turn to the right. Avoid this turn and continue straight ahead (northeast) on FR 799. In 5 miles, cross Canelo Pass and continue about 0.5 mile down the other side to a large parking area on the left (west) side of the road. The trail toward Patagonia departs from the right side of a kiosk; the trail arriving from Passage 2 is on the left side of the kiosk.

From the town of Sonoita, follow AZ 83 south for 18 miles to a turnoff on the right for FR 799. Continue 2.9 miles to a parking area on the right that is marked with AZT signs.

PASSAGE 3

Canelo Hills: West

KEY INFO

LOCATION Canelo Pass to Patagonia

DISTANCE 16.6 miles one-way

DAY-TRIP OPTION See turnaround note in the trail description.

SHUTTLE RECOMMENDATION Not applicable

DIFFICULTY Moderate

LAND MANAGER Coronado National Forest, Sierra Vista Ranger District, **www.fs.usda.gov/coronado,** 520-378-0311

RECOMMENDED MONTHS September–May

GATEWAY COMMUNITY See Patagonia (page 305).

GEOLOGY HIGHLIGHTS Not applicable

OVERVIEW

Rolling grasslands mixed with Upper Sonoran Desert define this passage. Hundreds of plant and animal species thrive in the nearby Patagonia–Sonoita Creek Preserve, owned and managed by The Nature Conservancy. This preserve's 275 species of birds

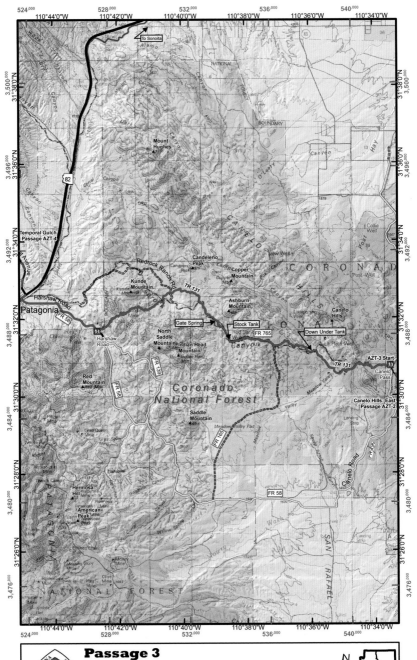

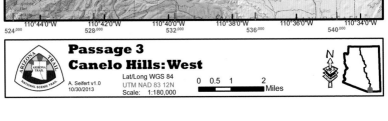

Passage 3
Canelo Hills: West

A. Seifert v1.0
10/30/2013

Lat/Long WGS 84
UTM NAD 83 12N
Scale: 1:180,000

0   0.5   1   2
Miles

N

attract tens of thousands of bird enthusiasts each year. You might catch a glimpse of a rare violet-crowned hummingbird, northern beardless-tyrannulet, or gray hawk.

Passage 3 does not feel as isolated as the first two passage, but it is rarely used—despite its proximity to the preserve. Novice backpackers might enjoy a one- or two-night shuttle hike starting at Canelo Pass and ending at the Harshaw Road Trailhead (see the map and alternate access instructions). Plan hikes to avoid camping between mile 5.5 and about mile 6.3, where regulations prohibit overnight stays.

ON THE TRAIL

Two singletracks lead away from the kiosk in the Canelo Pass Trailhead parking lot (5,330 feet). Follow the one on the right, to the west, climbing slightly. (The trail on the left is the end of the AZT's Passage 2.) Pass through a gate in a saddle at mile 1.1 (5,600 feet), and descend fairly steeply through three switchbacks to the north edge of Meadow Valley at mile 2.1. The trail soon turns left (southwest) onto an old jeep road.

At an intersection at mile 2.4, turn right and follow the road over a small hill to the intersection with a more heavily traveled road (FR 765). Cross the road and continue a bit more than a mile on a singletrack section that gradually slopes to the northwest taking you into Redrock Canyon and terminating at the southeast end of the Down Under Tank dam. You rejoin the ranch access road at the northwest end of the dam.

If there is no water in Down Under Tank, check in the streambed below the dam—within the first 200 yards. (And always remember to follow water-purification protocol in the wilderness; see "Contaminated Water," page 10.) Continue descending through the pleasant, open oak savannah.

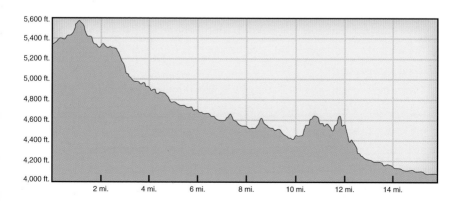

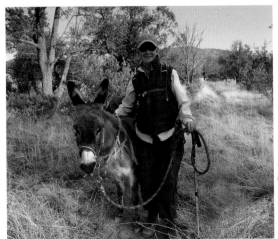

Photo: Leigh Anne Thrasher

Hikers not wanting to carry a fully-loaded backpack often rely on pack stock–donkeys, mules, llamas, goats, and horses–to help bear the burden.

TURNAROUND NOTE: At about mile 5.9, you reach a broken windmill where signs indicate camping is prohibited. This marks a great place to turn around and head back to your car if you're doing an out-and-back hike for the day.

The road veers right (north) to continue descending through Redrock Canyon, and near mile 6.3, it passes a north-facing no-camping sign (indicating you're leaving the no-camping zone). To continue on the trail, proceed on a charming old road to a fork at mile 7.5. Bear right (north) to cross the drainage and pass the windmill at Red Bank Well. If there's no visible water, try lowering the float in the trough to activate the flow. Pass through a corral as the road ends and continue down canyon to the north on a clear singletrack.

You pass near Gate Spring at mile 8.3, which is down the hillside about 150 yards to the south. Do not linger in this area because it is within the habitat of threatened and endangered species.

Turn right (north) at a fork at mile 9.3, pass through a gate at mile 9.4, and, in 50 yards, follow a trail that leaves the drainage bottom to the left (northwest). A brief climb leads into a gnarly forest of mesquite. Continue straight across a road to the west at mile 10.0. At mile 10.5, pass through a wash and turn southwest to parallel the wash for 80 yards. Follow the trail left (south) out of the wash, and climb through switchbacks to mile 11.9.

Pass through a gate, and then reach a saddle at mile 13.2 that offers a view of the Harshaw Creek Valley winding northwest to Patagonia. Several switchbacks lead down to Harshaw Road (FR 58) at mile 13.7. If you left a car here, cross the road and follow singletrack a few yards to the parking lot.

If you left your car in Patagonia—or if you're thru-hiking the AZT—turn right (northwest) and follow the road. Pass Patagonia RV Park at mile 16.3. At mile 16.6, the road winds to the left and enters the town. In another 0.1 mile, turn right at the post office, and walk to Naugle Avenue (AZ 82), the main drag through town. Turn right and follow the road to First Avenue. This is the end of Passage 3; Passage 4 turns left onto First Avenue and continues northwest.

Mountain Bike Notes

This passage of the AZT provides almost continuous riding for more advanced riders. It has short stretches of difficult terrain, with some rocky, steep sections, but most of the passage is accessible to those with honed singletrack skills. *For more information about mountain biking along the Arizona National Scenic Trail, visit* **aztrail.org.**

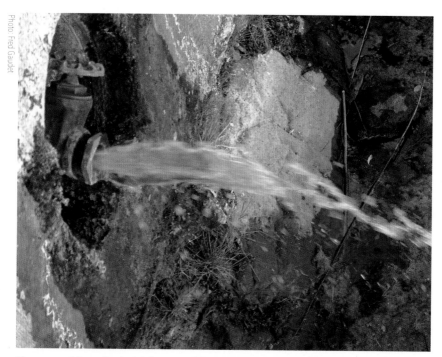

Photo: Fred Gaudet

The seasonal Down Under Tank is one of the most coveted water sources along Passage 3.

SOUTHERN ACCESS: Canelo Pass Trailhead

From the town of Patagonia, follow Harshaw Road (FR 58) east 14 miles to an intersection with FR 799. Traveling north on FR 799 for 5 miles, cross Canelo Pass and continue about 0.5 mile down the other side to a large parking area on the left (west) side of the road. The trail toward Patagonia departs from the right side of a kiosk; the trail arriving from Passage 2 is on the left side of the kiosk.

From the town of Sonoita, follow AZ 83 south for 18 miles to a turnoff on the right for FR 799. Continue 2.9 miles to a parking area on the right that is marked with AZT signs.

NORTHERN ACCESS: Patagonia

If you want to hit the trail from here, please follow the trail description in reverse order. While Passage 3 ends in the town of Patagonia, most trail users park at the Harshaw Road Trailhead to avoid the last 3.2 miles of this passage, which is along roads with motor vehicles. From Patagonia, take Harshaw Road (FR 58) east for 2.8 miles. You will see the trailhead on the left and a large parking area on the right.

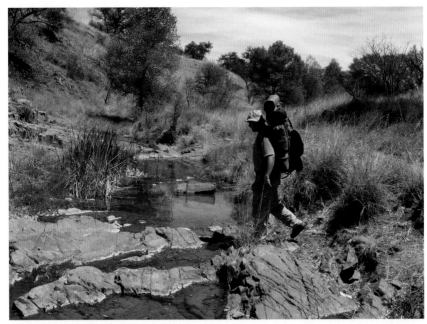

After winter snowmelt and summer monsoon storms, the canyons along Passage 3 hold water for a few weeks, turning the otherwise-dry hills into a pleasant paradise for trail users.

PASSAGE 4

Temporal Gulch

LOCATION Patagonia to Gardner Canyon Road (FR 92)

DISTANCE 22.3 miles one-way

DAY-TRIP OPTION See turnaround note in the trail description.

SHUTTLE RECOMMENDATION Temporal Gulch Trailhead (passage mile 7.0)

DIFFICULTY Strenuous

LAND MANAGER Coronado National Forest, Nogales Ranger District, **www.fs.usda.gov/coronado,** 520-281-2296

RECOMMENDED MONTHS March–November

GATEWAY COMMUNITIES See Patagonia (page 305) and Sonoita (page 306).

GEOLOGY HIGHLIGHTS Not applicable

OVERVIEW

The first part of this passage follows Temporal Canyon Road, a graded-gravel road extending 7 miles north from Patagonia to the Temporal Gulch trailhead, then traces 6.1 miles of high-clearance doubletrack to the trailhead at Upper Walker Tank. Temporal Canyon Road offers outstanding views of the Santa Rita Mountains and surrounding grasslands. This passage starts in a grassland ecosystem and climbs through oak savannah to reach the thick oak–pine forest on the edge of the Mount Wrightson Wilderness.

Passages 4 and 5 offer an interesting contrast, as the route passes through remote, relatively untouched wilderness and then enters one of southern Arizona's most productive former mining regions. The Greaterville Mining District, which the Arizona National Scenic Trail (AZT) enters shortly after exiting the wilderness, drew hundreds of Mexican and U.S. prospectors after gold was discovered here in 1874. Interpretive signs describe the extensive water-diversion project that took water uphill from Gardner Canyon into Boston Gulch for high-pressure hydraulic mining. As is the nature of boom-and-bust operations, the mine failed soon after it was started.

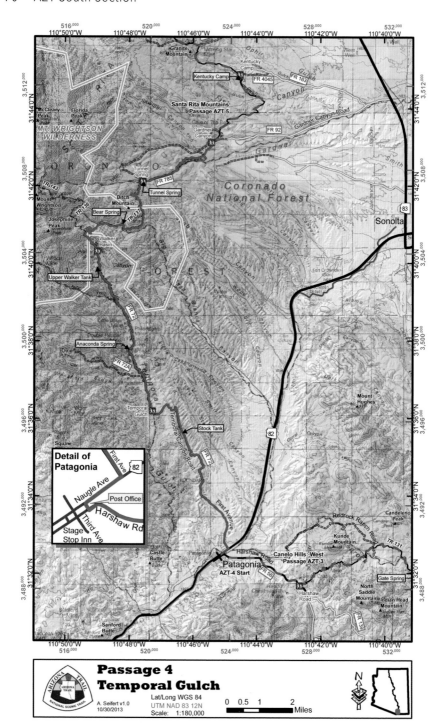

Passage 4
Temporal Gulch

Lat/Long WGS 84
A. Seifert v1.0   UTM NAD 83 12N
10/30/2013   Scale: 1:180,000

0   0.5   1   2
Miles

The jewel of the trail user's view of the Santa Rita Mountains is the Mount Wrightson Wilderness, whose summit rises to 9,453 feet. A side trip up this peak (although off the AZT) is incredible—there is nothing like standing on top of one of the most visible landmarks in southern Arizona. The rugged wilderness that surrounds the peak is home to rare birds and some plants that occur nowhere else north of Mexico.

In early spring, snow blankets the higher reaches of the AZT, making some hills difficult to traverse. Early-season travelers should wear sturdy boots, take their time on the snow, and travel with companions. Never underestimate the Santa Rita Mountains.

ON THE TRAIL

From the intersection of First Avenue and AZ 82 (Naugle Avenue), travel northwest along First Avenue for less than 1 mile (4,067 feet). Please respect private residences. After crossing a cattle guard at mile 0.5, the road turns to dirt. Avoid turning onto any side roads. At mile 0.8, the trail bends left, crosses a wash, and starts climbing. At a fork at mile 2, avoid a left turn to the landfill. In 0.4 mile, a sign indicates that you are on FR 72. The stony face of Mount Wrightson's summit dominates the horizon directly in front of you.

Stay on the main graded dirt road. After you pass a sign indicating you are entering public lands, there are plenty of places to camp along the road. Pass a sign at mile 6.8 that says ARIZONA TRAIL TRAILHEAD ¼ MILE, avoiding a fork to the left. In 0.2 mile, cross a cattle guard and follow a right fork to the trailhead (mile 7). Motorists must have a four-wheel-drive vehicle to proceed beyond this point.

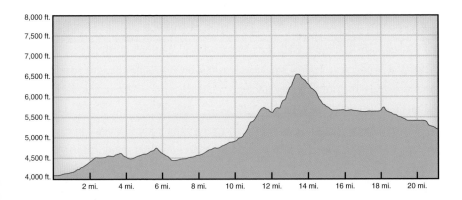

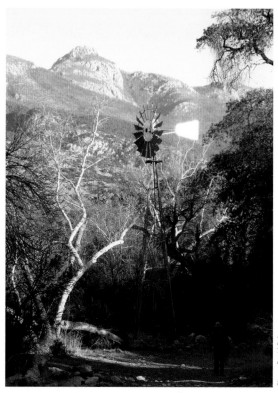

Photo: David Baker

The granite crown atop Mount Wrightson (9,453 feet) remains in view for much of Passage 4.

Follow the road west through a small wash and then bend to the right to parallel the wash to the north. You may find water here during spring runoff. Just after the trail crosses the wash again, you'll see several nice campsites. From here on, flat ground is rare, but you might improvise a camping spot at the Walker Basin Trailhead.

Brown carsonite posts mark the rest of the passage. Avoid the occasional fork, such as FR 72A or the singletrack Temporal Trail. You'll reach a small parking area for the Walker Basin Trailhead. Walk the rocky road as it continues north into the Mount Wrightson Wilderness. Follow singletrack as it switchbacks up the lower reaches of Josephine Peak. The stunning views behind you reach far into Mexico and the myriad mountain ranges within Sonora.

The trail forks at a saddle (6,560 feet), where you might find a place to camp but no water. A metal sign labeled ARIZONA TRAIL marks this intersection, the high point of Passage 4.

TURNAROUND NOTE: If you're just out for the day and have started near the Walker Basin Trailhead, this is a great spot to soak up the views and return to your vehicle.

To continue on the trail, turn 90 degrees to the right (east), and follow a side trail as it descends through several switchbacks into Big Casa Blanca Canyon. The trail meanders to the north and reaches the Tunnel Spring Trailhead and a dirt road (5,640 feet).

You soon pass the first of many interpretive signs describing the elaborate flume intended to transport water to Boston Gulch for gold mining in the early 1900s. Turn right (east) onto the road (FR 785), pass through a gate, continue 1.2 miles to a side road that breaks off sharply to the left (west), and turn onto it. This turn is easy to miss—there is a sign here, but it faces the opposite direction along the road. Cross the stream and pick up a clear singletrack turning back to the right (north). Follow this popular mountain bike segment across FR 785. After crossing a cow pasture, two gates, and a wash, you reach the road again; turn right (northeast), walk about 100 yards, and pick up the trail branching off to the left. Continue 0.3 mile to the Gardner Canyon Trailhead and the end of Passage 4.

Mountain Bike Notes

Most of this passage is unsuitable for biking, unless you want to combine the northern part of it with the southern part of Passage 5. While you may ride the easy, then difficult 13.1-mile Temporal Canyon Road, bikes are prohibited north of Walker Basin Trailhead. Instead, skip this southern portion of the trail by biking (or driving and then biking) AZ 82 north to Sonoita. Turn left (north) onto AZ 83, ride about 1.3 miles, and turn left (west) onto FR 4104.

Ride about 7 miles on an occasionally difficult road to FR 785, turn left, and continue west less than 2 miles to a sign on the right that marks the AZT, at the Tunnel Spring Trailhead. From this point and north through Passage 5 to AZ 83 provides excellent, moderate singletrack riding. You can ride point-to-point by leaving a vehicle at one of the access points, or do an out-and-back from a particular trailhead. *For detailed information about scenic mountain biking routes around wilderness areas,* visit **aztrail.org.**

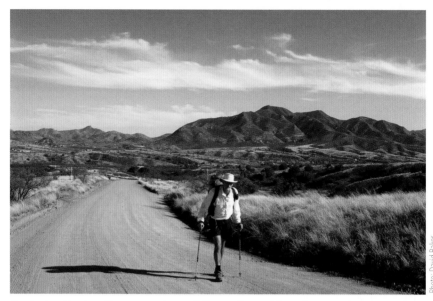

For the first 7 miles of Passage 4, the AZT follows a dirt road from the town of Patagonia into the dense forest of the Santa Rita Mountains.

SOUTHERN ACCESS: Temporal Gulch Trailhead

Take AZ 82 to the town of Patagonia. At the north end of town, south of the high school, First Avenue heads northwest from the highway. The AZT follows First Avenue (later FR 72) for the next 7 miles before it becomes a rugged four-wheel-drive road.

ALTERNATE ACCESS: Walker Basin Trailhead

Follow the same directions to Temporal Gulch Trailhead (above). From here, four-wheel-drive vehicles can continue 6.1 miles along very rough FR 72 to a small parking area at the trailhead.

NORTHERN ACCESS: Gardner Canyon Trailhead

If you want to hit the trail from here, please follow the trail description in reverse order. From Sonoita, follow AZ 83 north 4 miles, and turn left (west) onto Gardner Canyon Road (FR 92). Avoid turning onto any side roads. You reach the northern terminus for Passage 4, Gardner Trailhead (not to be confused with Gardner Canyon Trail, which is farther west), 5.5 miles from the highway on the right (north) side of the road. There is a large parking area here.

ALTERNATE NORTHERN ACCESS: Tunnel Spring Trailhead

If you want to hit the trail from here, please follow the trail description in reverse order.
From Sonoita, follow AZ 83 north 4 miles, and turn west (left) onto Gardner Canyon Road (FR 92). Avoid turning onto any side roads. You reach the Gardner Canyon Trailhead (the terminus for Passage 4), 5.5 miles from the highway on the right (north) side of the road. Continue another 0.8 mile and turn left (east) onto FR 785 at a sign for Gardner Canyon Trail. Continue 2.7 miles (crossing the AZT twice) to a small parking area at the Tunnel Spring Trailhead. The northbound trail continues down the road you just drove up. The southbound stretch heads into the trees to the southwest on singletrack.

PASSAGE 5

Santa Rita Mountains

KEY INFO

LOCATION Gardner Canyon Road to Oak Tree Canyon

DISTANCE 13.5 miles one-way

DAY-TRIP OPTION See turnaround note in the trail description.

SHUTTLE RECOMMENDATIONS Kentucky Camp Trailhead (passage mile 3.7), Forest Road 62 (passage mile 10.8)

DIFFICULTY Moderate

LAND MANAGER Coronado National Forest, Nogales Ranger District, **www.fs.usda.gov/coronado,** 520-281-2296

RECOMMENDED MONTHS September–May

GATEWAY COMMUNITY See Sonoita (page 306).

GEOLOGY HIGHLIGHTS Not applicable

OVERVIEW

Anyone who spends time in the Santa Rita Mountains comes to appreciate the rich biodiversity that exists within the sky islands. Black bears and bobcats are common sightings, and in 2012 a remote sensor camera captured images of a jaguar. If the theory holds that large mammals are excellent indicators for overall ecosystem health, the Santa Ritas make up a vibrant oasis in southern Arizona.

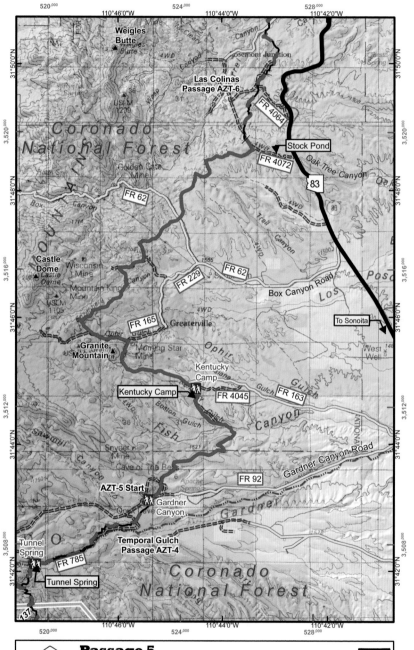

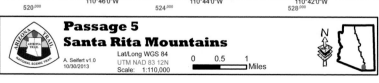

Passage 5
Santa Rita Mountains

A. Seifert v1.0
10/30/2013

Lat/Long WGS 84
UTM NAD 83 12N
Scale: 1:110,000

0   0.5   1
Miles

N

Like the terrain in the previous passage, these hills are rich in mining history, as you can observe from the trail. After gold was discovered in 1874, the town of Greaterville sprang up and soon boasted saloons, dance halls, stores, a jail, and a public school. Many of the original buildings still stand, and some are inhabited by descendants of the early Mexican residents. The town, whose buildings are private and not open to visitors, is just a mile off the Arizona National Scenic Trail (AZT).

The landscape around this passage might look significantly different if mining plans just after the turn of the 20th century had come to fruition. After gold production around Greaterville fell off in the early 1880s, the boomtown quieted, and most of its residents moved on to more promising venues. But there was a revival in 1904, when a well-financed Californian named James Stetson came to Greaterville with the idea of using hydraulic mining to reach previously inaccessible gold deposits in Boston Gulch. This system employed vast quantities of pressurized water to blast away the earth, revealing ore concealed beneath the surface. In order to ensure enough reliable water in Boston Gulch, Stetson built a system of pipes to carry water over a ridge from nearby Gardner Canyon, which is fed by the snowpack on Mount Wrightson. There is plenty of evidence of this aqueduct along the AZT, and frequent interpretive signs describe aspects of the project, including the physics of moving water uphill without a pump.

Much of Stetson's legacy remains in the form of Kentucky Camp, a collection of buildings constructed as a base for the mining operation. The AZT passes right through the camp, which is under renovation by the U.S. Forest Service and a dedicated group of volunteers called Friends of Kentucky Camp. The historic cabin is available for rent and makes for a deluxe camping experience.

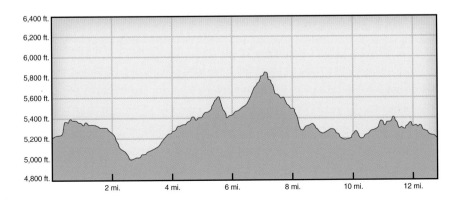

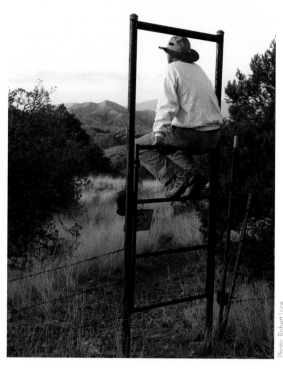

Looking back on the accordion-like ridges of the Santa Ritas

Photo: Robert Luce

Although a century has passed since mining activity was at its peak, the ground beneath the AZT remains rich with copper, molybdenum, and other minerals. An open-pit copper mine proposed for the Rosemont area (see "Future Impacts," page 84) may affect the AZT route within the next decade.

ON THE TRAIL

From the Gardner Canyon Trailhead, the AZT skirts the north side of the parking area (at 5,228 feet) and then makes a steep climb to the northeast. Top out in 0.2 mile after a few formidable switchbacks. Cross a minor high point and pass through a fence. The trail follows an old water-diversion ditch to the northeast. Turn right (east) onto FR 4110 and follow it along a high finger of land, where a trail departs to the left. Descend to the north and cross FR 4085 in less than a mile. Follow the trail through a meadow as it swings back to the west to reach historic Kentucky Camp (5,125 feet). Easy-to-follow AZT signs lead you through this area, which has running water, a modern outhouse, and a rental cabin. For information about the cabin, contact the Nogales Ranger District at 520-281-2296.

TURNAROUND NOTE: If you're hiking an out-and-back route from Gardner Canyon, Kentucky Camp makes a great destination and turn-around location. You'll have 7.5 miles under your boots by the time you return to your car at Gardner Canyon.

To continue on the trail, climb away from Kentucky Camp on the dirt road heading north. Pass through a fence in 0.3 mile, continue 50 yards, and turn left (west) onto FR 163. Climb steadily to a fork in the road, and stay right (north) on FR 163. Bear left at the next fork, staying on FR 163 until you reach the intersection with FR165 at the bottom of a very steep hill.

Turn left (southwest) onto FR 165, and follow it for 0.7 mile uphill to a small parking area and trailhead on the right. Pick up the singletrack that climbs to the north.

A stock pond just west of the trail here may have surprisingly clear water. To reach it, travel 0.1 mile along the AZT beyond the trailhead to a flat spot, and turn left (west) to bushwhack over a hill 0.1 mile to the pond.

The AZT soon joins an old roadbed and climbs gradually. Pick up singletrack with a sharp turn to the right. The trail reaches a high point in 0.5 mile and then begins descending to the north-northeast. Steep switchbacks lead to a drainage. The trail turns left (west-northwest) to join an old jeep road, then turns right (east) onto a second road. Watch for a 90-degree bend to the left (north).

The AZT crosses FR 62; look for a gate on the other side of the road and singletrack continuing to the northeast. In 0.1 mile, the trail turns left (north) onto an old road and climbs for the next 0.5 mile. Join another road and turn left (north). Make a sharp turn to the right (southeast) in 0.1 mile, then climb a ridge for 0.1 mile before taking off to the left (east) on singletrack.

After a short distance, join a road and turn left (north). Where the road appears to fork, avoid the clear road bending right (southeast) and turn left to follow a narrow track through a fence to the north. Continue to the top of a small knoll and take the right fork to the northeast. Pass through another gate, climb steeply for 100 yards, and turn left (northeast) onto a singletrack. The trail rejoins the narrow track and continues east and northeast. Join FR 4072 and turn left (north). The road descends 50 yards before bending right (east) in front of a water tank.

Continue east-northeast for 0.5 mile to junction and the end of Passage 5. Passage 6 is to your left (north); the right fork (east) connects in 0.8 mile to the small pullout and access point on AZ 83.

Mountain Bike Notes

This entire passage provides excellent singletrack riding. You can ride point-to-point by leaving a vehicle at one of the access points, or do an out-and-back from a particular trailhead or the junction with FR 62. *For more information about mountain biking along the Arizona National Scenic Trail, visit* **aztrail.org.**

SOUTHERN ACCESS: Gardner Canyon Trailhead

From Sonoita, follow AZ 83 north 4 miles and turn left (west) onto Gardner Canyon Road (FR 92). Avoid turning onto any side roads. You'll reach the Gardner Canyon Trailhead (not to be confused with Gardner Canyon Trail, which is farther west) 5.5 miles from the highway on the right side of the road. The trailhead has a large parking area.

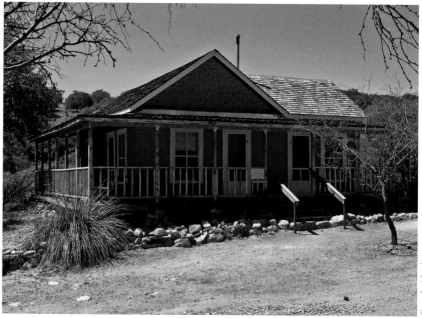

Photo: Fred Gaudet

Beautifully restored, this historic mining cabin at Kentucky Camp is available for rent through the Coronado National Forest.

ALTERNATE SOUTHERN ACCESS: Kentucky Camp

On AZ 83 at about mile marker 37.2, watch for signs pointing to Gardner Canyon and Kentucky Camp. Turn west onto FR 92, continue west for 1 mile to FR 163, and look for a sign on the north side of the road that points to Kentucky Camp. Take FR 163 for 5 miles to the gate for Kentucky Camp and FR 4085. The trailhead parking lot is clearly visible at this intersection; Kentucky Camp is about 0.3 mile down the hill. Please respect the private property owners' rights-of-way granted for public use.

NORTHERN ACCESS: AZ 83

If you want to hit the trail from here, please follow the trail description in reverse order. From the intersection of I-10 and AZ 83, drive south on AZ 83 approximately 16.5 miles to 0.8 mile past milepost 44. Pull off to the right (west) onto an unmarked road (FR 4072), and park near a locked metal gate. (Plans for an official trailhead at this location are under way.) Climb over the gate and follow the two-track road about 0.8 mile west up Oak Tree Canyon; watch for the trail on your right as it leaves the road and heads north.

PASSAGE 6

Las Colinas

KEY INFO

LOCATION Oak Tree Canyon to Lakes Road

DISTANCE 13.3 miles one-way

DAY-TRIP OPTION See turnaround note in the trail description.

SHUTTLE RECOMMENDATION Forest Road 231 (passage mile 3.2)

DIFFICULTY Moderate

LAND MANAGER Coronado National Forest, Nogales Ranger District, **www.fs.usda.gov/coronado,** 520-281-2296

RECOMMENDED MONTHS October–May

GATEWAY COMMUNITY Not applicable

GEOLOGY HIGHLIGHTS Not applicable

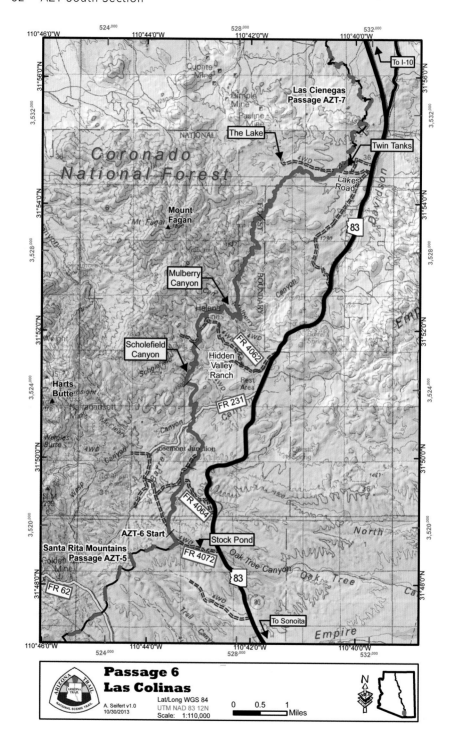

Passage 6
Las Colinas

Lat/Long WGS 84
UTM NAD 83 12N
Scale: 1:110,000

A. Seifert v1.0
10/30/2013

0   0.5   1
Miles

N

OVERVIEW

This beautiful passage rolls across the foothills of the Santa Rita Mountains with grand vistas to the west and the Empire Mountains to the east. Mount Wrightson dominates the south, while views of the majestic Rincon Mountains to the north foretell adventures ahead.

ON THE TRAIL

This passage begins on FR 4072 in Oak Tree Canyon. Singletrack heads north-northwest through semiopen country. There is a gate just past the 0.2-mile mark on top of a slight rise. From here the trail veers away from an old doubletrack and begins working its way downhill. At mile 1.6, you cross FR 4064. After a short section that heads due north, the trail turns to the northeast and passes through another gate at mile 2.0.

Climb a short ways and the trail turns to the northwest, presenting a view down into Barrel Canyon. After descending about 150 vertical feet and following the bottom of this large flat drainage for a short distance, arrive at FR 231, a well-maintained dirt road and the access route from AZ 83 to Rosemont Junction. The trail crosses at a slightly northbound angle and then works its way up and out of the canyon through a pleasant forest of ocotillo. Just before a high point, the trail passes through another gate at mile 4.4.

From the high point, the trail drops fairly steeply into Scholefield Canyon, where hikers have reported water but only in very wet seasons. Cross this drainage and then a smaller side drainage, and proceed to another gate at mile 5.5. Just past this gate, the trail curls around an unnamed drainage and then up to FR 4062 at mile 5.9. The trail climbs moderately up to a saddle and then turns to the east and descends first into Papago Canyon and then Mulberry Canyon.

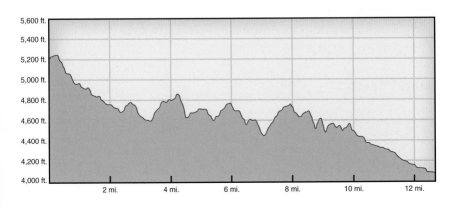

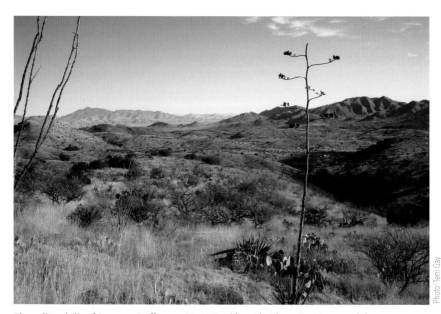

Photo: Terri Gay

The rolling hills of Passage 6 offer respite to tired legs that have just traversed the Santa Rita Mountains.

TURNAROUND NOTE: The aforementioned drainages make for a pleasant turnaround spot if you're day-tripping and you haven't arranged a car shuttle to the north.

To continue on the trail, climb out of Mulberry Canyon for about 250 feet over a distance of 0.7 mile. Traveling north, the trail turns north-northeast and begins crossing a series of small drainages and contouring around the hills between them. It passes through a gate at mile 10.5. Cross a road in 1.2 miles and continue 1.6 miles to the end of Passage 6, just southwest of the Twin Tanks stock tanks on Lakes Road.

Future Impacts

Rosemont Copper has plans to develop an open-pit copper mine in the northern region of the Santa Rita Mountains. If the U.S. Forest Service approves their proposal, mining operations would severely affect the current Arizona Trail route. Trail professionals and the ATA have designed a reroute of approximately 10 miles that will be implemented if the mine becomes reality.

Mountain Bike Notes

The entire passage provides decent singletrack. The grade of a portion of the trail is too steep to be completely enjoyable, but once you're out of the accordion-like features of the foothills, the trail improves dramatically. You can ride point-to-point by leaving a vehicle at one of the access points, or you can do an out-and-back ride from either the southern or northern access points. *For more information about mountain biking along the Arizona National Scenic Trail, visit* **aztrail.org.**

SOUTHERN ACCESS: AZ 83

From the intersection of I-10 and AZ 83, drive south on AZ 83 for 14 miles, to 0.8 mile past milepost 44. Pull off on the right (west) at an unmarked road (FR 4072), and park near a locked metal gate. Climb over the gate and walk about 0.8 mile west up Oak Tree Canyon, to an AZT trailhead sign.

NORTHERN ACCESS: Lakes Road

If you want to hit the trail from here, please follow the trail description in reverse order. From the intersection of I-10 and AZ 83, drive about south 7.2 miles on AZ 83 to 0.4 mile past milepost 51. Turn right (west) and pass through a gate on a rough, unmarked dirt road about 0.6 mile to the AZT trailhead sign. This road requires a high-clearance four-wheel-drive vehicle, but you could instead park near AZ 83 and walk or ride in (recommended).

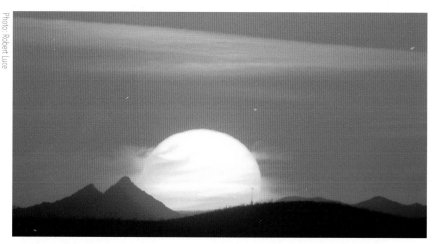

The sunsets of southern Arizona may be one of the state's greatest natural resources.

Photo: Robert Luce

Las Cienegas

KEY INFO

LOCATION Lakes Road to Gabe Zimmerman Trailhead

DISTANCE 13 miles one-way

DAY-TRIP OPTION See turnaround note in the trail description.

SHUTTLE RECOMMENDATION Sahuarita Road (passage mile 6.2)

DIFFICULTY Easy

LAND MANAGERS Pima County, **pima.gov,** 520-877-6000; Arizona State Land Department, **azland.gov,** 602-542-4631

RECOMMENDED MONTHS October–May

GATEWAY COMMUNITY See Sonoita (page 306) and Vail (page 308).

GEOLOGY HIGHLIGHTS Not applicable

OVERVIEW

This passage traverses the valley between the Santa Rita and Rincon Mountains. It offers spectacular views and, but for a few climbs, mostly involves a gentle descent to the north. The trail travels through low underpasses at AZ 83 and I-10. Equestrians should evaluate these before heading out; an equestrian bypass is available (and signed) under I-10 to avoid the cement culvert, which can be stressful for equines.

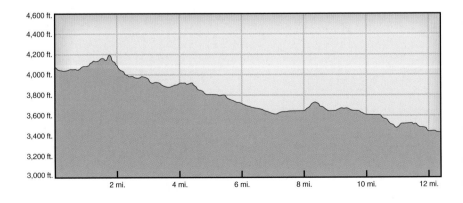

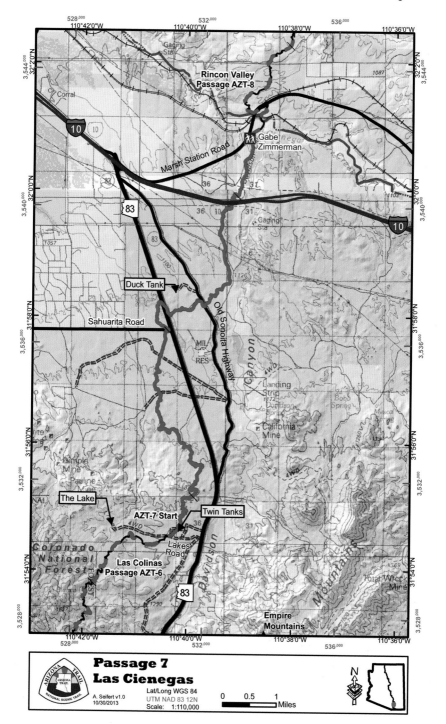

Passage 7
Las Cienegas

A. Seifert v1.0
10/30/2013

Lat/Long WGS 84
UTM NAD 83 12N
Scale: 1:110,000

0   0.5   1
Miles

N

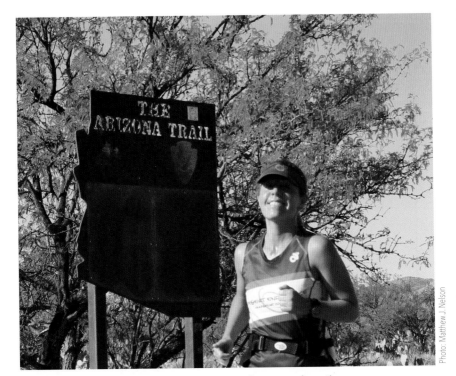

The gentle terrain of Passage 7 makes it a premier destination for trail runners.

As you approach Davidson Canyon and the Gabe Zimmerman Trailhead, you'll likely notice that the landscape is covered with creosote bush. After cattle-ranching operations decimated the native grasses and shrubs through here in the late 1800s, creosote moved in, and because it contains oils that are indigestible to cattle, it has become the dominant plant. The plant is highly medicinal and was used traditionally for respiratory ailments, to heal bruises and broken bones, and as a purgative. Whenever rain falls on the desert, the smell that rises from the earth is the sweet aroma of creosote. Crush a few of the oily green leaves between your fingers, and inhale for a refreshing experience.

ON THE TRAIL

This passage begins on a doubletrack known as Lakes Road. From there the trail heads north, with Twin Tanks visible to the east between the trail and AZ 83. At mile 0.2, cross a doubletrack that accesses the dirt-tank water of Twin Tanks. North of Twin Tanks, the trail enters a gentle rolling contour along low hills. Cross another doubletrack at mile 0.7. Reach a gate at a small saddle at mile 1.5.

After the gate, the benched trail affords great views north to the Rincon and Santa Catalina Mountains. The trail contours through fields of ocotillo, with the Empire Mountains to the east. Eventually the trail rolls in and out of several minor washes to reach a doubletrack at mile 2.7. Cross a flat area at 3.3 miles, a small drainage at mile 3.6, and a dirt road at mile 3.9. The trail stays nearly level and crosses a rough double-track at mile 5.3.

Reach a gate and Sahuarita Road at mile 6.8. Cross this paved road with caution, and pick up the trail on the north side of Sahuarita Road (look for a brown carsonite sign just a few feet down the trail).

TURNAROUND NOTE: If you haven't arranged a car shuttle, return to Lakes Road from Sahuarita Road for an out-and-back distance of 13.4 miles.

To continue on the trail, note that it stays on the west side of AZ 83 before crossing underneath the highway in a culvert at mile 7.6. Continue in the wash, and look for a cairn marking the exit from the wash off to the right. Take this path south, parallel-ing, but now east of AZ 83 until the trail starts to head east.

At mile 8.3 cross a seldom-used doubletrack, and then at mile 8.9 crest a small rise to cross paved Old Sonoita Highway, and go through the gate on the east side. Soon the trail, which has been traveling in a northeasterly direction, takes a turn to head north. Cross under a set of power lines at mile 10.3.

The trail turns east and descends into a wash, crossing a set of buried power lines right before reaching a gate. Cross underneath I-10 through a long, dark tunnel at about mile 11.5.

A cairn to the north marks where the trail continues through an area thick with creosote bushes. Go through a gate at mile 11.8, and cross a road at mile 12. Continue north along the west bank of Davidson Canyon, picking up a doubletrack before reach-ing the impressive Gabe Zimmerman Trailhead and the end of Passage 7. Equestrians should follow the signs and cairns to the east to avoid the I-10 culvert. This equestrian bypass rejoins the main AZT route near the Gabe Zimmerman Trailhead.

Gabriel "Gabe" Zimmerman, for whom the trailhead is named, was among six people killed when a gunman opened fire at a community event in Tucson, held by then–U.S. Representative Gabrielle Giffords (D–AZ) on January 8, 2011. At that time, Zimmerman was an aide to the congresswoman. This area celebrates his life—and those of everyone who was affected by that tragedy. Take a few moments to experience

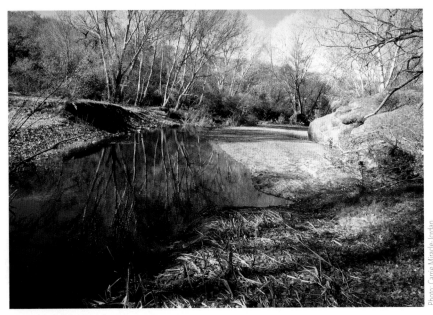

The AZT crosses through Cienega Creek Nature Preserve, a riparian corridor that supports a diverse population of plants, trees, insects, fish, reptiles, and mammals.

the contemplation bench, at the end of a short trail southeast of the trailhead, with views of Davidson Canyon, Cienega Creek, and the surrounding mountains.

Mountain Bike Notes

The entire passage provides excellent, moderate singletrack. You can ride point-to-point by leaving vehicles at one of the access points, or you can do an out-and-back ride from one of the trailheads. At the Gabe Zimmerman Trailhead, you can use the unique bike rack—in the form of a snake. *For more information about mountain biking along the Arizona National Scenic Trail, visit* **aztrail.org.**

SOUTHERN ACCESS: Lakes Road Trailhead

From the intersection of I-10 and AZ 83, drive about 7.2 miles south on AZ 83 to 0.4 mile past milepost 51. Turn right (west) and go through a gate on a rough, unmarked dirt road about 0.6 mile to a brown carsonite post. This road requires a high-clearance four-wheel-drive vehicle to access the trailhead, but you could instead park near AZ 83 and walk or ride in (recommended).

ALTERNATE SOUTHERN ACCESS: Sahuarita Road

From the intersection of I-10 and AZ 83, drive 3.4 miles south to Sahuarita Road. Park on the northwest corner of the intersection in the large dirt lot, and locate the trail where it discreetly crosses Sahuarita Road, 150 feet to the west.

NORTHERN ACCESS: Gabe Zimmerman Trailhead

If you want to hit the trail from here, please follow the trail description in reverse order. Take Exit 281 off I-10 and drive north to follow Marsh Station Road (frontage road) for 3 miles to a parking area, on the right (east) side of the road.

PASSAGE 8

Rincon Valley

KEY INFO

○ **LOCATION** Gabe Zimmerman Trailhead to Saguaro National Park

DISTANCE 14.8 miles one-way

DAY-TRIP OPTION See turnaround note in the trail description.

SHUTTLE RECOMMENDATION Colossal Cave Mountain Park (passage mile 4.7)

DIFFICULTY Easy

LAND MANAGERS Saguaro National Park, **nps.gov/sagu,** 520-733-5158 for headquarters; Colossal Cave Mountain Park, **colossalcave .com/welcome.html,** 520-647-7275; Pima County, **pima.gov,** 520-877-6000; Arizona State Land Department, **azland.gov,** 602-542-4631

RECOMMENDED MONTHS September–April

GATEWAY COMMUNITY See Vail (page 308).

GEOLOGY HIGHLIGHTS See "The Karst of Colossal Cave" (page 338).

OVERVIEW

This passage takes you through Cienega Creek, a lush riparian corridor that has perennial water and harbors a population of native fish. Autumn in the creek offers some of the

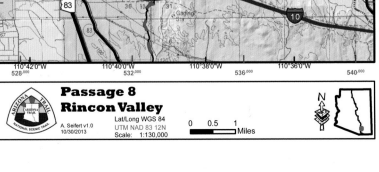

Passage 8
Rincon Valley

Lat/Long WGS 84
A. Seifert v1.0
10/30/2013

UTM NAD 83 12N
Scale: 1:130,000

0   0.5   1
Miles

N

best colors imaginable. The geology is dramatic and beautiful, and this passage is popular among equestrians, mountain bikers, and trail runners. The Arizona National Scenic Trail (AZT) through Cienega Creek Nature Preserve is open to all nonmotorized users, but exploring the preserve outside the trail corridor requires a permit from Pima County.

Passage 8 also passes through Colossal Cave Mountain Park, a privately operated Pima County Park that is home to one of southern Arizona's most accessible and impressive cave formations. This may be your only opportunity to go underground while on the AZT (culverts and underpasses don't count), and the perspective of seeing a completely different world just below the surface should not be missed.

Inspiring views of the Rincon Mountains define this passage, and as you enter Saguaro National Park (one of only two national parks that allow mountain bikes on dirt trails), you'll experience a vegetative transition from desert scrub to lush saguaro forests. Enjoy easy trail miles as you explore this wonderful singletrack, because an arduous ascent into the Rincon Mountains lies ahead.

ON THE TRAIL

The trail begins at the kiosk on the east side of the parking lot and follows a clear path northeast 0.3 mile where it drops into an arroyo and turns north. It runs through the sandy drainage, crosses Cienega Creek, passes under a trestle, and then quickly climbs out of the main wash in a side channel on the right (east) side. Follow this channel to the northeast a short distance to a doubletrack, and take a sharp turn to the west for 0.25 mile to reach Marsh Station Road.

Carefully cross the paved road, go under the train trestle, and pick up the trail on the other side of the fence. Mountain bikers and equestrians should go around the

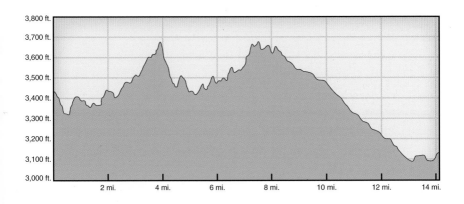

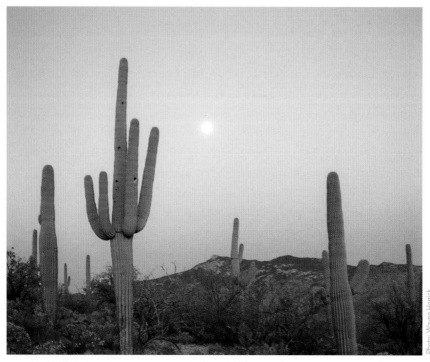

Photo: Wayne Herrick

The Sonoran Desert comes alive at night, and an experience along the AZT wouldn't be complete without a hike or mountain bike ride under the full moon.

end of the guardrail, while hikers can just step over it. Equestrians should walk their animals across Marsh Station Road.

The trail heads west for a very short distance, with views of Cienega Creek before resuming its path to the north. About 0.5 mile past the trestle, the trail passes through a fence and continues northeast on the south side of a wash before reaching a pipeline road and a power line. Continue north, passing through a gate, and crossing into Colossal Cave Mountain Park.

Take in the views at the saddle before descending the big sweeping switchbacks toward La Posta Quemada Ranch. A side trail leads from the AZT to the ranch where limited services, including camping, a gift shop, and snacks, are available.

TURNAROUND NOTE: If you're doing an out-and-back day hike from the south, Colossal Cave Mountain Park is a perfect destination and turnaround spot.

To continue on this passage, the trail contours northeasterly along Posta Quemada Canyon toward La Selvilla Picnic Area before bearing left out of the canyon bottom and turning north. It crosses four doubletracks in quick succession on its northern route to Pistol Hill Road. Shortly after Pistol Hill Road, it passes through a gate and makes its way along pleasant singletrack en route to X9 Ranch Road and then continues to the north-northwest to the attractive riparian areas of Rincon Creek. This area makes for fine camping before you enter Saguaro National Park, which requires permits for its limited camping areas.

The park boundary lies 0.2 trail mile north of Rincon Creek. Just 0.7 mile beyond is Hope Camp, a historic ranching site and the end of Passage 8.

Mountain Bike Notes

The entire passage provides excellent, moderate singletrack. You can ride point-to-point by leaving a vehicle at one of the access points, or you can do it as an out-and-back from any of them. The X9 Ranch Road crossing is the northernmost bike-friendly vehicle-access point on the passage; alternatively, park at the Loma Alta Trailhead and

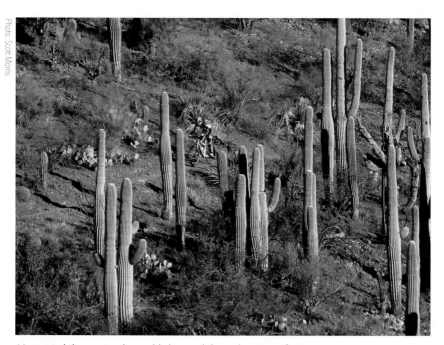

Photo: Scott Morris

Mountain bikers enjoy the world-class trail through saguaro forests near Colossal Cave Mountain Park.

ride 2.5 miles along the Hope Camp Trail to access the AZT. *For more information about mountain biking along the Arizona National Scenic Trail, visit* **aztrail.org.**

SOUTHERN ACCESS: Gabe Zimmerman Trailhead

Take Exit 281 off I-10 and follow Marsh Station Road (frontage road) 3 miles southeast, then north, to the parking area on the east side of the road.

NORTHERN ACCESS: Hope Camp

If you want to hit the trail from here, please follow the trail description in reverse order. There is no vehicle access for the 3 miles required to reach the beginning of the Hope Camp Trail. On Old Spanish Trail, travel approximately 7 miles southeast of the Saguaro National Park Visitor Center, or go 4 miles northwest of Colossal Cave Mountain Park on Old Spanish Trail and then turn north on Camino Loma Alta. Go about 2.5 miles until the road ends at a small trailhead and parking area. Travel 3 miles east on Hope Camp Trail to historic Hope Camp.

PASSAGE 9

Rincon Mountains

KEY INFO

LOCATION Saguaro National Park to Italian Trap

DISTANCE 21.6 miles one-way

DAY-TRIP OPTION See turnaround note in the trail description.

SHUTTLE RECOMMENDATION Not applicable

DIFFICULTY Moderate to difficult

LAND MANAGERS Coronado National Forest, Santa Catalina Ranger District, **www.fs.usda.gov/coronado,** 520-749-8700; Saguaro National Park, **nps.gov/sagu,** 520-733-5158

RECOMMENDED MONTHS March–November

GATEWAY COMMUNITY See Tucson (page 310).

GEOLOGY HIGHLIGHTS See "The Mighty Santa Catalina and Rincon Mountains" (page 339).

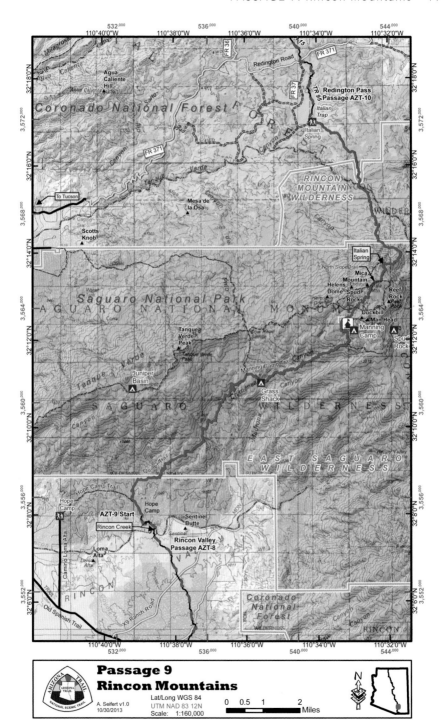

Passage 9
Rincon Mountains

A. Seifert v1.0
10/30/2013

Lat/Long WGS 84
UTM NAD 83 12N
Scale: 1:160,000

0 0.5 1   2
Miles

N

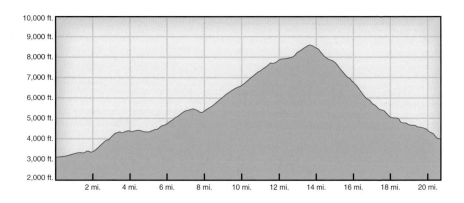

OVERVIEW

Saguaro National Park is home to the richest stands of saguaro cactus anywhere in the world, and you'll travel beneath these giant sentinels of the desert for the first few miles of this passage. If you're here in early summer you may be treated to their brilliant white blooms—the Arizona state flower—which attract nighttime pollinators to sip sweet nectar from the tops of the tall cacti. If pollinated, the saguaro produce ruby-red fruits in June that sustain almost every desert critter. A staple food source for native people, saguaro fruit is still harvested in the traditional way by the Tohono O'odham.

In addition to the saguaro forests at lower elevations, Saguaro National Park also contains high-elevation peaks where deep snow might cover the mountaintops four months of the year. Like the state of Arizona, this passage offers up diversity that you have to see (and hear and smell and feel) in order to believe.

Because the pine–fir forest community atop the Rincon Mountains is similar to forests of southern Canada, the 20.5-mile traverse of the park, including a 6,169-foot climb to the high point of Passage 9, at 8,602 feet, features the botanical equivalent of a 5,000-mile walk to Canada and back. Adventurers on the Arizona National Scenic Trail (AZT) will pass through six distinct biotic communities, each occupying a certain elevation range: desert scrub, desert grassland, oak woodland, pine–oak woodland, pine forest, and mixed-conifer forest. This variety of biomes supports 986 different species of plants.

Saguaro National Park prohibits backcountry camping and requires permits and reservations for overnight stays. Call or visit Saguaro National Park's East Visitor Center to get a permit. Same-day walk-in permits are issued before noon, depending on availability. The campgrounds rarely fill during the week. To guarantee a spot, you may

The banded gneiss of the Rincon Mountains is visible throughout Passage 9.

request a permit up to two months in advance. Some thru-hikers purchase permits for multiple days around their anticipated stay in the park to ensure that they have a permit should their trip plans change.

ON THE TRAIL

From Hope Camp the trail heads north for 0.5 mile to the beginning of the Quilter Trail, which heads north-northeast to a sharp right turn at mile 1.2. It goes east across more-or-less level terrain until mile 1.4 where it crosses a drainage, goes over a slight rise to another drainage, and then begins its relentless ascent toward the summit of Mica Mountain. Trail aficionados will appreciate the impressive rock work that makes this trail sustainable (and possible!) up the slopes of this rugged range. Flecks of mica, a naturally occurring mineral, adorn the trail, sparkling like tiny mirrors in the sunlight.

It's a tough slog up the steep terrain, dipping in and out of small drainages, and the views to the south improve with every foot of elevation you gain. At mile 5.3 the trail joins the Manning Camp Trail about 1.5 miles north of the Madrona Ranger Station (closed) and turns left (north) to continue its ascent.

TURNAROUND NOTE: Day-hikers attempting an out-and-back of this challenging passage will want to turn around near the junction with the Manning Camp Trail or Grass Shack Campground.

To continue on this passage, follow to where the AZT passes a trail junction at mile 7.6 and drops a bit into Grass Shack Campground, which has three campsites (permit required), an outhouse, and seasonal water in Chimenea Creek. From Grass Shack the trail climbs 2,657 feet through changing terrain and plant communities en route to Manning Camp. The trail follows a ridgeline between Chimenea and Madrona Canyons. Stay left at a trail junction about 3.5 miles from the campground, and continue across Chimenea Creek and up to Manning Camp at mile 12.8.

Manning Camp has six tent sites (permit required). A faucet with seasonal running water is on the east side of the main ranger building; the Park Service recommends treating the water before using it. The campground also has an outhouse.

To continue on the AZT, turn right (east) from the junction at mile 12.9 and follow the Mica Mountain Trail. Numerous trails loop through this area, and GPS users will appreciate having the track loaded in their unit as they make their way through here. Trail users without GPS receivers can stay on course by heading northeast along the creekbed, avoiding side trails, for approximately 0.7 mile to the Spud Rock Trail junction, and then turning right onto the North Slope Trail. At mile 13.6, turn 90 degrees to the left (north) onto the North Slope Trail, which descends steeply through switchbacks to approximately mile 15, where it levels somewhat and fades among the remnants of a forest fire.

Trail users without GPS units can stay on course by heading northeast along the creekbed, avoiding side trails, for approximately 0.7 mile. At the T-intersection, turn right (east) for a short distance, then left (north) on a trail toward Italian Spring. Follow metal markers on trees past a flat point that offers sweeping views to the east. The trail then bends back to the left (northwest) and continues descending on switchbacks.

Follow cairns when the trees become sparse as you descend into the high desert. Pass through a fence at mile 19.2 and continue downhill for approximately 2.8 miles, passing occasional cairns.

Cross the broad sandy Tanque Verde Wash (normally dry) diagonally to a point just north of an old-growth tree that is 6 feet in diameter. Turn right on the signed trail in a mesquite forest, and pass a carsonite marker with a decal and the number 95. Within

Photo: David Baker

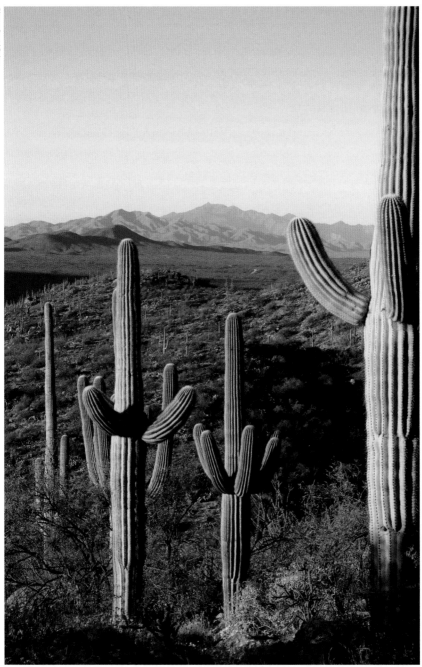

Passage 9 climbs incessantly toward the high domes of the Rincon Mountains, and views to the south reveal the Rincon Valley and Santa Rita Mountains.

100 yards you arrive at a metal AZT sign marking the boundary between Passages 9 and 10 (not visible from FR 37). This area is called Italian Trap, named for early settlers who constructed rock walls to assist with animal drives. Water is normally available in Italian Trap Tank in a fenced pasture less than 0.5 mile west off the trail.

Mountain Bike Notes

Bikes are prohibited in the East Saguaro Wilderness and Rincon Mountain Wilderness, which make up much of this passage. *For detailed information about scenic mountain biking routes around wilderness areas, visit* **aztrail.org.**

SOUTHERN ACCESS: Hope Camp

There is no vehicle access for the 3 miles required to reach Hope Camp and the Quilter Trail. From Old Spanish Trail in Tucson, travel approximately 7 miles southeast of the Saguaro National Park East Visitor Center, or go 4 miles northwest of Colossal Cave Mountain Park on Old Spanish Trail, then turn north on Camino Loma Alta. Go 2.5 miles until it ends at a small trailhead and parking area. Hike or ride 3 miles on Hope Camp Trail to Hope Camp.

NORTHERN ACCESS: Italian Trap

If you want to hit the trail from here, please follow the trail description in reverse order. From Tucson, head east on Tanque Verde Road, which becomes Redington Road after you leave the city. The road turns to dirt near mile marker 3. From that point, continue to just past mile marker 12 on Redington Road. If you are driving a passenger vehicle, park on the right at the top of a small ridge, as the remainder of the route is very rocky and bumpy. The AZT crosses Redington Road here as marked by signs. Those who wish to reach Italian Trap by high-clearance four-wheel-drive may descend the other side of the ridge to the south, and continue 2 miles. Park at a large metal AZT sign near the corrals and fences. The last stretch of Passage 9 arrives on the road from the east.

Redington Pass

KEY INFO

LOCATION Italian Trap to Gordon Hirabayashi Campground

DISTANCE 15.7 miles one-way

DAY-TRIP OPTION See turnaround note in the trail description.

SHUTTLE RECOMMENDATIONS Redington Road (passage mile 2.4), Bellota Ranch Road 36 (passage mile 6.7), Molino Basin Campground (passage mile 13.2)

DIFFICULTY Moderate

LAND MANAGER Coronado National Forest, Santa Catalina Ranger District, **www.fs.usda.gov/coronado**, 520-749-8700

RECOMMENDED MONTHS September–May

GATEWAY COMMUNITY See Tucson (page 310).

GEOLOGY HIGHLIGHTS See "The Mighty Santa Catalina and Rincon Mountains" (page 339).

OVERVIEW

This passage provides a link between Saguaro National Park and the Pusch Ridge Wilderness within the Santa Catalina Mountains. Oaks abound through this passage, and the nearby Bellota Ranch takes its name from the Spanish word for "acorn." The mountain biking through this passage is incredible.

There are two campgrounds near the terminus of this section. Molino Basin Campground closes for the summer (usually at the end of April), and the water is shut off at that time. Gordon Hirabayashi Campground is open year-round but has no water.

ON THE TRAIL

From the metal Arizona National Scenic Trail (AZT) sign at Italian Trap, follow the road's curve to the north. After 2 miles, crest a hill and avoid a side road on the right. Continue 0.1 mile past trail mileage signs to a maintained dirt road (Redington Road). Cross the road and head northeast past a large AZT sign. This easy-to-follow trail soon turns west and in 4 miles arrives at the Bellota Ranch Road. When approaching the

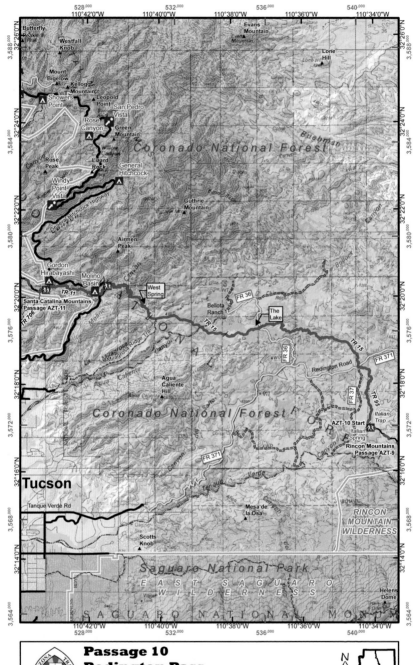

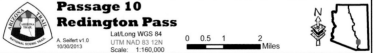

Passage 10
Redington Pass

Lat/Long WGS 84
A. Seifert v1.0   UTM NAD 83 12N
10/30/2013   Scale: 1:160,000

0   0.5   1   2
Miles

N

road, stay to the left of it—you'll pass a trail mileage sign—about 100 yards before crossing Bellota Ranch Road. Continue west across the road for 125 yards, where another large AZT marker greets you.

A feature known as The Lake (two water basins) is northeast of the AZT marker and about 100 yards off the trail. Bear left from the metal sign, follow a wash for about 100 yards, and then pick up the Bellota Trail (Trail 15), a singletrack that takes off to the left (southwest).

After about 8 miles, pass through a fence. The trail rolls through rocky hills and pleasant vegetation, descending to cross an upper finger of the Agua Caliente drainage at approximately mile 9, west-southwest of Bellota Ranch headquarters. A seasonal flow of water and the shade of large cottonwood trees offer a cool place to rest.

TURNAROUND NOTE: If you're on an out-and-back hike starting from Italian Trap, this spot is an ideal place to turn around and head back toward your vehicle.

Continuing, the trail turns left (west) onto a dirt road. Just beyond, stay on the trail to the right. (*Don't* take another cairn-marked trail, the Milagrosa Ridge Trail, on the left.) In 1.5 miles, pass through an old gate and climb out of a wash.

The road ends 0.4 mile later at a cement cistern that collects water from nearby West Spring (4,080 feet). Hop on a singletrack that departs to the west and then climbs steeply to the northwest. After plenty of switchbacks, the trail tops out in a saddle (4,846 feet). Mount Lemmon's sheer cliffs to the north-northwest are evidence of the rocky terrain waiting for you on Passage 11.

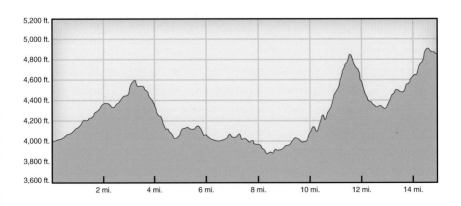

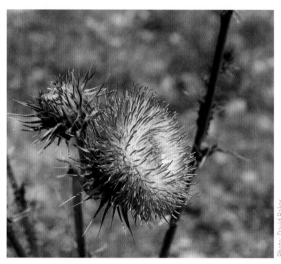

Photo: David Baker

The tall, purple flower heads of thistle *(Cirsium neomexica-num)* often adorn the trail.

The trail descends steeply to the west through many switchbacks, which can be hair-raising for cyclists. Reach the bottom of the drainage, and turn left (west) at a T-intersection. Carefully cross General Hitchcock Highway in 0.1 mile to enter Molino Basin Campground. From the highway, Tucson is 10.5 miles downhill to the left (west) for thru-hikers in need of supplies.

To continue from Molino Basin Campground, bear right, go around the bathroom facilities to the northwest corner of the parking lot, and find a trail marker for the singletrack Molino Basin Trail (Trail 11). Travel west on this trail about 50 yards to a T-intersection, turn right, and then make a quick left to avoid going through campsite 1. Descend through a wash, cross the road to the southwest, and continue on a trail that curves to the right (west).

The next 2.5 miles are popular with mountain bikers. While still in the campground, the trail crosses a road and begins a gradual climb to the northwest. Soon a sign indicates Upper Molino Basin Campground 0.1 mile to the right (north). Stay on the main trail. The AZT crests a small rise and begins to descend into an adjoining canyon. At a fork in 30 yards, take a left (southwest). As you gain elevation, it's easy to notice the effects of the Aspen Fire—a massive blaze that severely scorched these hills in 2003. Most of the manzanita are gone, but some of the old oaks remain. As you finish this passage, a spur trail leads right to the Gordon Hirabayashi Campground parking lot and the end of Passage 10. To stay on the AZT, continue straight (west).

Mountain Bike Notes

This entire passage is great, but beginning at West Spring Tank presents a challenging 1.5-mile climb. The ride from Bellota Trailhead past Molino Basin Campground and on to Gordon Hirabayashi Campground is classic, with everything from easy, flat spinning to lung-wrenching climbs and a crazy downhill. Passage 11 enters the Pusch Ridge Wilderness, so thru-riders must ride along the Bug Spring Trail (north of Gordon Hirabayashi Campground), Green Mountain Trail, Incinerator Ridge Trail, and other nonwilderness trails east of General Hitchcock Highway to reach the AZT at Oracle Ridge. *For detailed information about scenic mountain biking routes around wilderness areas, v*isit **aztrail.org.**

SOUTHERN ACCESS: Italian Trap

From Tucson, head east on Tanque Verde Road, which becomes Redington Road after you leave the city. The road turns to dirt near mile marker 3 and is slow going from there up. Continue to 0.5 mile past mile marker 12.

If you're driving a passenger vehicle, park on the right at the top of a small ridge, as the remainder of the route is very rocky and bumpy. The AZT crosses Redington Road here as marked by signs on both sides. Those who wish to reach Italian Trap by high-clearance four-wheel-drive may descend the south side of the ridge and continue 2 miles. Park at a large metal AZT sign near some corrals and fences. The last stretch of Passage 9 arrives on the road from the east.

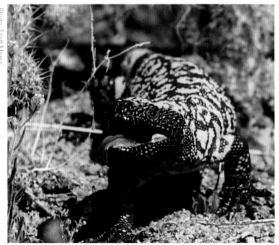

The gila monster *(Heloderma suspectum)* spends most of its life underground, so an encounter with one should be considered special . . . and enjoyed from a distance.

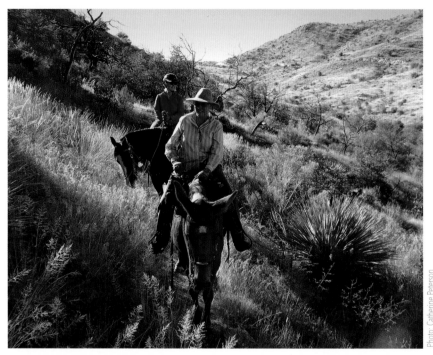

The oak-grassland of Redington Pass is a pleasant experience for equines and equestrians alike.

NORTHERN ACCESS: Gordon Hirabayashi Campground

If you want to hit the trail from here, please follow the trail description in reverse order. Follow Tanque Verde Road east from Tucson and turn left (north) on Catalina Highway. Drive about 9 miles and pass Molino Basin Campground. Continue 1.7 miles beyond the campground, and take the left (west) turn to Gordon Hirabayashi Campground. Drive 0.3 mile to a parking area. Follow a trail out of the south end of the parking lot for 40 yards to reach a T-intersection with the AZT.

Santa Catalina Mountains

LOCATION Gordon Hirabayashi Campground to Romero Pass

DISTANCE 11.7 miles one-way; 18.5 miles one-way to the summit of Mt. Lemmon

DAY-TRIP OPTION See turnaround note in the trail description.

SHUTTLE RECOMMENDATION Not applicable

DIFFICULTY Difficult to strenuous

LAND MANAGER Coronado National Forest, Santa Catalina Ranger District, **www.fs.usda.gov/coronado,** 520-749-8700

RECOMMENDED MONTHS Year-round

GATEWAY COMMUNITIES See Tucson (page 310) and Summerhaven (page 312).

GEOLOGY HIGHLIGHTS See "The Mighty Santa Catalina and Rincon Mountains" (page 339).

OVERVIEW

As with the other passages on the Arizona National Scenic Trail (AZT) that traverse sky islands, this section presents difficulties because of its extreme elevation ranging from 3,500 feet up to 8,500 feet, and the climate that comes with it.

It's hard to believe temperatures at the top of the mountain are 20 degrees cooler than in the valley. So, even though you may wear shorts and a T-shirt for the first part of this hike, be sure to throw in some warmer clothes for the high forests.

Hikers should also be prepared for strenuous trail miles. After leaving Hutch's Pool, the AZT climbs almost a vertical mile to reach the end of the passage. This undertaking is even more demanding if you're carrying supplies for the next passage, instead of stopping at the village of Summerhaven atop Mount Lemmon. The total distance from the beginning of this passage to the end of Passage 12, near Oracle, is about 34 miles. And although every step is beautiful, it's tough going.

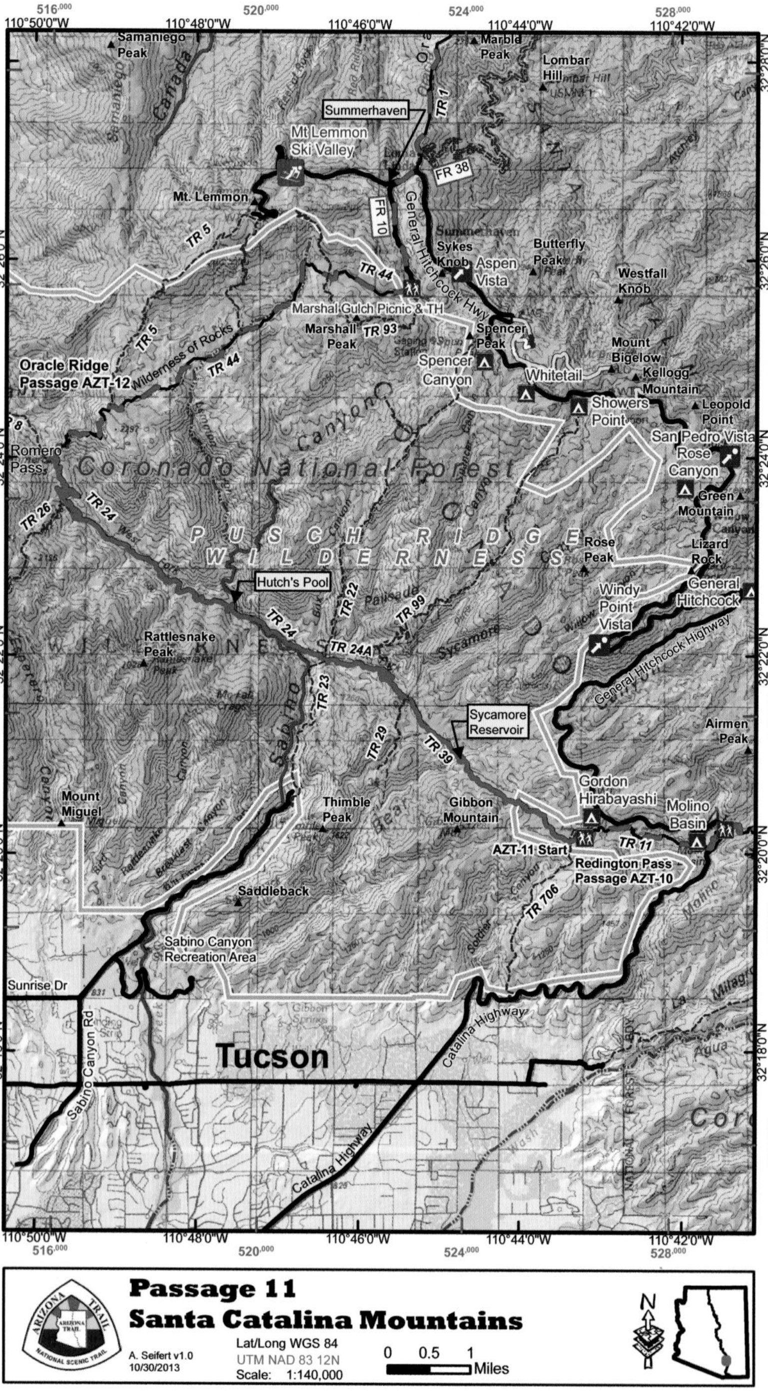

Passage 11
Santa Catalina Mountains
A. Seifert v1.0
10/30/2013
Lat/Long WGS 84
UTM NAD 83 12N
Scale: 1:140,000
0 0.5 1
Miles
N
Summerhaven
Mt Lemmon Ski Valley
Mt. Lemmon
Samaniego Peak
Marble Peak
Lombar Hill
FR 38
FR 10
TR 1
General Hitchcock Hwy
Sykes Knob
Aspen Vista
Butterfly Peak
Westfall Knob
TR 5
TR 44
Marshall Gulch Picnic & TH
Marshall Peak
TR 93
Spencer Peak
Spencer Canyon
Whitetail
Mount Bigelow
Kellogg Mountain
Showers Point
Leopold Point
San Pedro Vista
Rose Canyon
Green Mountain
Oracle Ridge Passage AZT-12
Wilderness of Rocks
Romero Pass
Coronado National Forest
PUSCH RIDGE WILDERNESS
TR 26
TR 24
Hutch's Pool
TR 22
TR 99
Rose Peak
Lizard Rock
Windy Point Vista
General Hitchcock
General Hitchcock Highway
Rattlesnake Peak
TR 24A
TR 23
Sycamore Reservoir
TR 29
TR 39
Airmen Peak
Gordon Hirabayashi
Mount Miguel
Thimble Peak
Gibbon Mountain
Molino Basin
AZT-11 Start
TR 11
Redington Pass Passage AZT-10
Saddleback
TR 706
Sabino Canyon Recreation Area
Sunrise Dr
Sabino Canyon Rd
Catalina Highway
Tucson

About halfway through this passage, you can enjoy the refreshing waters of Hutch's Pool. This large, deep swimming hole is a unique reward for the weary AZT hiker after a gritty hike through parched desert. This spot can attract a crowd on a hot spring or summer weekend, so if you're looking for solitude, try to plan your trip so you arrive on a weekday, especially if you want to camp nearby. Please practice Leave No Trace camping ethics to help Hutch's Pool retain its natural beauty.

Using techniques for properly storing your food in bear country is important along this passage. Hikers regularly report black bear and mountain lion sightings here, but these incidents are rare and should not cause undue concern—both animals are usually quite wary of humans. Nevertheless, keep your campsite clean and put all of your food in a bag or other container that can be hung high above the ground. For more information on safe travel in bear country, consult this U.S. Forest Service website: **ncrs.fs.fed.us/epubs/ht66.html.**

If you're planning to end your hike atop Mount Lemmon—the high point of the Santa Catalina Mountains—add 6.8 miles to the length of this passage, bringing it to 18.5 miles. Vehicle access is at Marshall Gulch Trailhead at the end of the Wilderness of Rocks and Marshall Gulch Trail, a component of Passage 12. Equestrians should not attempt this passage because of a very steep and rocky section near Romero Pass. Other trails in the Santa Catalina Mountains offer safer, more enjoyable routes to the top of the mountain.

ON THE TRAIL

Head right (west) from the intersection with the short access trail from Gordon Hirabayashi Campground (4,820 feet). Soon you follow an old dirt road downhill to

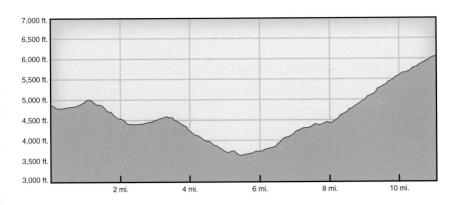

a confluence of roads. Walk straight (west-northwest), following a sign for Sycamore Reservoir Trail. The road immediately passes through a wash and then bends right (northwest). You'll find many nice places to camp in this shady, oak-lined valley.

This is the site of a former Japanese internment camp, and the campground and trailhead were called Prison Camp before being renamed in honor of Gordon Hirabayashi, a sociologist and educator best known for his resistance to the Japanese-American internment during World War II; he received the Presidential Medal of Freedom posthumously in 2012.

Although Hirabayashi at first considered accepting internment, he ultimately became one of three to openly defy it. In 1942 he turned himself in to the FBI and, after being convicted for curfew violation, was sentenced to 90 days in prison. He did this in part to appeal the verdict all the way to the U.S. Supreme Court with the backing of the American Civil Liberties Union. However, the court unanimously ruled against him in 1943. Because they would not pay for him to be sent to prison, he hitchhiked from Washington, D.C., to the Arizona prison where he was sentenced to reside. When new information surfaced 44 years later, Hirabayashi's case was reheard by the federal courts. In 1987, his conviction was overturned by the Court of Appeals for the Ninth Circuit.

Think of this history as you hike, and in less than 0.5 mile, the road turns into a wash. Continue along a gentle, winding climb. The trail leaves the wash to the south (left) and climbs to a metal AZT sign and the Pusch Ridge Wilderness boundary in a low saddle. Descend into the wilderness on the singletrack Sycamore Reservoir Trail (Trail 39).

As the trail reaches a road, watch for an obscure singletrack branching to the left (northwest). Follow this trail down a steep, rocky descent that lasts for 0.1 mile and ends in a lush valley of oak, willow, and riparian flora. At the bottom, you pass between a large boulder and the remnants of an old wall.

From here, you can make a side trip to Sycamore Reservoir by continuing straight ahead to the northwest for 100 yards. Although completely silted in, this small reservoir usually contains a reliable flow of surface water in the spring.

To continue on the AZT from the old wall, make a big U-turn to the right (southeast) and follow a singletrack trail 35 yards to a large cairn. The trail forks here. Turn left (northeast) and follow the trail as it bends farther to the left (north).

In another 0.2 mile, the trail disappears into a sandy wash. Follow cairns and traces of singletrack north, staying close to the slopes on the left. Keep your eyes open for a clear trail that exits this valley to the left (west-northwest). Avoid the temptation to stay in the valley as it ambles to the northeast.

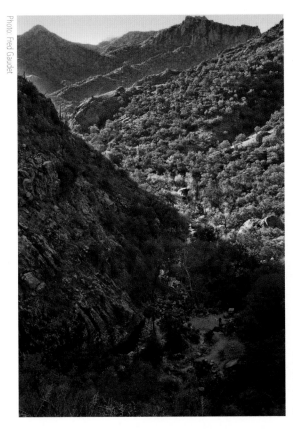

Daylight makes its way toward Hutch's Pool, an unforgettable destination along Passage 11.

Follow an old roadbed over a low ridge in 0.1 mile. On the other side, switchbacks lead into another lush valley of juniper, sycamore, and willow. At the bottom, turn sharply right (north) at a T-intersection to follow a clear singletrack. The trail parallels a seasonal streambed and then joins it. Bear left where the stream forks, following an intermittent trail. In 0.3 mile, avoid an obscure trail marked by cairns that breaks off to the left (west). Instead, continue straight (north). After passing through a thick forest of manzanita, the trail descends to the left to cross the rocky main drainage and then climbs to a saddle (4,590 feet). Take the right (north) fork here, and descend through countless switchbacks into the East Fork of Sabino Canyon.

At an intersection with the Palisades Trail (Trail 99), turn left (west) and continue to descend toward Sabino Canyon. Avoid Box Camp Trail at another intersection, continuing straight ahead (west) on the East Fork Trail. The AZT reaches a junction in a sycamore grove at the bottom of a side canyon. Saguaro cacti on the hillsides seem out of

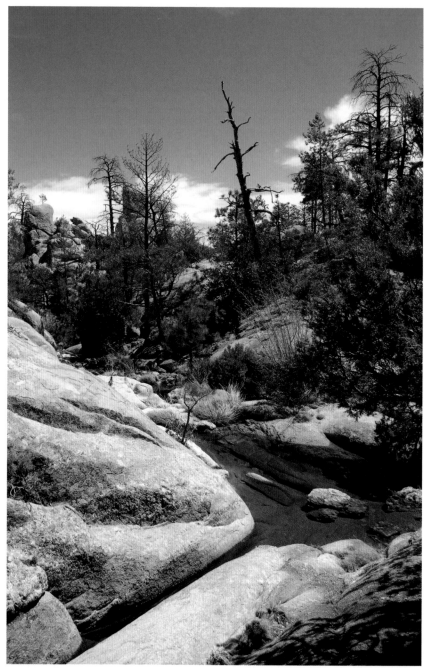

Water is abundant throughout the Santa Catalina Mountains . . . if you know where to look. See page 350 for water sources along the AZT.

place near this oasis. You may find a small amount of water here; if not, there is reliable water 1.7 miles ahead at Hutch's Pool. Turn right (north-northeast) toward the West Fork Trail (Trail 24). Watch for poison ivy and poison oak in the canyon over the next 8 miles. Cairns mark an immediate bend left to cross the East Fork of Sabino Canyon. Climb out along a rocky, dry streambed, and continue on a very clear singletrack into a veritable desert botanical garden, with saguaro, yucca, agave, mesquite, ocotillo, prickly pear, and dozens of desert species. You soon have a fleeting view down narrow Sabino Canyon with the Tucson sprawl in the background. Cross to the left (southwest) side of the drainage on large boulders.

At a junction, the AZT heads left (northwest), while the right fork descends north 100 yards and then climbs a short distance to Hutch's Pool. You have missed this cutoff to the pool if the main trail immediately switchbacks to the left (south) and climbs high above the canyon bottom.

TURNAROUND NOTE: Beautiful Hutch's Pool is a popular swimming hole for Tucsonans and tired AZT hikers, and is a picture-perfect destination if you are attempting an out-and-back adventure for the day. It's also the last source of water near the trail until the intermittent sources in the next passage about 8 miles away.

Hikers who are stopping at the parking area on Mount Lemmon have 12 miles of hiking and more than 5,000 feet of elevation gain remaining. At a trail intersection, avoid the Cathedral Rock Trail (Trail 26) and turn sharply right (east) to continue on the West Fork Trail (Trail 24). The scenery just keeps getting better as you reach an intersection at 6,080-foot Romero Pass with the Romero Canyon Trail and Mount Lemmon Trail (Trail 5) and the end of Passage 11.

Mountain Bike Notes

Passage 11 is almost entirely within the Pusch Ridge Wilderness, and bicycles are prohibited. Instead, follow a series of trails (including the Bug Spring, Green Mountain, Incinerator Ridge, and Butterfly Trails, to name a few) to Summerhaven, on the east side of General Hitchcock Highway. Even though more time on the dirt may be appealing, the elevation gain is so intense that you'll likely be walking your bike most of the time—pedaling up the pavement is always an option. *For detailed information about scenic mountain biking routes around wilderness areas, vi*sit **aztrail.org.**

SOUTHERN ACCESS: Gordon Hirabayashi Campground

Follow Tanque Verde Road east from Tucson and turn left (north) on Catalina Highway. Drive about 9 miles and pass Molino Basin Campground. Continue 1.7 miles after the campground and take the left turn to Gordon Hirabayashi Campground. Drive 0.3 mile to a parking area. Follow a trail out of the south end of the parking lot to reach a T-intersection with the AZT. Turn right and follow the trail description for this passage.

NORTHERN ACCESS: Romero Pass

If you want to hit the trail from here, please follow the trail description in reverse order. Even though this passage ends at Romero Pass, the closest vehicle access from Tucson is at the Marshall Gulch Picnic Area. Take Catalina Highway into the Santa Catalina Mountains. Near the top of the mountain range, bear left to the community of Summerhaven. Continue 1.5 miles south to the end of the road at Marshall Gulch Trailhead. The trail begins on the west side of the parking area. The Marshall Gulch Trail connects to the Wilderness of Rocks Trail, reaching Romero Pass in about 7 miles.

PASSAGE 12

Oracle Ridge

KEY INFO

LOCATION Romero Pass to American Flag Ranch

DISTANCE 22.1 miles one-way

DAY-TRIP OPTION See turnaround note in the trail description.

SHUTTLE RECOMMENDATION Oracle Ridge Trailhead (passage mile 8.9)

DIFFICULTY Difficult to strenuous

LAND MANAGER Coronado National Forest, Santa Catalina Ranger District, **www.fs.usda.gov/coronado**, 520-749-8700

RECOMMENDED MONTHS March–November

GATEWAY COMMUNITIES See Summerhaven (page 312), Oracle (page 314), and San Manuel (page 317).

GEOLOGY HIGHLIGHTS See "The Mighty Santa Catalina and Rincon Mountains" (page 339).

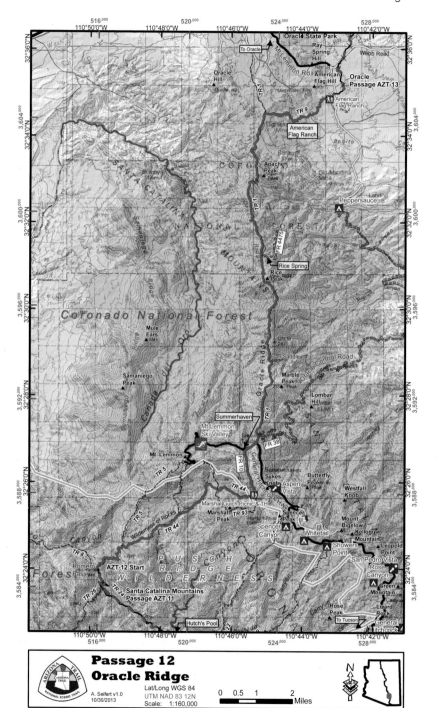

Passage 12
Oracle Ridge

A. Seifert v1.0
10/30/2013

Lat/Long WGS 84
UTM NAD 83 12N
Scale: 1:160,000

0   0.5   1   2
Miles

N

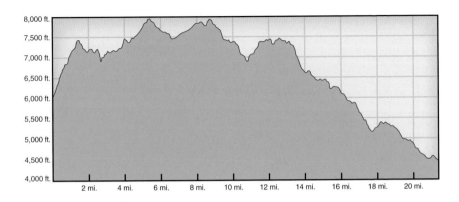

OVERVIEW

Long and arduous, Passage 12 includes a steep ascent from the remote southern end at Romero Pass, a rolling traverse along the Wilderness of Rocks Trail, a short road section and resupply opportunity in the mountaintop community of Summerhaven, and a long haul down Oracle Ridge to historic American Flag Ranch. The section begins in the Pusch Ridge Wilderness, passes through a small community, skirts a historic mining area, and drops into ranching country. The expansive views in all directions from this sky island passage, especially from Oracle Ridge, are astounding.

ON THE TRAIL

Follow the Mount Lemmon Trail (Trail 5) right (north) to a steep, rocky, difficult climb along the ridge. This is the stretch that deters pack animals on this passage—you may even have to use your hands to negotiate some spots. Soon, the climb peaks, and then you descend toward a saddle in a refreshing stand of ponderosa pines and a junction with the Wilderness of Rocks Trail at mile 1.7.

The relentless climb up to and beyond Romero Pass eases a bit on the Wilderness of Rocks Trail, but there are still plenty of ups and downs as the trail contours around to Marshall Gulch. It follows a drainage with intermittent water, depending on recent rainfall or snowmelt, for much of the way. Pine trees and oaks, as well as granite outcrops, dot the way. Tree cover is especially thick as the trail approaches Marshall Gulch at mile 6.8.

The trail emerges from the woods on the west side of the parking area and turns north up the main north-south road (FR 10, North Sabino Canyon Parkway) through the small community of Summerhaven. Follow the road through town. Services in

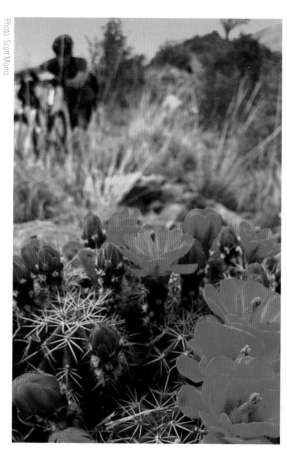

Photo: Scott Morris

A mountain biker trudges past blooming claret cup cactus (*Echinocereus coccineus*). Although the trail descends 3,500 feet from the Santa Catalina Mountains toward the town of Oracle, don't assume it's all downhill. Oracle Ridge presents some of the most arduous challenges in this part of the state.

Summerhaven are limited, but those who arrive during business hours may enjoy baked goods, warm meals, and resupply opportunities.

Approximately 1.3 miles north of the Marshall Gulch Trailhead, the paved road (and the Arizona National Scenic Trail) bends right (east), and 0.4 mile past the community center it arrives at Oracle Control Road, on the left. Here, the AZT turns left (north) and continues 0.25 mile past the fire station on the right to a parking area and AZT sign on the left. The Oracle Ridge Trail (Trail 1) leaves civilization and begins its long descent to American Flag Ranch and the desert beyond. During wet winters, the north side of the Santa Catalinas may be completely blanketed with snow, making route finding a serious endeavor. When the trail is obscured, relying on a GPS track or honed map and compass skills will be necessary. The trail goes to the left side of a small hill, and then stays on the sharp ridgeline to Dan Saddle at mile 11.2.

> **TURNAROUND NOTE:** If you're day-tripping from the Oracle Ridge Trailhead, Dan Saddle is the best place to turn around and reverse your route up the mountain.

To continue on the AZT, from Dan Saddle (6,910 feet) head northeast onto a singletrack that climbs away from the saddle. Don't be fooled into thinking the climbing ends at Dan Saddle. Soon, your extra effort on a steep trail earns you southwest views of the rugged Reef of Rock and, just behind that, the lush rift of Cañada del Oro. Farther north, in the lowlands just to the right of Samaniego Ridge, behind Cañada del Oro, you can see the white domes of Biosphere 2.

The AZT continues to climb and then descends steeply to a saddle before climbing again. Descend to cross through a gate, then turn left (north) onto a road. This road is open to motorized vehicles, but they are rarely seen. The road descends slightly until it forks. Take the left (westernmost) fork.

The steady descent continues to where FR 4475 leaves the AZT sharply to the right (southeast) to descend to Rice Spring, where water may be present. Head down this doubletrack approximately 100 feet, and descend into the gully to the left. There is a small dugout concrete bowl at the spring; you might have to shovel dirt out of it. Back on the AZT, continue north, where the road makes a sharp bend to the right. Just before that bend, leave the road by turning left (north) to pass through a fence, and follow the singletrack Oracle Ridge Trail.

The AZT rolls along the ridge for about 1.5 miles before passing through two gated fences to traverse along the steep west side of Apache Peak. The town of Oracle soon comes into view to the north. Looming beyond it in the distance are the peaks and ridges of Pinal County, including the Black Hills and Tortilla Mountains (Passages 14 and 15 of the AZT). After Apache Peak, the trail makes a long, steady descent through many switchbacks to a crossing of Trail 639. The trail then climbs, joins an old roadbed that is now a singletrack, and levels somewhat.

Pass a gate on the left that has an AZT marker on it, and continue straight (north-northeast) up the steep hill in front of you and top out. Ignore the occasional trails branching to the right until you reach an intersection with the Cody Trail (Trail 9). Take the right fork, as an AZT marker indicates, and begin a long, switchbacking descent to the east. (To reach the town of Oracle directly from here, continue north on Trail 1 for about 2 miles and then northwest on maintained roads for about 1 mile.)

In 1.1 miles, the switchbacks abate somewhat. The trail heads south-southeast another 0.4 mile to reach a fork with the trail to High Jinks Ranch, a rustic bed-and-breakfast that is on the National Register of Historic Places and has become a popular destination for thru-hikers. Continuing on the AZT, take the left fork into a switchback to the left (north-northeast), avoiding a couple of side trails. Descend through more switchbacks and cross a road.

All of this descending is interrupted by a 0.25-mile, 130-foot climb at mile 21.5. After a few more switchbacks, drop to the American Flag Ranch Trailhead and the end of Passage 12.

Mountain Bike Notes

The trail along Oracle Ridge is open to bikes and is a local proving ground for technically savvy riders. Steep, loose terrain composes most of the passage, and your brakes should be in excellent condition before you attempt these 13 hardcore miles. If you're fully loaded and concerned about surviving the descent, consider riding down the Oracle Control Road, just east of the trail. The dirt road is fast, fun, and drops more than 4,000 feet in 20 miles. *For detailed information about scenic mountain biking routes around wilderness areas, visit* **aztrail.org.**

SOUTHERN ACCESS: Romero Pass

Even though the passage starts at Romero Pass, the closest vehicle access from Tucson is at the Marshall Gulch Picnic Area. To get there, take the Catalina Highway into the Santa Catalina Mountains. Near the top of the mountain range, bear left to the community of Summerhaven. Continue 1.5 miles south to the end of the road at Marshall Gulch Trailhead. The trail begins on the west side of the parking area. The Marshall Gulch Trail connects to the Wilderness of Rocks Trail (Trail 44), reaching Romero Pass in about 7 miles.

NORTHERN ACCESS: American Flag Ranch Trailhead

If you want to hit the trail from here, please follow the trail description in reverse order. From Oracle, turn south at the eastern intersection of AZ 77 and East American Avenue, drive 1.5 miles on American Avenue, and then turn right onto Mount Lemmon Road. Continue 4 miles to American Flag Ranch Road and turn right (west) to reach the trailheads on both sides of the road, including parking areas near historic American Flag Ranch. The trail on the left (east) side of the road is the southern start of Passage 13; the northern end of Passage 12 arrives from the right (west).

Oracle

OVERVIEW

This short passage ambles through washes and across low ridges speckled with high-desert plants. They include yucca, prickly pear, cholla, the occasional juniper, and a variety of shrubs and grasses. The trail is clear except where it enters arroyos, but it is usually marked with rock cairns on either side. Local mountain bikers enjoy incorporating this stretch of the Arizona National Scenic Trail (AZT) into improvised loop rides.

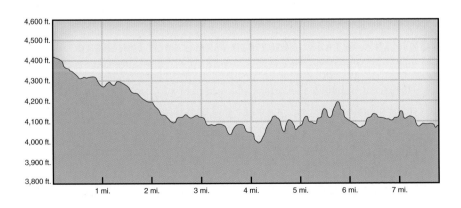

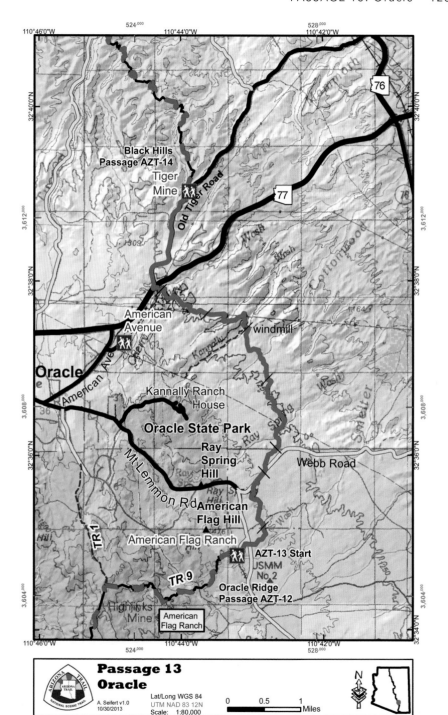

Passage 13
Oracle

A. Seifert v1.0
10/30/2013

Lat/Long WGS 84
UTM NAD 83 12N
Scale: 1:80,000

0   0.5   1
Miles

N

This passage is ideal for a point-to-point day hike. To avoid walking on a road, use a side trail that leaves the AZT at mile 6.3 to reach a convenient parking lot just outside the town of Oracle on American Avenue (see Alternate Southern Access, page 126). The AZT itself continues onto Old Tiger Road and into the Black Hills of Passage 14.

ON THE TRAIL

As of this printing, Oracle State Park is open on a limited basis due to state budget shortages. AZT users, however, may enter the park as long as they stay on the trail.

A clear singletrack leaves the parking area and immediately turns to the left (north). At mile 1.7, the trail reaches Webb Road and a fence. Turn right (north-northeast) to parallel the road for 0.4 mile before going through a gate. Cross the road and take another singletrack on the left (north).

Follow the trail mostly downhill and in and out of washes. At mile 4.4, the AZT turns left (northwest) onto an old road and descends sharply into a gully. In another 50 yards, the road meets a major drainage, Kannally Wash, where the tank at the windmill does not have water.

TURNAROUND NOTE: If you're just out for a day hike, the windmill is a great landmark to reach, then turn around and head back toward Oracle State Park. Once you arrive back at your vehicle, you'll have put nearly 9 miles on your legs.

To continue on the AZT, go straight across the wash, angling north-northwest on an old roadbed.

Follow the old roadbed into a sustained climb, followed by alternating climbs and descents. Pass through a junction at mile 5.6, and when the trail splits again, in about 100 yards, stay left and climb another old roadbed.

At mile 6.2, you come to the junction with the trail that leads to the American Avenue Trailhead. Continue on the main route until you reach a major wash next to AZ 77 at mile 6.5. To reach a low culvert that crosses under the highway, 30 yards to the northwest across the wash, you must go through a gate in a barbed-wire fence. On the other side of the highway, near the culvert, scramble to the right up a steep bank to dirt Old Tiger Road.

Head left (north) on the road. After 1.8 miles look for an unmistakable AZT gateway on the left (north) side of the road, where Passage 13 officially ends.

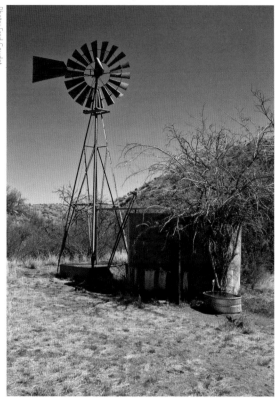

The windmill in Kannally Wash makes for a great day-tripping destination from Oracle State Park.

Mountain Bike Notes

This passage provides a fun ride that's great for entry-level riders. Where the AZT wanders into the deep sands, bypasses provide decent alternatives. Some of these are steep and rocky, but those sections are short. Most of the bypass intersections are marked with four-by-four AZT posts. Cyclists out for a day ride should take a detour at bike-mile 6.3 to reach the alternate trailhead near Oracle. *For more information about mountain biking along the Arizona National Scenic Trail, visit* **aztrail.org.**

SOUTHERN ACCESS: American Flag Ranch Trailhead

From Oracle, turn south at the eastern intersection of AZ 77 and East American Avenue, drive 1.5 miles on American Avenue, and then turn right onto Mount Lemmon Road. Continue 3.1 miles to American Flag Ranch Road, and turn right (west) to reach the trailheads on both sides of the road, including parking areas near the historic American

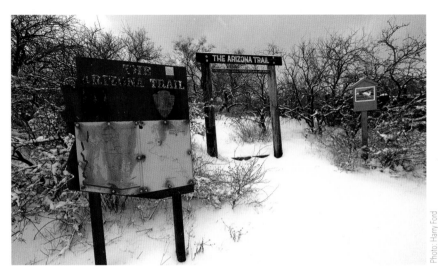

The trailhead at American Flag Ranch after an unexpected winter storm

Flag Ranch. The trail on the left (east) side of the road is the start of Passage 13; Passage 12 arrives from the west (right).

ALTERNATE SOUTHERN ACCESS:
American Avenue Trailhead

From the east intersection of AZ 77 and East American Avenue, turn south onto East American Avenue. Drive 0.25 mile, turn left (east), and continue 0.25 mile to a parking lot. A four-by-four post marks the trailhead on the south side of the parking lot. Follow this trail for 0.8 mile to meet the AZT at mile 6.3 of Passage 13.

Note: To continue toward American Flag Ranch Trailhead, turn right and follow the trail description *backward* from mile 6.3. To access Old Tiger Road toward the next passage, follow the trail description *forward* from mile 6.3.

NORTHERN ACCESS: Tiger Mine Trailhead

If you want to hit the trail from here, please follow the trail description in reverse order. From the east entrance to the town of Oracle, drive 0.8 mile east on AZ 77 to mile marker 105, and turn left (north) onto Old Tiger Road. After 1.5 miles on this road, look for an unmistakable AZT gateway on the left (north) side of the road. Parking is available on either side of the road.

Black Hills

KEY INFO

LOCATION Tiger Mine Trailhead to Freeman Road Trailhead

DISTANCE 27.4 miles one-way

DAY-TRIP OPTION See turnaround note in the trail description.

SHUTTLE RECOMMENDATIONS Tucson Wash Road (passage mile 4.2), Camp Grant Road (passage mile 12.0)

DIFFICULTY Moderate

LAND MANAGERS Pinal County, **pinalcountyaz.gov,** 520-866-6455; Arizona State Land Department, **azland.gov,** 602-542-4631

RECOMMENDED MONTHS February–May and October–December

GATEWAY COMMUNITIES See Central Copper Corridor (page 318).

GEOLOGY HIGHLIGHTS Not applicable

OVERVIEW

Ubiquitous cactus, sandy soil, and hot, dry weather characterize Passage 14. Here, visitors will find a rich, complex community of plants and animals in delicate coexistence. The opportunities for solitude are as limitless as the Arizona sky, and the whispers of wind and songs of cactus wrens are the only sounds. At night, you'll be treated to celestial entertainment unlike anything you've ever seen. This is one of the most seldom visited passages on the Arizona National Scenic Trail (AZT).

That is because—despite its beauty—Passage 14 serves up serious challenges associated with hiking, biking, and riding in the desert. Temperatures routinely top 100 degrees from June through September, and finding shade is nearly impossible (except when turkey vultures are circling overhead). In winter, temperatures plunge and torrents of water can fill the otherwise-dry washes in minutes. Precise planning is imperative to ensure a safe and successful trip, especially where water caches are concerned.

Water may present the single greatest planning challenge to the AZT traveler on desert passages. You need to drink up to a gallon of water per day, and there are few

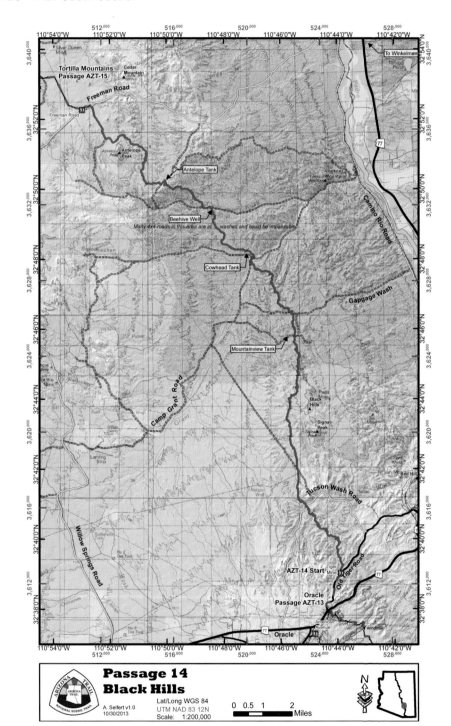

Passage 14
Black Hills

A. Seifert v1.0
10/30/2013

Lat/Long WGS 84
UTM NAD 83 12N
Scale: 1:200,000

0 0.5 1   2
Miles

N

reliable natural sources. All available water along this passage is owned by ranchers, whose permission you must secure before using it. You have two alternatives: either cache water along your route prior to your outing, or arrange for people to meet you along the way.

Note: *This passage crosses Arizona State Land, and you must have a permit to venture outside the 15-foot trail corridor.*

ON THE TRAIL

From the Tiger Mine Trailhead, the trail twists north-northwest for about 5.5 miles until it reaches a three-way pipeline road intersection. Over this section, en route to the pipeline, you descend into and cross several distinct washes, all of which are about a mile apart; eventually you reach the largest, Tucson Wash.

TURNAROUND NOTE: This is a moderate turnaround location for anyone day-hiking a portion of this remote passage. Mountain bikers may wish to continue on to Mountainview Tank before turning around.

To continue, climb out of Tucson Wash, the trail gently curves around to a true north direction as you traverse several ridges, one gate, and a dirt road and then arrive at the pipeline intersection. At this junction, a large white steel gate on the east side signifies private land owned by El Paso Gas.

To continue, follow singletrack as it twists north for approximately 10.5 miles to the confluence of Camp Grant and Bloodsucker Washes. Over this distance you traverse many drainages, unique rock formations, and panoramic views as you climb up

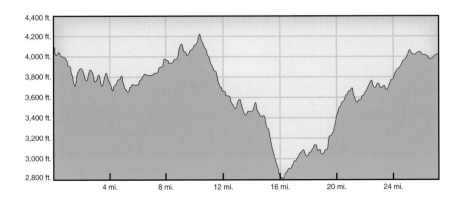

and over the ridgeline of the Black Hills. Antelope Peak is a prominent landmark, as are the Superstition and Pinal Mountains. To the east lie the entire Galiuro Mountains, the San Pedro River, and Mount Graham (10,720 feet). To the south you can see the Rincon and Santa Catalina Mountains. This vista helps you understand how expansive the Sonoran Desert is as it transitions from low to high desert.

Traversing this 10.5-mile section, you pass through three cowboy-style gates, cross five dirt ranch roads, and possibly observe many nearby old cattle tanks, broken windmills, and abandoned wells. Near the middle of this stretch and visible from long distances is Mountainview Tank. Water is pumped up to this 40,000-gallon tank from lower wells, which then gravity feeds to numerous smaller tanks across many miles of the cattle ranch. Once you are past the tank area, the trail crosses one more ranch road and winds around numerous drainages and smaller ridgelines for the next 2 miles.

There is ample signage, both cairns and carsonites, as the trail turns gently to the west and climbs to a high ridgeline, the final ridge before it drops to the confluence of Camp Grant and Bloodsucker Washes. At this point the trail descends directly into

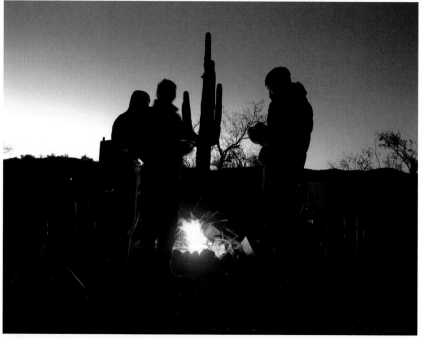

Photo: Terri Gay

Often overlooked because of its remote nature, Passage 14 offers outstanding opportunities for trail adventures and relaxation under star-filled skies.

the ever-changing wash, crosses to a vegetated island, and then traverses the rest of the confluence, dotted with numerous carsonite signs, until it reaches a doubletrack ranch road.

Continue on the road as it bends west, passing through several gates and eventually dropping down to Beehive Well and Tank, on the edge of Putnam Wash. The trail heads northwest in Putnam Wash for a short distance, exiting to the northeast, then crosses several ridges, descends into Dobson Wash, and passes near Antelope Tank. After another gate and road crossing, the trail continues northwest as it circles on the east and north sides of Antelope Peak, where it joins a doubletrack. It joins another doubletrack and heads north for approximately 1 mile, crosses Freeman Road and turns west, goes through one more gate, and then arrives at the Freeman Road Trailhead, marking the end of Passage 14.

Mountain Bike Notes

Although some of this passage follows roads that are easy to ride, most miles are on singletrack that will present difficulties for novice riders. For those with desert riding experience, Passage 14 is an outstanding point-to-point route if you can arrange a car shuttle. *For more information about mountain biking along the Arizona National Scenic Trail, visit* **aztrail.org.**

SOUTHERN ACCESS: Tiger Mine Trailhead

From the east entrance to the town of Oracle (East American Avenue), drive 0.8 mile east on AZ 77 to mile marker 105 and turn left (north) onto Old Tiger Road. After 1.5 miles on this road, look for an unmistakable AZT gateway on the left (north) side of the road. Parking is available on both sides of the road.

ALTERNATE SOUTHERN ACCESS: Mountainview Tank

This route is usually passable by high-clearance vehicles; a four-wheel-drive is recommended. On the north end of the town of Mammoth, turn west onto Camino Rio Road, which quickly turns north. Drive north on Camino Rio for 4.7 miles, then turn left (west) into unmarked Gapgage Wash. A two-track road runs up the wash. At mile 7.0, stay on the road as it continues west out of the wash.

Cross a wash at mile 9.9 and begin a wide, sweeping curve, first right and then left, ultimately turning south. At mile 14.4, watch for corrals on your right. Stay right and pass immediately next to the corrals, reaching a Y-intersection in a few hundred feet. Bear left (south-southwest). Do not make any sharp turns in the maze of old roads here. The road climbs a short distance out of the wash.

At mile 19.6 the road turns sharply right; the open area south of the road here is a popular camping spot for hunters and trail workers. The AZT crosses the road approximately 0.25 mile west of this corner. The 40,000-gallon Mountainview Tank is visible just beyond the trail crossing.

NORTHERN ACCESS: Freeman Road

If you want to hit the trail from here, please follow the trail description in reverse order. The trailhead is quite remote and many miles from common landmarks.

From the south, drive north from Oracle Junction on AZ 79 and turn right (east) on Freeman Road 0.8 mile past milepost 111. After 14 miles, continue past Barkerville Road, which joins from the left (north). At approximately 15.5 miles, notice the sign for Willow Springs Road, which joins from the right (south), but bear left and continue on Freeman Road, which becomes Barkerville Road. Note Haydon Ranch Road on the left (north) at approximately mile 16.8 and then a power line at 18.7, followed quickly by an underground pipeline crossing at 18.9. Slow down and watch for an obscure double-track joining the road on the left (north) at mile 19.5. Turn left and follow this road to immediately encounter the AZT trailhead.

PASSAGE 15

Tortilla Mountains

KEY INFO

LOCATION Freeman Road Trailhead to Gila River

DISTANCE 28.4 miles one-way

DAY-TRIP OPTION See turnaround note in the trail description.

SHUTTLE RECOMMENDATION Tecolote Ranch Road (passage mile 8.5)

DIFFICULTY Moderate

LAND MANAGERS Pinal County, **pinalcountyaz.gov**, 520-866-6455; Arizona State Land Department, **azland.gov**, 602-542-4631

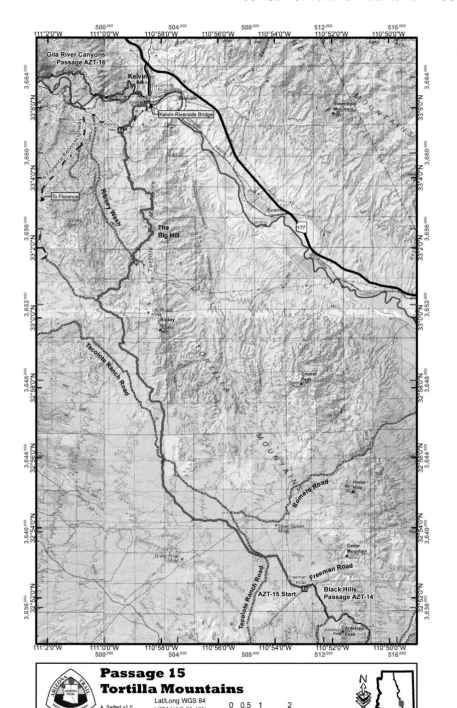

Passage 15
Tortilla Mountains

A. Seifert v1.0
10/30/2013

Lat/Long WGS 84
UTM NAD 83 12N
Scale: 1:200,000

0   0.5   1   2   Miles

N

RECOMMENDED MONTHS February–May and October–December

GATEWAY COMMUNITIES See Central Copper Corridor (page 318) and Florence (page 321).

GEOLOGY HIGHLIGHTS Not applicable

OVERVIEW

Moderate trail miles along singletrack and doubletrack make for easy travel through rolling desert terrain. The trail eventually climbs into the foothills of the Tortilla Mountains before descending toward the Gila River. A combination of carsonite signs and rock cairns marks the trail, but cattle trails crossing the passage sometimes obscure the route.

Although this passage crosses Arizona State Land, no permit is required to travel on the trail or camp within the 15-foot Arizona National Scenic Trail (AZT) corridor. Trail users, however, must respect all livestock operations in this area and close all gates along the trail unless they are intentionally wired open.

ON THE TRAIL

From the Freeman Road Trailhead, the route heads northwest on singletrack crossing several drainages and one larger wash. At 0.6 mile, the trail arrives at a pipeline road and turns right (north), following this road. After about 50 yards the trail follows the road on the left at a Y-junction. The trail continues on this road about 1 mile and then follows the singletrack that exits to the left (west).

The trail meanders through more drainages and a wash for 0.3 mile where it crosses a road and continues on for another 0.2 mile where it crosses Tecolote Ranch Road (Haydon Ranch Road) at mile 2.2. The trail begins to head northwest, goes under

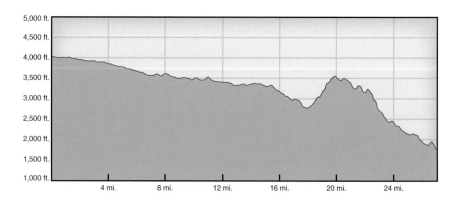

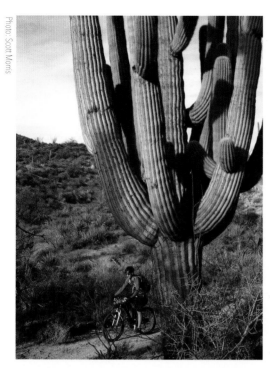

Photo: Scott Morris

The descent through Ripsey Wash and its forest of swollen saguaros is one of the many hidden treasures along Passage 15.

some high-tension power lines at mile 2.5, crosses two doubletracks, and then crosses a pipeline road at about mile 3.7.

Shortly after crossing the pipeline road, the trail crosses a large wash and then turns to the west where it begins following a fence line on the right. About 1.8 miles from the pipeline road is a gate next to a fence corner. After going through the gate, the trail turns to the northwest and passes several more boulders, a very large boulder pile, the first saguaro cactus on this passage, and a few more boulders. From here the trail crosses several arroyos and then a doubletrack road about 1.2 miles from the gate. After passing through more small drainages, the trail turns north, heads up more small washes, climbs up a hill and passes through another gate just before Tecolote Ranch Road.

TURNAROUND NOTE: Because of the remote nature of this passage, out-and-back day-hikers should not go beyond this road, which makes for a 17-mile round-trip from Freeman Road Trailhead.

Moving forward, after crossing Tecolote Ranch Road, the trail keeps to the north, crossing more washes, passing under the same high-tension power lines, and joining

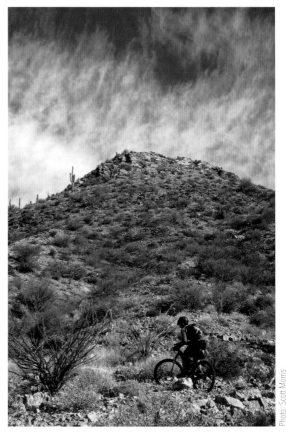

Climbing "The Big Hill" requires strong legs and lots of determination.

Photo: Scott Morris

a road 1.9 miles from Tecolote Ranch Road. It turns left onto this road, stays to the right at a road junction 0.4 mile along it, and continues on it for almost 2 miles. Leaving the road, the route heads across desert terrain before joining another road. From here the trail turns north, passes through a gate and several road junctions, and then leaves the road (left) and climbs to a gate on a hill.

The trail descends the northeast side of this hill, follows a drainage, and then joins a road for a very short distance up a steep hill. After leaving the road (left), the trail follows singletrack south just above the east side of Ripsey Wash. It turns left into the wash and follows a path marked by large cairns to the east side of the wash, where it turns left (north) again to a tributary wash coming in from the right (east).

The trail then turns right and follows a tributary wash for about 0.4 mile. It passes through a gate and begins climbing up what is called The Big Hill. After about 1 mile, the trail begins a series of switchbacks on the southwest side of the peak. It skirts the west side of the peak and continues to a ridge. The trail follows this ridgeline to the north-northwest. After about 0.8 mile, the trail turns to the right (east), and after another 0.4 mile, it turns left (north). In 0.6 mile, the trail crosses a saddle and turns left (west) again. After another 0.6-mile stretch, the trail crosses a high point and begins a descent to the north. Numerous switchbacks snake through this section, and the trail eventually reaches the bottom of a deep arroyo. After crossing several washes, the trail reaches singletrack leading to Florence–Kelvin Highway. It crosses the highway (currently a dirt road that will soon be paved) and heads north-northeast. After crossing a large wash, it curves around and down to the Gila River and the end of Passage 15.

Accommodations and supplies are available 6 miles to the southeast on AZ 177 in the town of Kearny and about 17 miles north in Superior on AZ 177.

Future Impacts

One of Arizona's largest mining corporations, ASARCO, has purchased a large tract of Arizona State Land for the purpose of storing excess tailings from nearby mining operations. Although it may be many years before waste rock is piled in the area near Ripsey Wash, the project will severely affect the current AZT. The ATA is currently developing a scenic and sustainable reroute for the northern portion of this passage.

Mountain Bike Notes

The first 11 miles of this passage are largely on singletrack through rolling desert terrain, offering an excellent mountain biking experience for most skill levels. The next section often follows old doubletrack roads and becomes more challenging as the trail climbs into the Tortilla Mountains. *For more information about mountain biking along the Arizona National Scenic Trail, visit* **aztrail.org.**

SOUTHERN ACCESS: Freeman Road Trailhead

The southern-access trailhead is quite remote and many miles from common landmarks. From the south, drive north from Oracle Junction on AZ 79, and 0.8 mile past milepost 111 turn right (east) onto Freeman Road. At about 14 miles, continue past Barkerville Road, which joins from the left (north). At approximately 15.5 miles, notice the sign for Willow Springs Road, which joins from the right (south), but bear left and continue on Freeman Road, which becomes Barkerville Road. Note Haydon Ranch

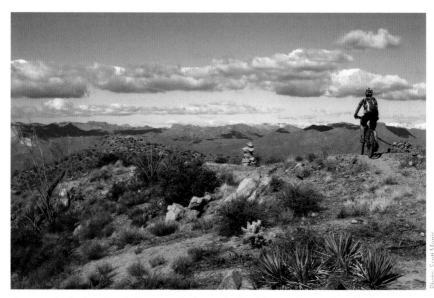

Cresting the high point of Passage 15 before a thrilling descent toward the Gila River

Road on the left (north) at approximately mile 16.8 and then a power line at 18.7 followed quickly by an underground pipeline crossing at 18.9. Slow down and watch for an obscure doubletrack joining the road on the left (north) at mile 19.5. Turn left and follow this road, and immediately encounter the AZT trailhead.

NORTHERN ACCESS: Kelvin-Riverside Bridge

If you want to hit the trail from here, please follow the trail description in reverse order.
From the town of Superior, take AZ 177 south 15.5 miles, and then turn right (south) toward the town of Kelvin. Continue 1.2 miles to the bridge. Passage 14 approaches the bridge from the south. From Florence, drive 1.5 miles south on AZ 79, and turn left (east) on the dirt Florence–Kelvin Highway. Continue 31 miles to the town of Kelvin and a historic bridge over the Gila River.

From the towns of Hayden and Winkelman, drive northwest on AZ 177 about 16 miles, and then turn south (left) on the Florence–Kelvin Highway toward Kelvin. Continue 1.2 miles to the bridge.

AZT Central Section

Passages 16 through 27

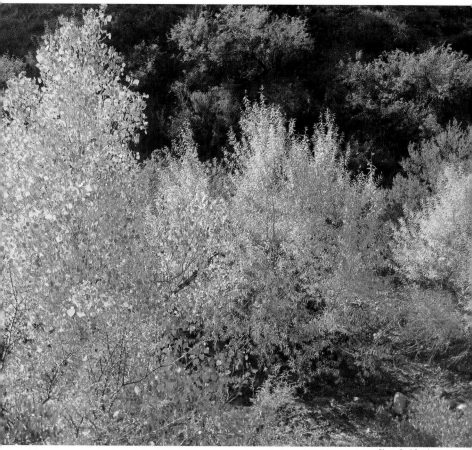

Whitford Canyon displays brilliant autumn colors. (See Passage 8, page 152.)

Photo: Fred Gaudet

Gila River Canyons

LOCATION Gila River to Tonto National Forest boundary

DISTANCE 25.2 miles one-way

DAY-TRIP OPTION See turnaround note in the trail description.

SHUTTLE RECOMMENDATION Drive north on Cochran Road from Florence–Kelvin Highway until it meets the Gila River. (*Warning:* Depending on the amount of water being released upstream, the Gila may be dry, knee-deep, or navigable only by kayak.) Park, cross the river, and walk 0.25 mile east to the AZT.

DIFFICULTY Moderate

LAND MANAGERS U.S. Department of the Interior, Bureau of Land Management (BLM), **blm.gov/wo/st/en.html** (Arizona State Office, 602-417-9200); Arizona State Land Department, **azland.gov,** 602-542-4631

RECOMMENDED MONTHS October–April

GATEWAY COMMUNITIES See Central Copper Corridor (page 318) and Florence (page 321).

GEOLOGY HIGHLIGHTS See "Supervolcanoes of the Superstition Mountains" (page 341).

OVERVIEW

This passage was the last segment of the Arizona National Scenic Trail (AZT) to be completed, with the final singletrack constructed in spring 2012. The first 16 miles follow the

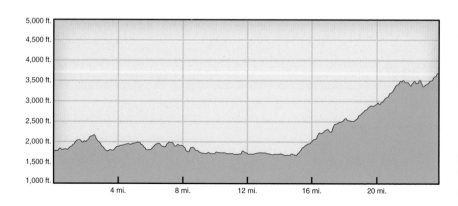

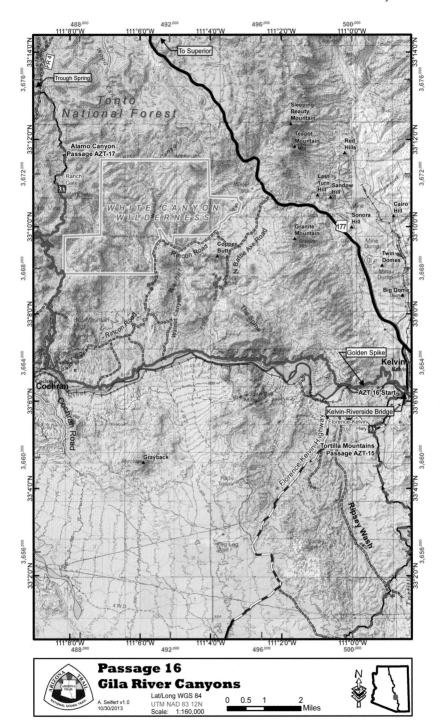

Passage 16
Gila River Canyons

A. Seifert v1.0
10/30/2013

Lat/Long WGS 84
UTM NAD 83 12N
Scale: 1:160,000

0   0.5   1   2
                        Miles

N

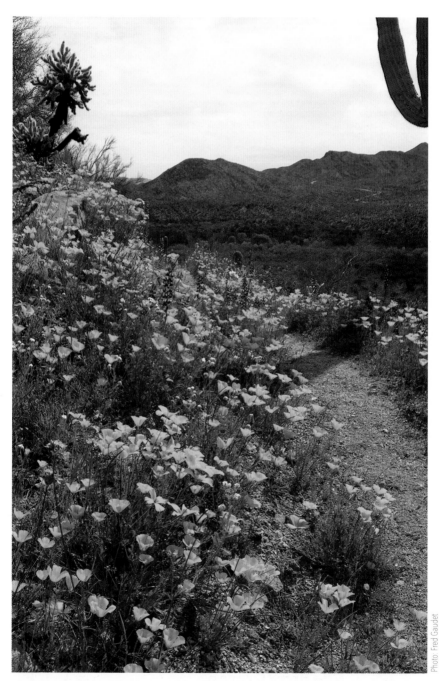

Photo: Fred Gaudet

The Gila River Canyons boast some of the best wildflower displays in Arizona, including dramatic displays of Mexican gold poppies, bluedicks, and purple lupines.

Gila River, offering views unlike anywhere else along the AZT. The final 9 miles penetrate some of the most spectacular gorge scenery outside the Grand Canyon.

ON THE TRAIL

This passage consists of two distinct corridors. The first is the Gila River section (almost 16 miles long), and the second is the Canyons (9-plus miles). The trail starts on the south side of the Kelvin–Riverside Bridge, heads north across the bridge, and quickly turns left (west) on Centurion Road. This dirt road crosses Mineral Creek, passes some private homes, and follows newly constructed trail for the next 2 miles. After gaining a few hundred feet in elevation, the trail arrives at a scenic viewpoint. Nearby is the "golden spike" of the AZT, marking the historic location where the last mile of trail was officially completed in 2012. The initials DS are inscribed in the concrete to honor Dale Shewalter, the "father of the Arizona Trail." It continues west, winding downhill toward a railroad bridge as it passes through numerous boulder formations.

Once the trail is near a railroad bridge, it passes through a mesquite forest until it arrives at a gate. For the next 8 miles it consistently gains and loses elevation as it parallels the Gila River. Expect some great views to the north, south, and along the river.

TURNAROUND NOTE: If you're day-hiking, it's challenging to turn around while along this portion of the trail for fear of missing what beauty lies ahead, but the farther along the river you walk, the longer your day will be. Another option for out-and-back hiking is arranging a car shuttle at the historic townsite of Cochran, on the southern bank of the Gila River, 0.25 mile downstream of where the Arizona Trail heads north up Rincon Road. Cochran Road is accessible from Florence–Kelvin Highway. It's a 16-mile hike from the Kelvin–Riverside Bridge to Cochran and requires you to cross the Gila River from north to south near Cochran. *Note:* Depending on the flow of the Gila, this crossing may or may not be possible. Exercise extreme caution when attempting to cross the river.

Continuing west, you'll pass several arroyos from the mountainous terrain to the north and eventually arrive at Walnut Canyon at mile 11.3. To the north, but mostly out of view from the trail, are formations that define the Gila River Canyons, including The Spine and The Rincon. Much farther north are Copper Butte and the White Canyon Wilderness, both of which drain down through the narrows of Walnut Canyon. If you're looking for a side trip in this area, head north up Walnut Canyon for 3.5 miles to an artesian well.

After crossing Walnut Canyon and passing through a gate, the trail hugs the river closely for the next 4.5 miles. Depending upon recent rains, this section could have a few short muddy sections, but having close proximity to the river, it offers several nice camping areas. The river section ends at the junction of Rincon–Battle Axe Road.

Heading north, the trail uses the rocky Rincon Road for 0.3 mile to the point where the road turns east and new singletrack begins its climb through the canyons to the north. The grade through the canyons will vary between 6 and 18 percent, but the epic scenery distracts you from the steepness of the climb.

After 2 miles, a prominent rhyolite pinnacle, among the defining features of this passage, rises to the west. As you continue north, the shape of the pinnacle changes dramatically. Although currently an unnamed feature, some AZT users have referred to it as Dale's Butte, in honor of Dale Shewalter, the "Father of the Arizona Trail."

Climbing to the northwest, the trail presents remarkable views of deeply cut canyons. This area is prime habitat for bighorn sheep, mountain lions, and Gila monsters. At the westernmost point of the trail, Martinez Canyon comes into view. Because of its remote location, few could have gazed into this natural wonder before this part of the trail was constructed.

Continuing north and east, the trail contours along some severe slopes with switchbacks and passes several deep chasms with natural water catchments that hold water for a short time after recent rains. On the final stretch, the trail crosses an undefined border between Tonto National Forest and BLM lands, and then it crosses the abandoned Ajax Mine Road as it arrives at a ranch gate and the northern end of Passage 16.

Mountain Bike Notes

For the experienced rider, this entire passage is mountain-bike-friendly and may be some of the best singletrack along the AZT. *For more information about mountain biking along the Arizona National Scenic Trail, visit* **aztrail.org***.*

SOUTHERN ACCESS: Kelvin-Riverside Bridge

From the town of Superior, take AZ 177 south for 15.2 miles (milepost 152.1). Turn right (south) onto Florence–Kelvin Highway (next to the railroad crossing), continue

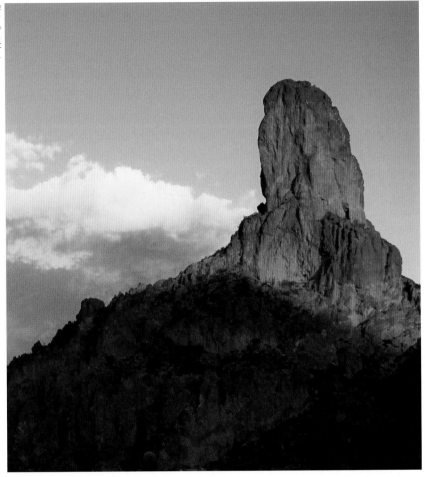

The northern half of Passage 16 showcases dramatic geology in a relatively unexplored part of Arizona.

1.2 miles through the community of Kelvin, and cross the Kelvin–Riverside Bridge, which spans the Gila River. The passage begins on the south side of the bridge, along Centurion Road. There is a large parking area at the junction of Riverside Road and Florence–Kelvin Highway, just across the road from the trailhead. The best parking and access, however, are at the Florence–Kelvin Trailhead, 2 miles south of the Gila River on Passage 15.

NORTHERN ACCESS: Tonto National Forest–Ranch Gate

If you want to hit the trail from here, please follow the trail description in reverse order. The closest way to access the north end of Passage 16 is to hike in on Alamo Passage from either the Picketpost Trailhead (11.5 miles) or to drive in on FR 4 from Superior (Mary Road) for 7 miles. (Caution: FR 4 is extremely rocky and accessible only with a high-clearance four-wheel-drive vehicle and a very confident driver.) There is room to park and camp where the trail crosses FR 4. From this point, you still need to travel south for 4 miles to the ranch gate that divides the north end of Passage 16 from the south end of Passage 17.

PASSAGE 17

Alamo Canyon

KEY INFO

LOCATION Tonto National Forest boundary to Picketpost Trailhead

DISTANCE 11.5 miles one-way

DAY-TRIP OPTION Not applicable

SHUTTLE RECOMMENDATION Not applicable

DIFFICULTY Moderate

LAND MANAGERS Tonto National Forest, Globe Ranger District, **www.fs.usda.gov/tonto,** 928-402-6200,

RECOMMENDED MONTHS October–April

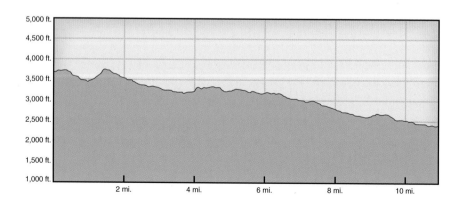

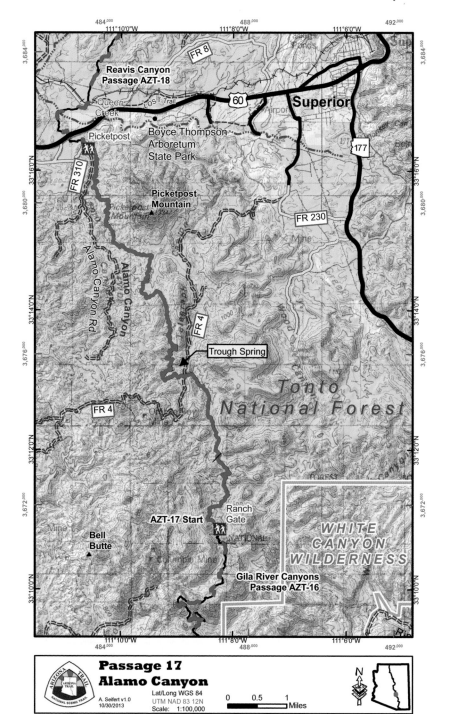

Passage 17
Alamo Canyon

Lat/Long WGS 84
UTM NAD 83 12N
Scale: 1:100,000

A. Seifert v1.0
10/30/2013

0   0.5   1
Miles

N

GATEWAY COMMUNITIES See Globe (page 319), Florence (page 321), and Superior (page 322).

GEOLOGY HIGHLIGHTS See "Supervolcanoes of the Superstition Mountains" (page 341).

OVERVIEW

The rugged desert, mountains, and canyons that characterize most of this passage are as isolated as they are beautiful. Because of its difficult access for day-trippers, this passage is, overall, most approachable by multiday adventurers or those willing to put in long miles between Passages 16 and 17. Springtime brings an abundance of wildflowers to this region, and seeing Alamo Canyon in full bloom is breathtaking.

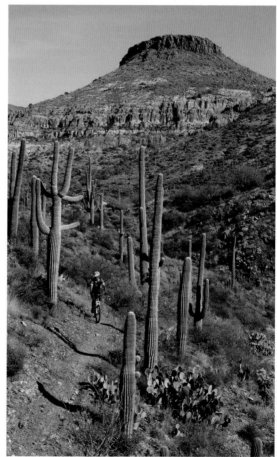

Passage 17 has become one of Arizona's hot spots for mountain bikers with strong singletrack skills.

Photo: Matthew J. Nelson

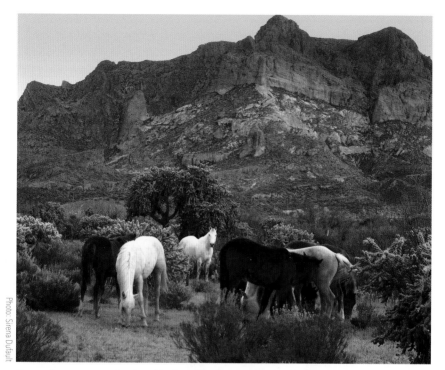

Horses forage on a springtime blanket of fresh greens near Picketpost Mountain.

The termination point, Picketpost Trailhead has become increasingly popular with day-hikers, trail runners, equestrians, and mountain bikers alike. And for good reason—it has ample parking, a bathroom, horse-trailer parking, and hitching rails, and it provides access to an amazing part of the Tonto National Forest.

ON THE TRAIL

This passage lies entirely within Tonto National Forest and begins at a ranch gate about 0.3 mile north of the national forest and BLM boundary. From this gate the trail heads north for 1 mile before dropping into an old narrow doubletrack drainage (once used as a trail) where signs lead toward Picketpost. A small seasonal earthen water tank sits only a few feet away on the southwest side at this location. Continue north (uphill) to a saddle; after crossing the saddle, the trail heads downhill across a few drainages and lush hillsides.

After passing through a ranch gate, the trail gently drops down close to the head-waters for Telegraph Canyon, which it parallels until it reaches FR 4. After crossing FR 4, the trail winds to the west and north through hills and valleys as you work your way toward Picketpost Mountain. Trough Spring, the only viable water source along this passage, is 0.25 mile down Telegraph Canyon. As you approach Picketpost, the trail wraps around on the west side and tends to parallel Alamo Canyon drainage, until it reaches the trailhead. This large trailhead has a bathroom and plenty of parking, but water is unavailable. Approximately 3.3 miles south of Picketpost, a connecting trail leads east to FR 4, which has become popular with equestrian groups that like to make a loop around Picketpost Mountain.

Additionally, the Legends of Superior Trail (LOST), a side trail, heads east to the town of Superior. This 5-mile trail connects the AZT and the Gateway Community of Superior, and it passes through the remains of the historic mining town of Pinal City.

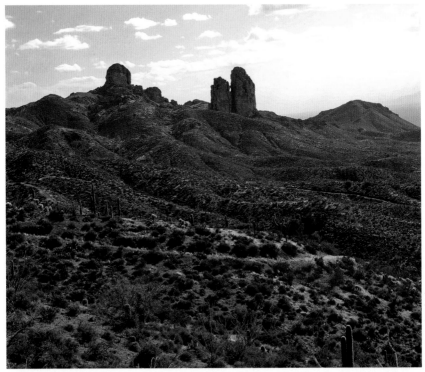

Photo: Sue and Mark Johnson

Rhyolite hoodoos near Alamo Canyon are weathered remnants of Arizona's volcanic past. (See "Supervolcanoes of the Superstition Mountains," page 341, for more information.)

Currently the trail terminates at the Superior airport on the west end of town. To access the LOST from the AZT, you must continue north from the Picketpost Trailhead for 1.6 miles on Passage 18 to near the junction with Hewitt Station Road and follow the signage.

Mountain Bike Notes

The entire passage features high-quality singletrack. If you link Passages 16 and 17 as a long day trip or an overnight bikepacking trip, you'll ride some of the Arizona National Scenic Trail's (AZT) highest-quality miles for mountain bikers. *For more information about mountain biking along the Arizona National Scenic Trail, visit* **aztrail.org.**

SOUTHERN ACCESS: Tonto National Forest–Ranch Gate

The closest access to the south end of Passage 17 is to hike in on Alamo Passage from either Picketpost Trailhead (11.5 miles), or drive in on FR 4 from Superior (Mary Road) for 7 miles. (*Caution:* FR 4 is extremely rocky and accessible only with a high-clearance four-wheel-drive vehicle and a very confident driver.) There is room to park and camp where the trail crosses FR 4. From this point, you still need to travel south for 4 miles to a ranch gate that divides the Passages 16 and 17.

NORTHERN ACCESS: Picketpost Trailhead

If you want to hit the trail from here, please follow the trail description in reverse order. From Florence Junction, drive east on US 60 for 9 miles. After mile marker 221, continue 0.5 mile and turn right (south) onto FR 231. (This point is 4 miles west of the town of Superior, on US 60.) Drive 0.4 mile and turn left onto FR 310. Continue 0.6 mile, then turn right at a sign for Picketpost Trailhead. You'll see a large metal AZT sign marking the trailhead in 0.1 mile. There is no vehicle access to the Tonto National Forest boundary from here.

Reavis Canyon

LOCATION Picketpost Trailhead to Rogers Trough Trailhead

DISTANCE 18.6 miles one-way

DAY-TRIP OPTION See turnaround note in the trail description.

SHUTTLE RECOMMENDATIONS Southern and northern access

DIFFICULTY Moderate

LAND MANAGER Tonto National Forest, Globe Ranger District, **www.fs.usda.gov/tonto,** 928-402-6200

RECOMMENDED MONTHS October–May

GATEWAY COMMUNITIES See Globe (page 319) and Superior (page 322).

GEOLOGY HIGHLIGHTS See "Supervolcanoes of the Superstition Mountains" (page 341).

OVERVIEW

This passage links the desert canyons of Passage 17 to the higher elevations on the east side of the Superstition Wilderness. The trail features beautiful Sonoran Desert landscapes with panoramic views of the Superstition Mountains to the northwest, Picketpost Mountain to the south, and the Apache Leap formation to the east. Lucky hikers may see a variety of wildlife, including deer, rabbits, javelinas, quail, rattlesnakes, and

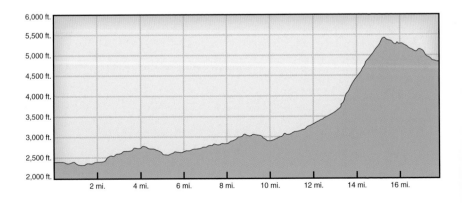

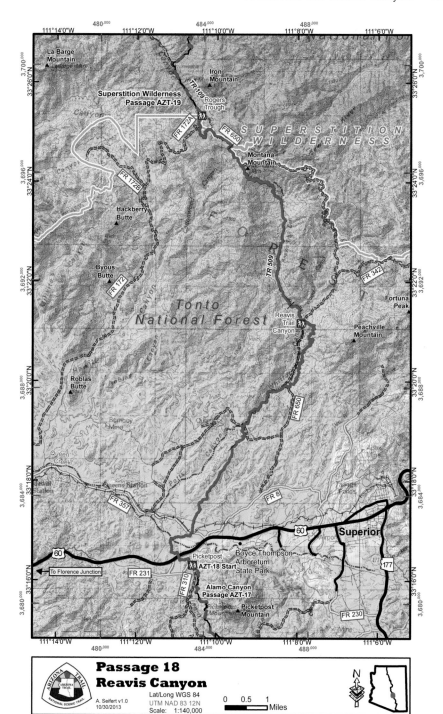

Passage 18
Reavis Canyon

A. Seifert v1.0
10/30/2013

Lat/Long WGS 84
UTM NAD 83 12N
Scale: 1:140,000

0   0.5   1
Miles

N

the elusive Gila monster. *Note: Whitford Canyon and Reavis Trail Canyon are notorious flash-flood paths; be aware of the weather forecast, and don't hike through these canyons when rain is imminent.*

ON THE TRAIL

From the Picketpost Trailhead sign, the trail heads straight north through the parking area and veers left (near the entrance to the parking area) and on to singletrack marked by trail signs. Continue until you cross an old paved road; crest a hill in 100 yards, and continue west on singletrack marked by cairns. The trail descends to a wash and turns right (north) toward US 60. Go through the culverts under the highway, and pass through a fence on the opposite side.

Continue 30 yards along the wash, then turn left (west) onto singletrack at a cairn and wooden AZT marker. The trail soon heads north along a hill to a wooden AZT marker at a barbed-wire fence. Descend to cross Queen Creek, a major wash, and head for a wooden sign that marks the trail's continuation on the other side.

In the next 120 yards, the trail curves right and then left before reaching a place where you cross a fence by going through two gates within 6 feet of each other. Continue through heavy vegetation, heading just slightly south and east. Follow a faint tread, and frequent cairns, generally east and northeast.

When you reach a fence line, turn right (east) and continue 0.1 mile until you pass a fence line perpendicular to the one you're following. Turn left (north) to pass through the second (easternmost) of two gates, follow the perpendicular fence line 20 yards, and then pick up the trail heading to the right (northeast). It continues on to FR 357 and then crosses the railroad tracks. *Watch for trains.*

At this point the Legends of Superior Trail (LOST) connects the historic mining town of Superior with the AZT. From its junction at Hewitt Station Road, follow the signposts for 5-plus miles to the east. The LOST terminates at the Superior airport, 1 mile west of town.

Continuing on the AZT, cross a dirt road, pass under the power lines and then climb up to a ridgeline and follow it. The trail now tracks northeast up a roughly cut switchback and then up and down a ridgeline with eight crests over the next 2 miles.

From this ridge you have excellent views in all directions. From the sixth crest, you can see the impressive volcanic monolith called Weaver's Needle in the Superstition Mountains to the northwest. As the trail begins descending the ridge to the northwest, it passes just east of a stone structure called Barnett Camp.

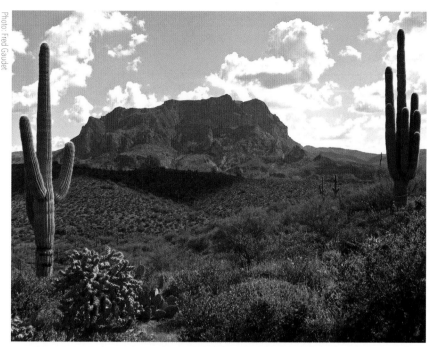

As the AZT climbs higher into the Superstition Mountains, the hulking mass of Picketpost Mountain to the south becomes increasingly dramatic.

TURNAROUND NOTE: The AZT now enters Whitford Canyon, which it follows for the next 1.8 miles and exits near FR 650. For day-hikers who haven't arranged a car shuttle, Whitford Canyon makes for a nice turnaround spot.

To continue on the trail, cross FR 650, the AZT continues on singletrack for the next 3.2 miles, paralleling Whitford Canyon and then crossing FR 650 again. It joins a doubletrack for a short distance down to the well-marked Reavis Trail Canyon Trailhead.

Here, you're on the historic Reavis Trail (Trail 509), which passes through an old ruin that offers some nice, flat camping spots along with numerous remnants of early European American artifacts. Follow cairns as the trail weaves in and out of the drainage. The canyon and the trail soon bend sharply to the northwest, leaving the drainage as you head for higher elevations. After passing through a gate, it becomes a rather long and arduous climb to a saddle with numerous switchbacks up long grassy slopes. Fires damaged these slopes in 2011, and they may be rerouted in the future.

At the higher elevations, the spectacular view to the south is an interesting perspective on Picketpost Mountain as you gaze down on the flat mountaintop that towered over the beginning of this passage. Once on the ridgeline, the trail joins FR 650, only this time you remain on FR 650 for almost 2 miles to the end, which is the T-intersection with FR 172A. Continue north on FR 172A for 0.4 mile to the Rogers Trough Trailhead and the beginning of Passage 19.

Mountain Bike Notes

The terrain on this part of the Arizona National Scenic Trail (AZT) varies greatly, from flat dirt roads to steep singletrack that only highly skilled riders will enjoy. This passage terminates at the boundary of the Superstition Wilderness—where bikes are prohibited. *For detailed information about scenic mountain biking routes around wilderness areas, vi*sit **aztrail.org.**

SOUTHERN ACCESS: Picketpost Trailhead

From Florence Junction, drive east on US 60 for 9 miles. After mile marker 221, continue 0.5 mile and turn right (south) onto FR 231. (This point is 4 miles west of the

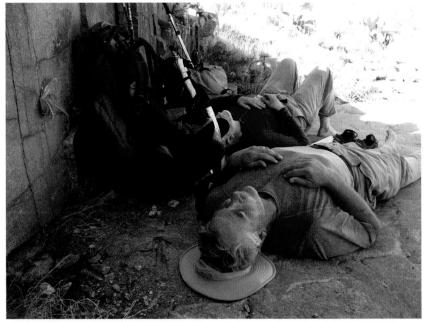

Shade is among the most precious resources along the desert passages of the AZT.

Photo: Robert Luce

town of Superior on US 60.) Drive 0.4 mile and turn left onto FR 310. Continue 0.6 mile, then turn right at a sign for Picketpost Trailhead. You'll see the large metal AZT sign marking the trailhead in 0.1 mile.

ALTERNATE ACCESS: Reavis Trail Canyon Trailhead

From Florence Junction, travel east on US 60 for 10 miles. After mile marker 222, continue 0.4 mile east, then turn left (north) onto a dirt road at an unmarked intersection. Continue about 50 yards, and turn right (east) onto FR 8, which is poorly marked with an old sign. At mile 1.8 (mileages given from the highway), bear left at a Y-intersection onto FR 650.

At mile 2.1, avoid a left fork and descend to the right on the better road. This road gradually worsens, soon requiring a four-wheel-drive vehicle. The road jogs in and out of a wash that may have water running through it in the spring. At mile 6.2, the road climbs steeply along the right side of the drainage. Just after it tops out, take a left fork down to an Arizona National Scenic Trail (AZT) marker and a ROAD CLOSED sign at mile 6.3. From here, a singletrack continues up Reavis Trail Canyon.

NORTHERN ACCESS: Rogers Trough Trailhead

Note: This access usually requires a high-clearance vehicle. If you want to hit the trail from here, please follow the trail description in reverse order.

From Florence Junction, travel east on US 60 for 1.8 miles, turn left (north) onto Queen Valley Road, continue 1.8 miles, and turn right (east) on FR 357. Drive 3 miles and turn left (north) onto FR 172 at a sign for Rogers Trough Trailhead. (You'll see a sign for FR 172 about 20 yards after the turn.) Continue 9.2 miles to a fork and bear right onto FR 172A. Follow this road 3.7 miles, bear left at an intersection with FR 650 and continue 0.4 mile to a very large parking area. The trail departs from the north end of the parking lot.

From Superior, travel west about 3 miles on US 60, 0.6 mile west of mile marker 223, turn right (north) at an unmarked intersection onto a dirt road, which is FR 357. Follow it 5 miles to a right turn onto FR 172, which is marked as such only about 20 yards after the turn. (A sign on FR 357, facing the opposite direction, indicates that this is the turn for Rogers Trough Trailhead.) Continue 9.2 miles to a fork and bear right onto FR 172A. Follow this road 3.7 miles, bear left at an intersection with FR 650, and continue 0.4 mile to a very large parking area. The trail departs from the north end of the parking lot.

Superstition Wilderness

KEY INFO

LOCATION Rogers Trough Trailhead to Theodore Roosevelt Lake

DISTANCE 28.7 miles one-way

DAY-TRIP OPTION See turnaround note in the trail description.

SHUTTLE RECOMMENDATIONS Reavis Mountain School (hike along Trail 117 to AZT), Tule Canyon Trailhead off FR 449

DIFFICULTY Strenuous

LAND MANAGERS Tonto National Forest, Mesa Ranger District, 480-610-3300, and Tonto Basin Ranger District, 928-467-3200; **www.fs.usda.gov/tonto**

RECOMMENDED MONTHS September–April

GATEWAY COMMUNITIES See Globe (page 319) and Roosevelt and Tonto Basin (page 323).

GEOLOGY HIGHLIGHTS See "Supervolcanoes of the Superstition Mountains" (page 341).

OVERVIEW

Although the Superstition Wilderness is heavily traveled, this passage still gives trail users a genuine sense of wilderness as it traverses the east side, farthest from Phoenix, and the trailheads require long drives on four-wheel-drive roads. This sense of solitude certainly seems to have appealed to Elisha Reavis, who settled here along a reliable

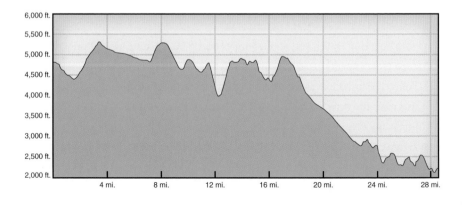

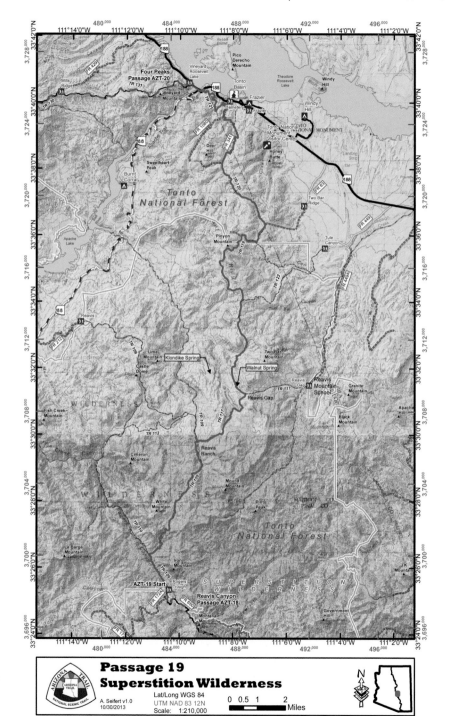

Passage 19
Superstition Wilderness

A. Seifert v1.0
10/30/2013

Lat/Long WGS 84
UTM NAD 83 12N
Scale: 1:210,000

0   0.5   1   2
Miles

N

creek around 1874. Rich soil and a favorable climate helped Reavis grow apples and vegetables, which he sold at mining towns in the area. The Arizona National Scenic Trail (AZT) passes the site of the old Reavis Ranch—still a pastoral place with a few apple trees remaining from the orchard. If you walk the grounds, which are now managed by the U.S. Forest Service, you will see pieces of rusting farm implements and foundations of the original homestead.

The final miles of this passage are at low elevations that are quite hot in summer. Campsites are plentiful on this passage, especially near Walnut Spring, at mile 12.3. Camping near Pine Creek is delightful, and water is often available, depending on the season. Camping is limited before you crest a ridge at mile 4.1. There's very little camping between mile 18.0 and mile 23.0, and it's limited again during the final few miles, starting at mile 26.6.

ON THE TRAIL

Follow the trail out of the north end of the Rogers Trough trailhead by using the Reavis Ranch Trail (Trail 109). In 1.3 miles the trail reaches an intersection with Trail 110. The AZT turns northeast onto the Reavis Ranch Trail, and then it travels up to Reavis Saddle and then to the ruins of Reavis Ranch. The trail descends along Reavis Creek—avoid a sharp right turn onto the Fire Line Trail—and continues north on the same Reavis Ranch Trail.

TURNAROUND NOTE: If you're just out for the day and attempting an out-and-back hike of this passage, Reavis Ranch is a great turnaround location–*before* you reach Reavis Creek. By the time you're back at your car, you'll have 13.6 miles under your boots.

To continue on the trail, at mile 7.9 follow the right-hand option of the two trails paralleling one another. At mile 8 the trail forks just before a fence; take the faint option to the east. The last place you can camp legally in the ranch area is near the creek crossing.

The AZT merges with the Reavis Gap Trail (Trail 117) here. Cross the stream and follow the route along the southern flanks of Boulder Mountain until it tops out. A descent into the Pine Creek drainage leads to a tributary crossing of the creek. Climb north-northeast to a saddle, and cross into another drainage at mile 10.2. Then continue around the top of the drainage to the intersection at mile 10.5, where the AZT leaves the Reavis Gap Trail and turns left (west) onto the Two Bar Ridge Trail (Trail 119).

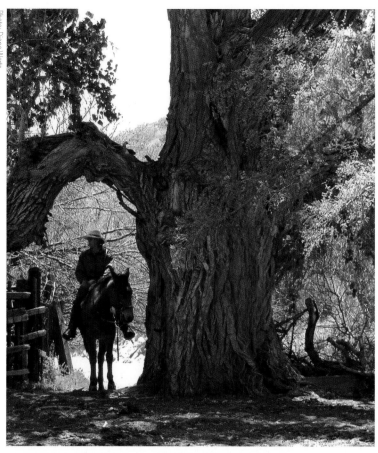

An ancient cottonwood tree (*Populus fremontii*) near Reavis Ranch

As the AZT continues down on Two Bar Ridge, frequent cairns mark it until it reaches Walnut Spring at mile 11, and then it gradually climbs to the north to cross a ridge. The trail tends to fade here, but cairns show the way to the north-northwest before descending the other side. Cairns again mark a strenuous climb through a healthy population of prickly-pear cacti, often crowding the tread on the way to a saddle. The trail turns north to follow the trail's namesake land formation, Two Bar Ridge.

Continue north on Two Bar Ridge. At the junction with Tule Canyon Trail (Trail 122), the AZT continues north past the junction until it veers to the west, descending gradually before making an abrupt turn to the right (north) at mile 17.4. It descends into a pine forest with some nice camping spots without water. After a low point, the AZT climbs steeply and peaks on a southwest ridge of Pinyon Mountain. Trend north and east to exit the wilderness at mile 17.8. After walking around to the northeast slopes, drop abruptly to the south edge of the parking area for the Two Bar Ridge Trailhead.

Just beyond Pinyon Mountain, Two Bar Ridge Trail ends at FR 83 (Black Bush Ranch Road). The trail follows this doubletrack to the junction with Cottonwood Canyon Trail (Trail 120) at mile 19.7. The AZT currently uses the 3-plus-mile stretch of Cottonwood Canyon for the passage until it reaches FR 341. The canyon is beautiful, but it is narrow, extremely rocky, and tends to flood during the summer monsoons. Often the flooding causes severe washouts and extensive damage, along with brush overgrowth throughout the entire length. Hikers rarely have difficulty with this section, but equestrians and mountain bikers should not attempt it.

Once you are through the canyon and arrive at FR 341, turn right (north) and continue on the doubletrack. The road climbs above the Cottonwood Creek drainage and reaches a high point with views of Theodore Roosevelt Lake, as well as the blue-roofed Visitor Center building.

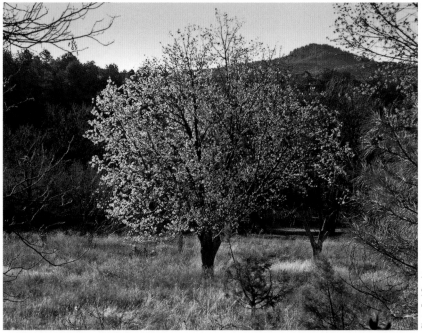

Photo: Fred Gaudet

Some of the fruit trees planted by Elisha Reavis in the 1870s still produce apples near the historic Reavis Ranch.

At mile 25.5, the road drops to cross Cottonwood Creek. Just before the creek crossing, turn west (left) and cross the creek (the spur to the right is the 1.2-mile spur to the Frazier Trailhead). The road ascends to a junction with FR 1080. Cross this road and pick up the singletrack Thompson Trail (Trail 121), which is also a popular day-hiking trail.

The trail soon reaches another junction, this time with the Cemetery Trail, a 0.25-mile trail that leads through a fence to the right to the Cemetery Trailhead, which is directly across the highway from the Roosevelt Lake Visitor Center and Marina. The marina is a good place to access very limited services in this area.

After passing this junction, continue to the northwest and follow the signage for a new alignment that was developed for shared use. It wraps around a hillside and drops into a drainage crossing with a water tank, and then climbs to a saddle. After several more drainage contours, it descends to reach a trailhead just before AZ 188. Cross the suspension bridge by walking on the far left side, and pick up the trail where the cement guardrail ends on the west side. A large parking area is on the right (east) side of the highway.

Mountain Bike Notes

Bikes are prohibited for most of this passage as the majority is within the Superstition Wilderness. Refer to the Arizona Trail Association's (ATA) *Mountain Bike Databook* for preferred routes around the wilderness. (Download the book from **aztrail.org/mtn _bikers.html**.) Seasonal storms render Cottonwood Canyon unfriendly to bikes, and equestrians are warned to avoid the area. *For detailed information about scenic mountain biking routes around wilderness areas, visit* **aztrail.org.**

SOUTHERN ACCESS: Rogers Trough Trailhead

Note: This access usually requires a high-clearance four-wheel-drive vehicle.

From Florence Junction, travel east on US 60 for 1.8 miles and turn left (north) onto Queen Valley Road. Continue 1.8 miles and turn right (east) on FR 357. Drive 3 miles and turn left (north) onto FR 172 at a sign for Rogers Trough Trailhead (There is a sign for FR 172 about 20 yards after the turn.) Continue 9.2 miles to a fork and bear right onto FR 172A. Follow this road for 3.7 miles, bear left at an intersection with FR 650, and continue 0.4 mile to a very large parking area. The trail departs from the north end of the parking lot.

From Superior, travel west about 3 miles on US 60, 0.6 mile west of mile marker 223, and turn right (north) at an unmarked intersection onto a dirt road, which is FR

357. Follow it 5 miles to a right turn onto FR 172, which is marked as such only about 20 yards after the turn. (A sign on FR 357, facing the opposite direction, indicates that this is the turn for Rogers Trough Trailhead.) Continue 9.2 miles to a fork and bear right onto FR 172A. Follow this road for 3.7 miles, bear left at an intersection with FR 650, and continue 0.4 mile to a very large parking area. The trail departs from the north end of the parking lot.

ALTERNATE ACCESS: Two Bar Ridge Trailhead

From the suspension bridge near Roosevelt Dam, follow AZ 188 east for 5.5 miles and turn right onto a dirt road, which is marked as FR 83 a short distance off the highway. The following mileages are from the highway turnoff: Drive 2.8 miles to a gate at Black Bush Ranch and bear left, continuing on FR 83. At a gate and fork at mile 3.9, take the left fork, go about 30 yards to another fork, and bear right.

At mile 4.1, you'll see Trail 120 on the right (north), the path of the AZT along Cottonwood Creek. Continue southwest on the "main" road (and the AZT), which becomes quite steep. Make a left turn at mile 5.6, just before the road crosses an earthen dam. Drive the final steep 0.1 mile to the trailhead.

ALTERNATE ACCESS: Frazier Trailhead

This trailhead is recommended for trail users towing horse trailers. From the suspension bridge near Theodore Roosevelt Dam, follow AZ 188 east for 2 miles and turn right, into the trailhead parking area. The AZT is 1.2 miles up the trail.

ALTERNATE ACCESS: Cemetery Trailhead

From the suspension bridge by Roosevelt Dam, follow AZ 188 east for 1.4 miles, then turn right into an RV park across the highway from the Roosevelt Marina and Visitor Center. Make another immediate right into the Cemetery Trail parking area. The AZT is 0.25 mile up the trail.

NORTHERN ACCESS: Theodore Roosevelt Lake

If you want to hit the trail from here, please follow the trail description in reverse order. This is near Roosevelt Dam, where AZ 88 and AZ 188 meet. The parking area is at the north end of the suspension bridge, on the east side of the highway.

Four Peaks

KEY INFO

● **LOCATION** Theodore Roosevelt Lake to Lone Pine Saddle

DISTANCE 19.5 miles one-way

DAY-TRIP OPTION For the highest quality trail miles, drive to Mills Ridge Trailhead, hike northwest along the AZT to Granite Spring, and then return.

SHUTTLE RECOMMENDATION Mills Ridge Trailhead

DIFFICULTY Strenuous

LAND MANAGER Tonto National Forest, Tonto Basin Ranger District, **www.fs.usda.gov/tonto,** 928-467-3200

RECOMMENDED MONTHS March–May; September–November

GATEWAY COMMUNITIES See Roosevelt and Tonto Basin (page 323).

GEOLOGY HIGHLIGHTS See "Amazing Mazatzals" (page 342).

OVERVIEW

This passage has several striking aspects, including great views of Roosevelt Lake and the dam that created it, close-up views of the magnificent Four Peaks, and the startling effects of an intense forest fire.

Roosevelt Dam was completed in 1911, following President Theodore Roosevelt's 1902 edict to divert and store water to spur development of the West. In 1984, engineers determined that the dam might be inadequate to withstand the greatest possible earthquake that could occur in the area, and also that a large flood could overwhelm the dam. A $410 million project to reconfigure the dam began in 1989 and was completed in 1996. The dam's height increased from 280 to 357 feet, the length of the crest grew from 723 to 1,210 feet, and the lake's surface gained 1,862 acres, an increase of almost 10 percent.

Another human-made feature that defines this passage was less carefully planned and executed. Careless campers started a wild conflagration called the Lone Fire near Pigeon Spring on April 28, 1996. In a week, it consumed 60,000 acres, making it the

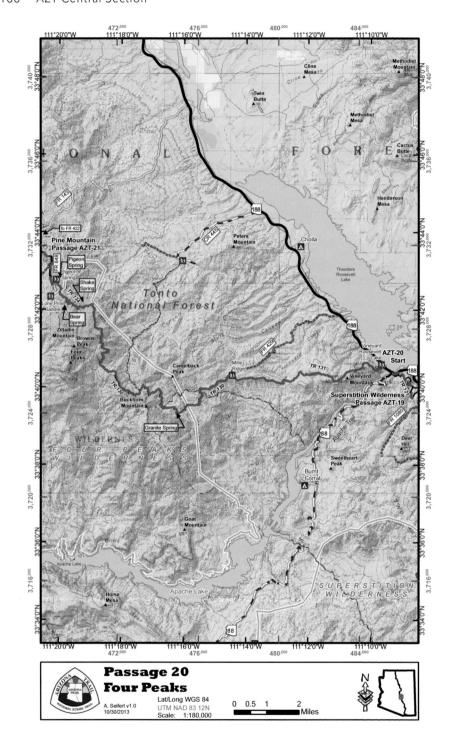

Passage 20
Four Peaks

A. Seifert v1.0
10/30/2013

Lat/Long WGS 84
UTM NAD 83 12N
Scale: 1:180,000

0   0.5   1   2
Miles

N

largest fire in Arizona history at that time. The Arizona National Scenic Trail (AZT) goes through the heart of this burn area, presenting some unique challenges to the hiker. Cairns mark the trail in these areas, but they are frequently inadequate. Adding to the peril are burned-out snags that can topple at any time.

As of March 2013, the passage corridor has been completely cleared and is passable along the entire length of the trail, but there are a few sections that have annual brush encroachment. Water conditions vary throughout the year. The trail traverses some high ridges with significant elevation gains, and the loss of benching tends to make the cross slopes slippery. It is recommended only for equestrians with extensive trail riding experience.

ON THE TRAIL

From the parking area on the east side of AZ 188, walk southwest across the highway near the suspension bridge, and look for a trail that climbs to the southwest: the Vineyard Trail (Trail 131), marked with an AZT carsonite sign. Wind up the ridge, and after 0.5 mile make a sharp turn to the right as another spur continues straight to the south (this spur leads a short distance to a bird's-eye view of Roosevelt Dam).

The trail's initial climb soon gives way to rolling ups and downs along a prominent ridge, with stunning views of Apache Lake to the south. Soon you reach an old double-track that is marked by AZT stickers on carsonite posts. Turn right (west) and follow a slight descent.

The ridge dwindles away and the trail fades somewhat as it bends right (northwest) to climb pretty steeply onto another ridge. As you walk due west along this ridge, you feel like you're near the top of the world, with astounding views in all directions, even

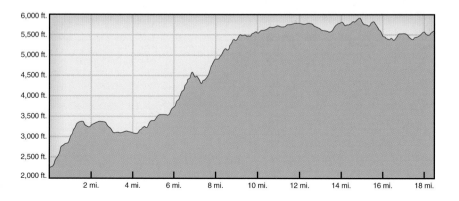

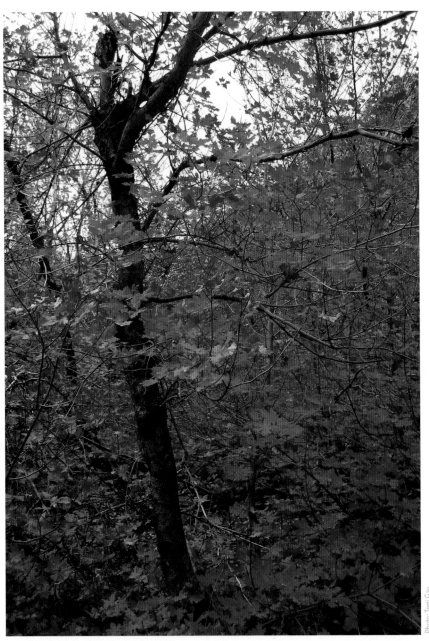

Photo: Terri Gay

Autumn brings gorgeous colors to Passage 20, including the Halloween hues of bigtooth maple (*Acer grandidentatum*) leaves.

though you're only about 3,400 feet above sea level. Upon reaching a parking area at Mills Ridge Trailhead, walk west across the parking area to pick up the AZT at a sign for Trail 130. A relatively steep climb leads to a ridge crest in 0.5 mile, followed by a knob. The trail drops into Buckhorn Creek and then goes up again, passing Hackberry Creek and finally reaching unreliable Granite Spring. From here, Four Peaks Trail (Trail 130) heads north and then west, skirting Buckhorn Peak.

Continuing north, you reach an intersection with the Alder Creek Trail (Trail 82). Stay on Trail 130 to the right (west) for about 10 yards, and then follow it as it makes a right (north) turn to continue contouring along this steep hillside. The trail becomes very clear. At the intersection with Oak Flat Trail (Trail 123), turn left (northwest). You soon reach unreliable Shake Spring. Continue on past Bear Spring on Pigeon Trail (Trail 134) until you arrive at Pigeon Spring.

To go to the popular trailhead at Lone Pine Saddle, continue up the trail to the south, and later west-northwest, about 2 miles. After crossing a streambed, the trail fades near some unusually flat terrain. Bear right (east) of the flat point, and the trail is soon apparent.

In less than a mile, crest a small ridge and exit the Four Peaks Wilderness at a marker. Next you reach Pigeon Spring. From the sign for Pigeon Spring, the trail climbs southwest on an old roadbed. The trail reaches Pigeon Trailhead on FR 648, and the end of Passage 20.

Mountain Bike Notes

Most of this passage is inside the Four Peaks Wilderness, where bikes are prohibited. *For detailed information about scenic mountain biking routes around wilderness areas, visit* aztrail.org.

SOUTHERN ACCESS: Theodore Roosevelt Lake

The southern access area for this passage is near Theodore Roosevelt Dam, where AZ 88 and AZ 188 meet. The parking area is at the north end of the suspension bridge, on the east side of the highway.

ALTERNATE ACCESS: Mills Ridge Trailhead

From the Roosevelt suspension bridge, drive 2.5 miles northwest on AZ 188 and cross a bridge. Turn left (west) onto the dirt road (which connects to FR 429). The following mileages are from AZ 188: Follow the road's curve to the right, then turn left (west) onto FR 429 at mile 0.4. Stay on FR 429 until you reach a parking area and trailhead at mile 4.9. The AZT arrives from the east (downhill side) on the Vineyard Trail and departs to the west (uphill) on Trail 130.

NORTHERN ACCESS:
Pigeon Spring and Lone Pine Saddle Trailheads

If you want to hit the trail from here, please follow the trail description in reverse order. From the suspension bridge near Roosevelt Dam, drive north on AZ 188 for 11 miles and turn left (west) at mile marker 255 onto El Oso Road. At 4.4 miles from the highway, the road appears to fork. Take the sharp right turn and follow the road as it climbs. Continue another 4.2 miles to an intersection with FR 422, which is the path of the AZT to the north. The AZT arrives from the southeast (left) on FR 143. Drive 1 mile on FR 143 to an intersection, bear left onto FR 648, and continue almost another mile to Pigeon Spring Trailhead on the left.

Alternatively, to reach a larger, more developed parking area and trailhead at Lone Pine Saddle, continue 0.5 mile ahead. Parking here allows you to hike on singletrack into the Four Peaks Wilderness and meet the AZT in about 2 miles.

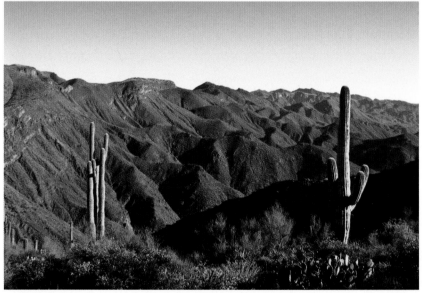

Photo: Robert Luce

Passage 20 features a diverse mix of desert and forest environments.

Pine Mountain

KEY INFO

LOCATION Lone Pine Saddle to Sunflower

DISTANCE 19.8 miles one-way

DAY-TRIP OPTION From the southern access point, hike as far as time and energy permit, and then return to Pigeon Spring Trailhead. From the northern access point, hike south for 7 miles to Boulder Creek, and then return.

SHUTTLE RECOMMENDATIONS Southern and northern access points

DIFFICULTY Moderate to difficult

LAND MANAGERS Tonto National Forest, Tonto Basin Ranger District, **www.fs.usda.gov/tonto,** 928-467-3200

RECOMMENDED MONTHS March–November

GATEWAY COMMUNITY See Roosevelt and Tonto Basin (page 323).

GEOLOGY HIGHLIGHTS See "Amazing Mazatzals" (page 342).

OVERVIEW

In spite of this passage's accessibility, it has a remote feel, and the singletrack in the Boulder Creek drainage offers beautiful views.

ON THE TRAIL

From the Pigeon Spring Trailhead, hike northwest on FR 648 for 1 mile until you reach an intersection with FR 143. Turn right (north) on FR 143, descend another mile, and take a left (northwest) fork onto FR 422. Follow AZT stickers on carsonite posts, and stay on the FR 422 doubletrack for approximately 9 miles. Bear right (east) at a fork and make your way through a ponderosa pine–oak forest.

Campsites are plentiful along this part of the passage. In 0.5 mile, the road reaches a high north-facing slope and bends to the left (west), offering spectacular 180-degree views. Continue on the primary road, avoiding the occasional faint fork. The road

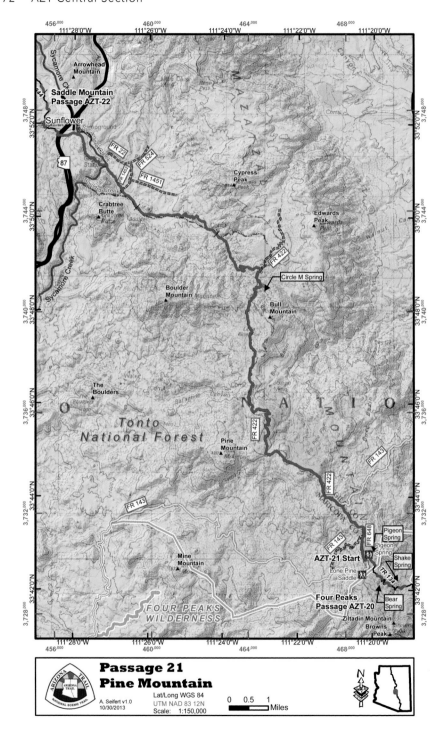

Passage 21
Pine Mountain

Lat/Long WGS 84
UTM NAD 83 12N
Scale: 1:150,000

A. Seifert v1.0
10/30/2013

0   0.5   1
Miles

N

begins a sharp, rocky descent and bottoms out in a saddle. Climb 0.1 mile northeast on the road; descend another 0.1 mile and look for singletrack climbing from the road on the left (west) side. After a brief climb, the trail begins to descend. Turn right (west) onto the trail in the drainage and continue your descent.

Continuing northwest, the trail follows the valley through thick manzanita and other vegetation crowding the passage. Descend steadily until the AZT climbs gradually out of the drainage to the right (north). Undulations through side washes lead to a 0.2-mile climb. During the steep descent that ensues, the trail becomes a primitive doubletrack. Follow this track due west along the crest of a ridge for the next 1.3 miles. Pass a junction with FR 1451 on your left, but continue straight west.

In 1 mile, you reach the junction of a second doubletrack (FR 1452), which crosses this east–west ridge from north to south. Turn left (south) to follow this doubletrack, which drops steeply to the valley floor of Boulder Creek. Before reaching Boulder Creek, the road levels where a carsonite post marks the return of the AZT to singletrack. Watch on your right (west) for the carsonite where the AZT leads directly west.

The trail begins a long, gradual westward climb to cross a saddle. Continue west as the trail gradually drops into the valley of Sycamore Creek and reaches the stream crossing. A cairn and carsonite sign mark the trail access to the crossing on each side of the floodplain. Look directly west for a cairn that marks a short, steep ramp leading up and out of the streambed. Water usually flows in Sycamore Creek at low levels during normal precipitation years.

After a climb south out of Sycamore Creek, the trail levels out and begins following a midslope contour as it parallels the valley formed by Sycamore Creek. There are many good campsites along Sycamore Creek below. After further descending and

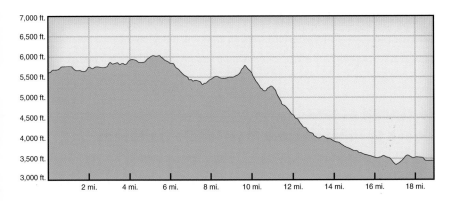

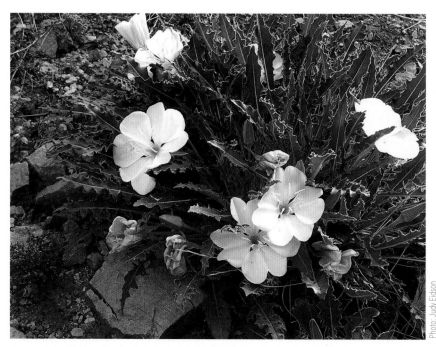

Photo: Judy Eidson

Opening in the evening and closing shortly after dawn, the flowers of evening primrose (*Oenothera caespitosa*) emit a delicious fragrance.

crossing Sycamore Creek, the trail works its way west. Follow the trail to a large AZT trailhead sign. At this point, the AZT continues west to Passage 22, or look to your right for a wire gate leading to the Sunflower Trail.

Mountain Bike Notes

Most of this passage is possible on a bike, but only about 20 percent of the Boulder Creek Trail is passable. The other 80 percent of that stretch resembles a bowling alley filled with cobbles of all shapes and sizes. In addition, note that the final 0.8 mile of this passage is not passable by bike. *For more information about mountain biking along the Arizona National Scenic Trail, visit* **aztrail.org.**

SOUTHERN ACCESS:
Pigeon Spring and Lone Pine Saddle Trailheads

From the suspension bridge near Roosevelt Dam, drive north on AZ 188 for 11 miles, and turn left (west) at mile marker 255 onto El Oso Road (FR 143). At 4.4 miles from the highway, the road appears to fork. Take the sharp right turn and follow the road as it climbs. Continue another 4.2 miles to an intersection with FR 422. FR 143 continues on to the south, which is also the path of the Arizona National Scenic Trail (AZT). The AZT arrives from the left (southeast) on FR 143. Drive 1 mile on FR 143 to an intersection, bear left onto FR 648, and continue almost another mile to Pigeon Spring Trailhead on the left.

To reach a larger, more developed parking area and trailhead at Lone Pine Saddle a bit farther on, continue 0.5 mile on FR 648. Parking here allows you to hike on single-track into the Four Peaks Wilderness and meet the AZT in about 2 miles.

NORTHERN ACCESS: Sunflower

If you want to hit the trail from here, please follow the trail description in reverse order. Take AZ 87 north to FR 22 (Bushnell Tanks Road). Park along the road just before the massive gate. Walk south on FR 22 about 0.5 mile until just after it turns left; watch for the trail descending to the right. (If you reach the cattle guard, you've gone too far.)

Turn right again at the bottom of the bank along the road and follow the drainage and carsonite signs about 300 yards to a grove of large sycamore trees along Syca-more Creek. This creek floods and changes course frequently; the trail may be obscure through the grove. Cross Sycamore Creek and take the short spur trail about 200 yards to the AZT. A large AZT sign marks the junction. Follow the trail west (right) of the sign through a tunnel under AZ 87 to hike north on the Sunflower Trail.

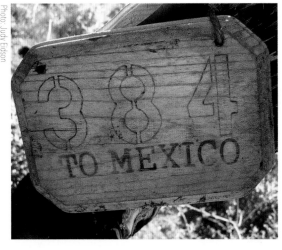

Photo: Judy Eidson

Mileage markers are found intermittently along the AZT.

Saddle Mountain

KEY INFO

LOCATION Sunflower to Mount Peeley

DISTANCE 16 miles one-way

DAY-TRIP OPTION See turnaround note in the trail description.

SHUTTLE RECOMMENDATIONS Cross F and Mormon Grove Trailheads

DIFFICULTY Strenuous

LAND MANAGER Tonto National Forest, Mesa Ranger District, **www.fs.usda.gov/tonto,** 480-610-3300,

RECOMMENDED MONTHS March–November

GATEWAY COMMUNITY Not applicable

GEOLOGY HIGHLIGHTS See "Amazing Mazatzals" (page 342).

OVERVIEW

This inconspicuous passage traverses some of the most beautiful places on the entire Arizona National Scenic Trail (AZT) and offers a stunning variety of landscapes over a relatively short distance. You're unlikely to see many people on the trail, and even fewer now that the Sunflower Fire of 2012 incinerated a large portion of the landscape.

This passage begins a long stint in the Mazatzal Wilderness, which continues through Passage 25. This diverse range is marked by serpentine canyons and craggy

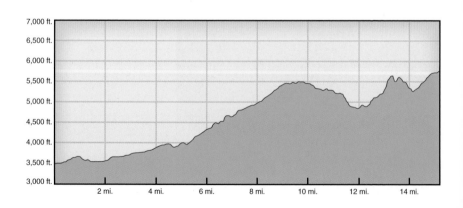

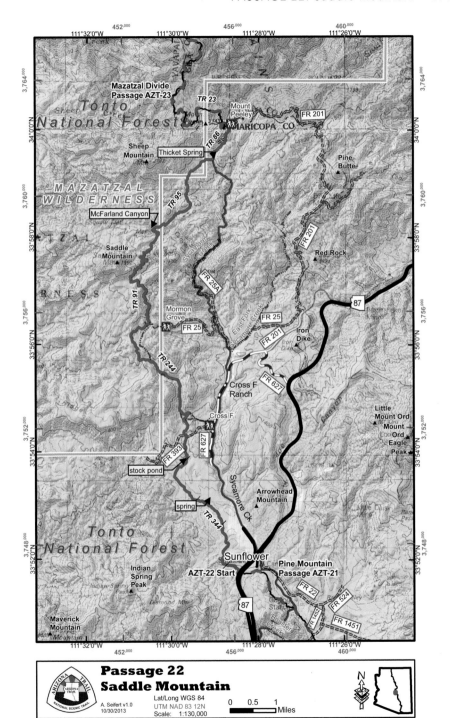

**Passage 22
Saddle Mountain**

A. Seifert v1.0
10/30/2013

Lat/Long WGS 84
UTM NAD 83 12N
Scale: 1:130,000

0   0.5   1
Miles

N

peaks, a perennial river farther ahead, and surreal high desert. Bring protective clothing and keep it accessible, as Arizona's formidable flora often crowds the trail.

ON THE TRAIL

From the sycamore grove under AZ 87 and the turnoff for Bushnell Tanks, follow the access trail about 0.25 mile to the AZT trailhead sign. Turn right (west) onto the AZT, where a carsonite post marks the trail about 30 yards away. The trail soon crosses an abandoned road; look for cairns on the opposite side and continue west. At this point, a tunnel under AZ 87 becomes visible. Follow the trail through the tunnel and pass through a wire gate on the west side of the highway. Specifically designed for the AZT, this tunnel is tall and wide enough to accommodate equestrians.

Continue west from the tunnel along the fence line for about 50 yards to where a cairn marks a right-hand (north) turn. A carsonite post marks the singletrack that soon climbs over a small ridge to the north. The trail veers left (northwest) to drop into a small wash. Pass through a gate and follow cairns west along a somewhat fainter trail. Stay off the dirt road on your right and follow Trail 344, a faint remnant of a doubletrack. Pass through another gate to the south side of the fence, and you are soon on a very clear singletrack. Crest a small hill and cross a wash on the other side. Cattle trails create multiple forks here, but the large cairns will keep you on the right path.

In 0.4 mile, pass through another gate and look due north for carsonite posts marking a clear doubletrack. The AZT follows a left (west) fork in the road. The right fork leads about 80 yards to a spring that seems to be reliable—to find the spring, make a 90-degree turn to the right when you reach a fence.

Take the right (north) fork and stay on Trail 344. Follow the faint singletrack that breaks off to the left (north) of the road, as signs indicate. Soon, you pass through yet another gate and a stock pond. Cairns guide you north-northwest; under power lines at the northern edge of the grassy field, the trail crosses FR 393.

Continue north through scrub oak, and more cairns, as the trail crosses a streambed in a charming valley under idyllic white cliffs. Near the 5-mile point, the trail intersects the Cross F Access Trail, which connects to the Cross F Trailhead.

TURNAROUND NOTE: This is an ideal spot for turning around if you're just out for the day.

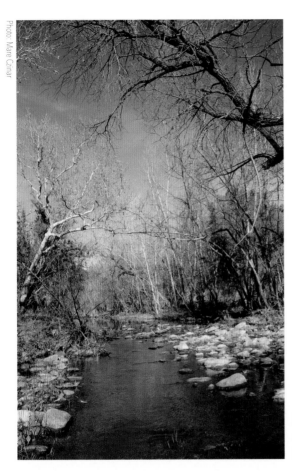

Sycamore Creek is a pleasant riparian corridor that parallels Passage 22.

To continue on the trail, take the left fork to wind north-northwest, following Little Saddle Mountain Trail (Trail 244). Pass through a gate and climb northward along a canyon that leads into the stunning Mazatzal Wilderness. After it climbs to the ridge above the canyon, the trail eventually intersects with the Mormon Grove Access Trail (near an abandoned corral) and becomes the Saddle Mountain Trail (Trail 91). The AZT continues on Trail 91, which is an old mining roadbed converted to singletrack, and passes through a flat saddle called the Potato Patch. Just beyond and to the northwest of the trail stands Saddle Mountain, at 6,535 feet.

Hiking on past Saddle Mountain, you pass the intersection with the trail to Story Mine; for the next mile or so brush tends to encroach on the trail from McFarland Canyon, which sometimes has water flowing or a few standing pools. After crossing

McFarland Canyon, the route becomes Trail 95 as it climbs up to Thicket Spring and the intersection with Cornucopia Trail (Trail 86), a great spot to take a break. From here it's a rather long and rocky climb on abandoned doubletrack, leading to the junction with the Mazatzal Divide Trail (Trail 23) and the end of the passage. To reach the Mount Peeley Trailhead, continue straight for 0.5 mile on the Cornucopia Trail.

Mountain Bike Notes

Most of this passage is in the Mazatzal Wilderness, where bikes are prohibited. *For detailed information about scenic mountain biking routes around wilderness areas, visit* **aztrail.org.**

SOUTHERN ACCESS: Sunflower

Take AZ 87 north to FR 22 (Bushnell Tanks Road) near milepost 218. Park along the road just before the massive gate. Walk south on FR 22 about 0.5 mile until just after

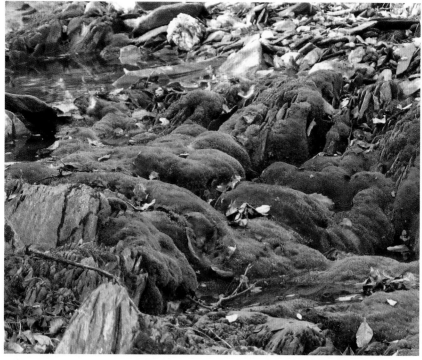

Photo: Robert Luce

The numerous springs, seeps, and creeks of the Mazatzal Mountains are a welcome contrast to the dry desert passages of the south.

it turns left; watch for the trail descending to the right. (If you reach the cattle guard, you've gone too far.) Turn right again at the bottom of the bank along the road, and follow the drainage and carsonite signs about 300 yards to a grove of large sycamore trees along Sycamore Creek. This creek floods and changes course frequently; the trail may be obscured through the grove. Cross Sycamore Creek and take the short spur trail about 200 yards to the AZT. A large AZT sign marks the junction. Follow the trail right (west) of the sign through a tunnel under AZ 87, and hike north on the Sunflower Trail.

ALTERNATE ACCESS: Mormon Grove Trailhead

Drive 4.8 miles north of the historic townsite of Sunflower and the turnoff for Bushnell Tanks on AZ 87 to mile marker 222.8. Turn left (west) onto a paved road (FR 627), opposite the Mount Ord turnoff. Follow FR 627 downhill 1.2 miles and then turn right, over a cattle guard, onto FR 201. The sign is visible after you make the turn. Follow FR 201 for 1.2 miles and turn left (west) onto FR 25. Continue on FR 25 for 4.7 miles to a corral and parking area. Hike up the access road, past the wilderness signage, for 0.5 mile to intersect the AZT and Saddle Mountain Trail (Trail 91).

ALTERNATE ACCESS: Cross F Trailhead

Drive 4.8 miles north of Sunflower on AZ 87 to mile marker 222.8. Turn left (west) onto paved FR 627, opposite the Mount Ord turnoff. Follow FR 627 downhill 3.4 miles to the signed trailhead, on your left. The access is on the opposite side of the paved road. Hike 0.7 mile to intersect the AZT and Saddle Mountain Trail.

NORTHERN ACCESS: Mount Peeley Trailhead

If you want to hit the trail from here, please follow the trail description in reverse order. Drive 4.8 miles north of Sunflower on AZ 87 to mile marker 222.8. Turn left (west) onto paved FR 627, opposite the Mount Ord turnoff. Follow FR 627 downhill 1.2 miles and then turn right, over a cattle guard, onto FR 201. Drive 9.3 miles on FR 201 to the Mount Peeley Trailhead, where you'll find a small parking area. The sign here says CORNUCOPIA TRAIL (TRAIL 86) and indicates a 0.5-mile hike to the Mazatzal Divide Trail (Trail 23) and AZT.

Mazatzal Divide

LOCATION Mount Peeley to The Park

DISTANCE 22.3 miles one-way

DAY-TRIP OPTION See turnaround note in the trail description.

SHUTTLE RECOMMENDATION Not applicable

DIFFICULTY Strenuous

LAND MANAGER Tonto National Forest, Payson Ranger District, **www.fs.usda.gov/tonto,** 928-474-7936

RECOMMENDED MONTHS March–November

GATEWAY COMMUNITY See Payson (page 325).

GEOLOGY HIGHLIGHTS See "Amazing Mazatzals" (page 342).

OVERVIEW

Before the Willow and Sunflower Fires severely ravaged this passage in 2004 and 2012, respectively, this route was considered one of the most beautiful segments of the Arizona National Scenic Trail (AZT). It traverses to near the top of the Mazatzal Mountains, including Mazatzal Peak, whose impressive west face towers 1,700 feet above the trail. The cool, thin air encourages the growth of beautiful trees, especially stands of ponderosa pines that are hundreds of years old. The fire was brutal, but some of these

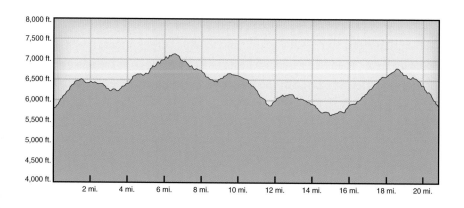

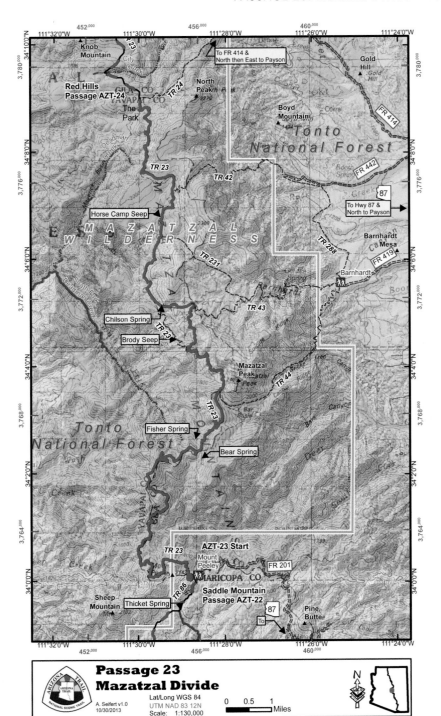

To FR 414 &
North then East to Payson

Gold
Hill

Knob
Mountain

Red Hills
Passage AZT-24

The
Park

TR 24

North
Peak

Boyd
Mountain

*Tonto
National Forest*

FR 414

TR 23

TR 42

FR 442

87

Horse Camp Seep

*M A Z A T Z A L
W I L D E R N E S S*

To Hwy 87 &
North to Payson

TR 288

Barnhardt
Mesa

TR 231

FR 419

Barnhardt

Chilson Spring

TR 23

TR 43

Brody Seep

Mazatzal
Peak

TR 44

TR 23

Fisher Spring

*Tonto
National Forest*

Bear Spring

TR 23

AZT-23 Start

Mount
Peeley

FR 201

TR 23

MARICOPA CO

TR 86

Saddle Mountain
Passage AZT-22

Sheep
Mountain

Thicket Spring

87

To

Pine
Butte

111°32'0"W   111°30'0"W   111°28'0"W   111°26'0"W   111°24'0"W

**Passage 23
Mazatzal Divide**

A. Seifert v1.0
10/30/2013

Lat/Long WGS 84
UTM NAD 83 12N
Scale: 1:130,000

0   0.5   1
Miles

N

ancient treasures remain. Farther north on the passage, red-rock canyons reflect sunset colors that would be difficult for any artist to recreate. This is the middle of the AZT's longest sojourn in a designated wilderness area, and you can feel it! Humans are infrequent visitors to these lonely ridges, and the land is much the same as it was hundreds of years ago when it was the domain of the Yavapai and Apache peoples.

Late spring is an ideal time to hike here, although summer temperatures are generally not unbearable. Snow is very likely in the winter months, making most of the Mazatzal Mountains impassable. Campsites are rare because of the precipitous terrain, but there are some nice spots at the following locations: mile 6.7, mile 9.4, mile 19.4, and mile 22.

ON THE TRAIL

From the parking area, hike 0.5 mile up the Cornucopia Trail (Trail 86) to reach the AZT. The Mazatzal Divide Trail (Trail 23) begins here with a steep climb up a number of switchbacks that may seem endless as the trail climbs the east side of Mount Peeley. The trail then levels off after 1.5 miles as it bends west to pass under the north slopes of the mountain as you enter the Mazatzal Wilderness. The views from here are incredible.

After 4.2 miles, the trail skirts very deep canyons across steep slopes. A saddle offers a rare place to camp, near the higher reaches of this long ridge, but no water. This elevated perch provides some awesome views to the west.

TURNAROUND NOTE: Day-hikers would be wise to turn around here—the next descent isn't something you'd want to hike back up.

The trail now descends sharp switchbacks, and Mazatzal Peak's intimidating west face dominates the immediate horizon. A second broad saddle, adorned with peaceful stands of ponderosa pines, provides another nice place to camp. In the next 0.1 mile, signs indicate two springs a short distance off the trail. Bear Spring is fairly reliable.

After 10.5 miles from the Mount Peeley Trailhead, the trail begins to switchback through the remains of old-growth ponderosa pine, alligator juniper, and scrub oak as it reaches a saddle, 0.5 mile farther, and crosses to the east side of the divide as it continues on singletrack trending north-northeast over gentle terrain. At the intersection with the Y Bar Trail (Trail 44), turn left (north) to stay on the Mazatzal Divide Trail (Trail 23). After passing under the steep cliffs of Mazatzal Peak, the trail climbs through some thick manzanita, making protective clothing helpful. Signs along the next 8 miles

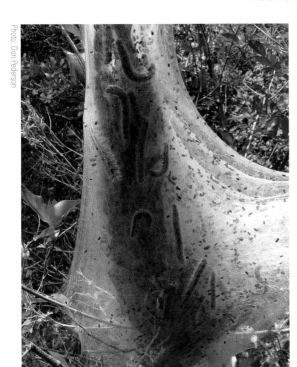

Photo: Dori Pederson

Bagworms spin their silk around trees and shrubs in the Mazatzal Mountains in preparation for their metamorphosis into moths.

may indicate turnoffs to several springs and seeps, such as Brody Seep, Chilson Spring, and Horse Camp Seep (a popular campsite); however, they may or may not have water. Conditions change rapidly, so always check with the ATA water-resource guide (**aztrail .org/watersources.html**). Usually the last person hiking through the area can provide the most accurate information, which makes hiking blogs very helpful.

Continuing on this stretch, you will notice numerous places with spectacular views as well as a couple of turnoffs, including Barnhardt Trail (Trail 43), Sandy Saddle Trail (Trail 231), and Rock Creek Trail (Trail 42). Hopi Spring is the turnoff for the Rock Creek Trailhead, but the Willow Fire mostly destroyed the spring—it even burned the spring box and piping. Approximately 1 mile past Hopi Spring, cairns guide you through a rocky section, with a high, rocky point offering expansive views of the valleys to the west and the low country along the East Verde River to the north-northwest. On a clear day, you can see the snowcapped San Francisco Peaks about 75 miles to the north.

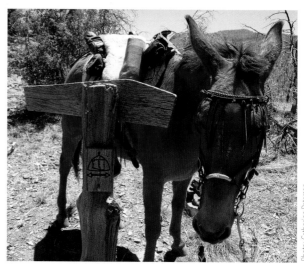

A mule finds an inconspicuous wooden AZT marker along Passage 23.

Photo: Catherine Peterson

From this point, turn right (northeast), walk about 50 yards, and follow a switch-back that descends to the left (south) underneath the rocky escarpment. Another switchback soon heads back to the north with a long, gradual descent leading to a T-intersection with the Willow Spring Trail (Trail 223). Turn right (north-northeast), as the signs indicate, and in 0.1 mile, watch for cairns marking the trail's crossing of a rocky streambed. Soon you'll arrive at a natural open area called The Park, marking the end of Passage 23. At this location, the North Peak Trail (Trail 24) breaks off to the northeast (right) and proceeds down to the Mineral Creek Trailhead. The AZT continues straight ahead (north) on the Red Rock Passage down to the East Verde River.

Mountain Bike Notes

Bikes are prohibited on this passage, which lies entirely within the Mazatzal Wilderness. *For detailed information about scenic mountain biking routes around wilderness areas, visit* **aztrail.org.**

SOUTHERN ACCESS: Mount Peeley Trailhead

Drive 4.8 miles north of Sunflower on AZ 87 to mile marker 222.8. Turn left (west) onto paved FR 627, opposite the Mount Ord turnoff. Follow FR 627 downhill 1.2 miles and then turn right, over a cattle guard, onto FR 201. Drive 9.3 miles on FR 201 to the Mount Peeley Trailhead, where you'll find a small parking area. The sign here says

CORNUCOPIA TRAIL (TRAIL 86) and indicates a 0.5-mile hike to the Mazatzal Divide Trail (Trail 23) and AZT.

ALTERNATE ACCESS: Barnhardt Trailhead

Take AZ 87 to mile marker 238.4 (about 11 miles south of Payson). Turn west onto FR 419 and drive almost 6 miles to the Barnhardt Trailhead. Then hike up the Barnhardt Trail (Trail 43) for 5.9 miles to the junction with the AZT and Mazatzal Divide Trail (Trail 23).

NORTHERN ACCESS: The Park

If you want to hit the trail from here, please follow the trail description in reverse order. From Payson on AZ 87 drive west on Main Street. Stay on the main road past a golf course, where the pavement ends and the road becomes FR 406. About 5.2 miles from AZ 87, turn left on FR 414 and continue another 5.2 miles. Turn right and continue 0.2 mile to a three-way fork in the road. Turn left and go about 100 feet to Mineral Creek Trailhead. Hike along the North Peak Trail for 4 miles to reach the AZT.

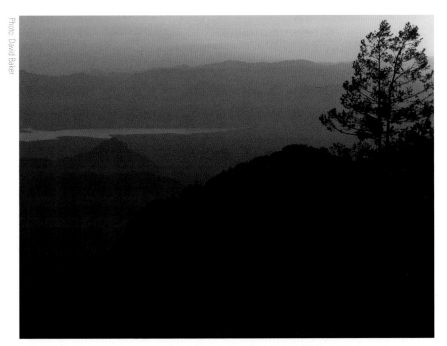

Sunset over Horseshoe Reservoir from deep within the Mazatzal Wilderness

Red Hills

KEY INFO

LOCATION The Park to East Verde River

DISTANCE 14 miles one-way

DAY-TRIP OPTION See turnaround note in the trail description.

SHUTTLE RECOMMENDATION Not applicable

DIFFICULTY Moderate

LAND MANAGER Tonto National Forest, Payson Ranger District, **www.fs.usda.gov/tonto,** 928-474-7936

RECOMMENDED MONTHS March–November

GATEWAY COMMUNITY See Payson (page 325).

GEOLOGY HIGHLIGHTS See "Amazing Mazatzals" (page 342).

OVERVIEW

The longest stretch of the Arizona National Scenic Trail (AZT) that is entirely within designated wilderness areas continues as the trail bends even deeper into this pristine, remote landscape. Thru-hikers will lose much of the elevation they gained over the previous few passages as the trail drops into the valley of the East Verde River. The elevation ranges from 6,284 feet on Knob Mountain to 3,277 feet at the passage's terminus near the river.

This elevation change offers the opportunity to see a variety of Arizona's biotic communities, from majestic stands of ponderosa pines to a lush riparian zone whose

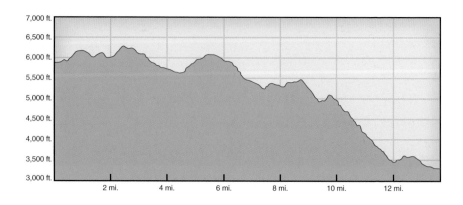

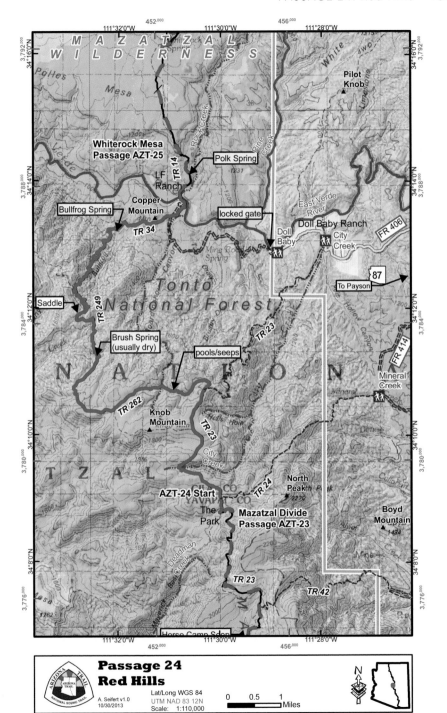

**Passage 24
Red Hills**

A. Seifert v1.0
10/30/2013

Lat/Long WGS 84
UTM NAD 83 12N
Scale: 1:110,000

0   0.5   1
Miles

N

denizens include turtles and rare birds. Because the flora is so thick in places that it obscures the trail, you'll want to wear protective clothing.

ON THE TRAIL

Starting from The Park at the junction with the North Peak Trail (Trail 24), head north on the Mazatzal Divide Trail (Trail 23), the route of the AZT. You soon bend northwest and climb to 6,170 feet, descend to cross two tributary canyons of City Creek, and then turn back to the northeast and climb again. From a high point on indistinct Knob Mountain (6,284 feet), you can look northeast for a clear view of the Mogollon Rim, the geographical dividing line between Arizona's lower-elevation southern half and the cooler, higher elevations to the north. Thru-hikers will climb onto the rim within a few days.

Soon you will reach an important trail intersection—where the AZT departs from the Mazatzal Divide Trail (Trail 23). The AZT goes left (west) on a combination of trails: Red Hills Trail (Trail 262), Brush Trail (Trail 249), and Bull Spring Trail (Trail 34). And the Mazatzal Divide Trail (Trail 23) makes a hard right turn and heads northeast down to the City Creek Trailhead. Continuing on the AZT and a few quick switchbacks, the trail turns left at a cairn-marked junction, descends to the west along a small drainage, and passes through an idyllic pine forest. In springtime, water is often present here. In a confluence of drainages, follow large cairns as the trail turns left, makes a few steep climbs to the southwest, and then levels just before a trail intersection.

TURNAROUND NOTE: Day-hikers should consider this their turnaround spot (5.5 miles from the start of the passage).

To continue, stay right (west) onto the Brush Trail. As the trail descends to the west and northwest, it then turns northeast along a drainage with nice views of the East Verde River Valley. The trail drops sharply on a rocky, red path. Thick vegetation occasionally obscures the trail, but cairns show the way.

The trail reaches a sign for the usually dry Brush Spring, which is about 50 yards to the northwest. There is a slightly overused place to camp here, the last site for 5 miles. From this sign, the trail bends right (east) to go upstream along an adjoining drainage. In 0.1 mile, the AZT climbs northwest out of the drainage and follows switchbacks along a swath cut through thick vegetation to reach the top of a steep hill.

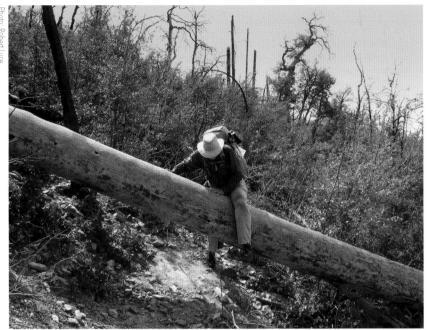

Downed trees present one of the greatest challenges along many of the AZT's mountain passages.

A brief descent leads through heavy brush as it crosses a fence in a saddle and climbs north 0.1 mile to an important but obscure trail junction. Make a sharp left (southwest) and climb a bit more. After wrapping around to the right, you top out in a saddle before beginning a steep descent, from which you can see the East Verde River in the valley bottom. You're now on the grounds of the historic LF Ranch, an active ranch with hiker-friendly facilities, including a bunkhouse and shower.

To exit the wilderness and AZT for the nearest road access, take the road 3.8 miles to the east to the Doll Baby Trailhead. If you're a long-distance trail traveler and you plan to continue along the AZT, head northeast on this road, walk 70 yards, and look for a sign on the right indicating the next passage of the AZT. The East Verde River awaits you and your water bottles.

Mountain Bike Notes

Bikes are prohibited on this passage, which lies entirely within the Mazatzal Wilderness. *For detailed information about scenic mountain biking routes around wilderness areas, visit* **aztrail.org.**

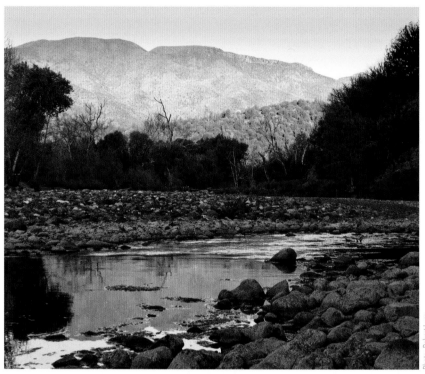

A highlight of Passage 24, the East Verde River is one of only four rivers that the AZT crosses between Mexico and Utah.

SOUTHERN ACCESS: The Park

Note: The Park is at the junction of Mazatzal Divide Trail (Trail 23) and North Peak Trail (Trail 24) via Mineral Creek Trailhead. From Payson on AZ 87 drive west on Main Street. Stay on the main road past a golf course, where the pavement ends and the road becomes FR 406. About 5.2 miles from AZ 87, turn left on FR 414 and continue another 5.2 miles. Turn right and continue 0.2 mile to a three-way fork in the road. Turn left and go about 100 feet to Mineral Creek Trailhead. Hike along the North Peak Trail for 4 miles to reach the AZT with 2,500 feet of elevation gain to reach The Park.

NORTHERN ACCESS:
East Verde River (LF Ranch) via Doll Baby Trailhead

If you want to hit the trail from here, please follow the trail description in reverse order. From the town of Payson, at the intersection of AZ 87 and Main Street, take Main

Street west for 2 miles, which turns into Country Club Drive. Near the end of Country Club Drive, the road passes a sanitation plant, crosses a creek, and continues another 6 miles on a newly paved road, referred to as Doll Baby Ranch Road or LF Ranch Road depending on which map you're using. At this point the road becomes a dirt double-track (FR 406). Continue on FR 406 for approximately 3 miles, passing the City Creek Trailhead and Doll Baby Ranch, eventually arriving at the locked gate that marks the Doll Baby Trailhead, where parking and camping are allowed. From the trailhead, walk around the gate and hike on the doubletrack for 3.9 miles. The road winds around the hills and eventually levels out in the valley near the ranch. The AZT intersects the road from the west as a faint singletrack.

PASSAGE 25

Whiterock Mesa

KEY INFO

LOCATION East Verde River to Twin Buttes

DISTANCE 11.4 miles one-way

DAY-TRIP OPTION See turnaround note in the trail description.

SHUTTLE RECOMMENDATIONS Southern and northern access points

DIFFICULTY Easy

LAND MANAGER Tonto National Forest, Payson Ranger District, **www.fs.usda.gov/tonto,** 928-474-7936

RECOMMENDED MONTHS September–April

GATEWAY COMMUNITY See Payson (page 325).

GEOLOGY HIGHLIGHTS Not applicable

OVERVIEW

This passage makes a consistent, gradual climb from the East Verde River Valley through high desert terrain characterized by juniper and piñon pine. The climb is constant: you will gain 2,661 feet while losing only 87 feet over the next 11.4 miles. Keep an eye out for animals that inhabit this ecosystem, including javelina and wild turkeys.

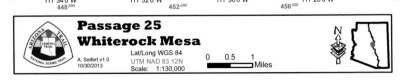

Passage 25
Whiterock Mesa

ARIZONA TRAIL
NATIONAL SCENIC TRAIL

A. Seifert v1.0
10/30/2013

Lat/Long WGS 84
UTM NAD 83 12N
Scale: 1:130,000

0   0.5   1
Miles

N

Because the climb away from the East Verde River to the top of the mesa is so rocky, it's wise to camp near the river. There is also a nice campsite in a drainage between Whiterock Mesa and Saddle Ridge. From there, the terrain is incredibly rocky again until near the end of the passage.

ON THE TRAIL

From the junction of the doubletrack coming from the Doll Baby Trailhead and the AZT singletrack, follow the road northeast 70 yards to a sign on the right with an AZT marker. This sign also indicates Polk Spring and Whiterock Spring. Leave the road here and follow a singletrack east on an old roadbed. Use cairns to follow the old roadbed through a bend to the left (northeast) and pass through a gate. In another 0.2 mile, avoid a singletrack cutting off toward the ranch to the left (northwest), continue about 10 yards to a rocky streambed on the left (due north), and follow it. If you miss this turn and continue straight ahead, you'll run into the river within about 100 yards, and you'll know you've gone too far.

Immediately after you cross through another drainage, the trail bends left (north-west) to parallel the river, which is 40 yards to the right. In less than 0.25 mile, several large cairns lead out of the right side of the drainage and over to the bank of the East Verde River. As you pass by a painted wooden sign for the ranch (which may be missing), look across the river for a trail climbing the opposite bank, just downstream from a solid-rock streambed where spring water flows into the river. The water depth varies depending on the season and recent weather—wade across at your own risk. Climb the bank on the north side of the river, pass through a fence, and follow the trail as it climbs to the north-northeast.

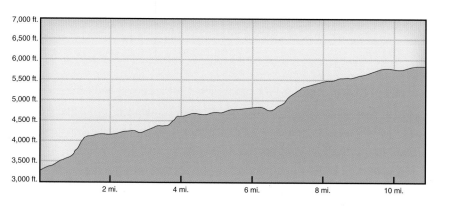

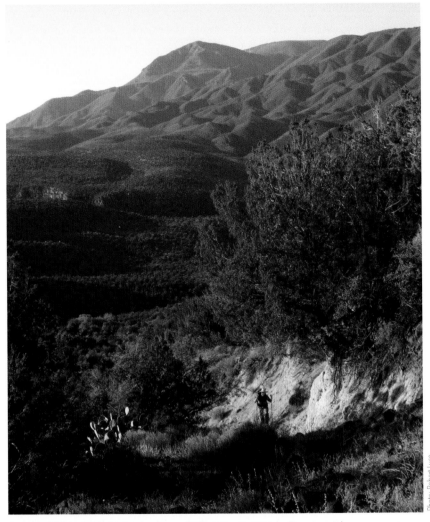

Photo: Robert Luce

Passage 25 is notable for its steady ascent from the East Verde River toward the Mogollon Rim.

Soon you'll find a sign for Polk Spring, about 30 yards away and behind a gigantic tree. If you walk a couple hundred yards southeast from here, you'll find an open meadow (the last one for at least 3 miles) that provides good camping. Just make sure to camp at least 200 feet away from the water.

From the sign for the spring, follow a singletrack to the left (northwest). This faint trail soon becomes much clearer—if you get confused, head for the high, rocky butte to the northwest. A very rocky road leads to and ascends Polles Mesa. The grade steepens considerably as the AZT climbs through loose volcanic rock and then flattens on the mesa. The trail virtually disappears here; bear north-northeast and look for the occasional cairn. They are there, often just below the high vegetation. The ground is so rocky that it would be difficult to find a place to camp.

The trail passes by the west side of Red Saddle Tank, which is usually dry. Cairns mark the trail as you continue north. In 1 mile, pass through a gate, and take a 90-degree turn to the right (east) in 0.1 mile at the base of Whiterock Mesa. At Whiterock Spring, the AZT makes a sharp turn to the left (northwest) for a brief, steep climb onto the aptly named Whiterock Mesa.

TURNAROUND NOTE: Day-trippers will enjoy this turnaround spot, which affords incredible views, a reliable water source, and moderate distance (3.8 miles from the beginning of the passage).

As you slowly gain elevation, a few pine trees start to make an appearance. Climb along the mesa to where the trail descends briefly to a drainage (usually dry) between Whiterock Mesa and Saddle Ridge. There is a nice place to camp here. The climbing resumes on the rocky trail as you make your way up Saddle Ridge, a spit of land above Rock Creek on the east and The Gorge on the west. Soon you leave the Mazatzal Wilderness, and cairns lead to a crossing of two fences. From here, you enter Saddle Ridge Pasture, a broad expanse sparsely covered with small trees.

The trail passes just to the right (east) of Saddle Ridge Pasture Tank. Finally, the trail reaches FR 194 at a T-intersection, the end of Passage 25.

Mountain Bike Notes

Bikes are prohibited on this passage, which lies entirely within the Mazatzal Wilderness. *For detailed information about scenic mountain biking routes around wilderness areas, visit* **aztrail.org.**

SOUTHERN ACCESS:
East Verde River (LF Ranch) via Doll Baby Trailhead

From the town of Payson, at the intersection of AZ 87 and Main Street, take Main Street west for 2 miles, which turns into Country Club Drive. Near the end of Country Club Drive, the road passes a sanitation plant, crosses a creek, and continues another

6 miles on a newly paved road, referred to as Doll Baby Ranch Road or LF Ranch Road depending on which map you are using.

At this point the road becomes a dirt doubletrack (FR 406). Continue on FR 406 for approximately 3 miles, passing the City Creek Trailhead and Doll Baby Ranch, eventually arriving at a locked gate that marks the Doll Baby Trailhead, where parking and camping are allowed.

From the trailhead, walk around the gate and hike on the doubletrack for 3.9 miles. The road winds around the hills and eventually levels out in the valley near the ranch. The AZT intersects the road from the west as a faint singletrack.

NORTHERN ACCESS: Twin Buttes (FR 194)

If you want to hit the trail from here, please follow the trail description in reverse order. From AZ 87, turn west into the town of Strawberry and continue west on Fossil Creek Road for 2.8 miles. Turn left (south) onto FR 428, continue for almost 1 mile, and then turn right onto FR 194. Follow FR 194 for 4.2 miles. AZT markers indicate the end of Passage 25 and the beginning of Hardscrabble Mesa, Passage 26.

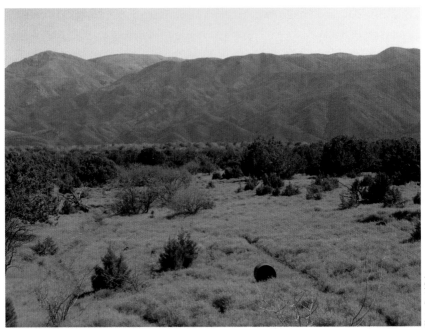

Photo: David Baker

Diversity defines the AZT experience. As the elevation changes, so do the biotic communities along the trail.

Hardscrabble Mesa

LOCATION Twin Buttes to Pine Trailhead

DISTANCE 12 miles one-way

DAY-TRIP OPTION See turnaround note in the trail description.

SHUTTLE RECOMMENDATIONS Southern and northern access points

DIFFICULTY Moderate

LAND MANAGER Tonto National Forest, Payson Ranger District, **www.fs.usda.gov/tonto,** 928-474-7936

RECOMMENDED MONTHS March–October

GATEWAY COMMUNITIES See Payson (page 325) and Pine and Strawberry (page 326).

GEOLOGY HIGHLIGHTS Not applicable

OVERVIEW

This passage uses existing roads and trails to travel from the north end of the Mazatzal Wilderness to the Pine Trailhead on AZ 87. Its relatively short length and trails provide a nice setting for a long day hike or a quick overnighter. Although this passage is entirely outside of designated wilderness, portions of it feel quite remote, and the lush zone through Oak Spring Canyon is beautiful. Trail users also enjoy frequent views of the Mogollon Rim, the massive and colorful escarpment that rises 1,500 feet above the Pine Valley.

ON THE TRAIL

From the AZT's intersection with FR 194, walk northeast on the road. (If you just drove to this trailhead from Strawberry, you'll be backtracking.) Walk 1.2 miles and turn right (southeast) to follow a faint rock-laden roadbed along a power line, as indicated by a brown carsonite post.

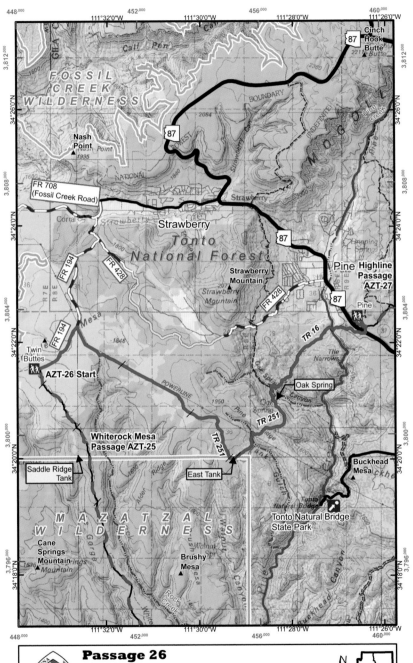

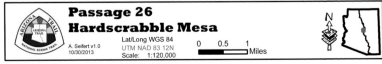

Passage 26
Hardscrabble Mesa

A. Seifert v1.0
10/30/2013

Lat/Long WGS 84
UTM NAD 83 12N
Scale: 1:120,000

0   0.5   1
Miles

N

Photo: Fred Gaudet

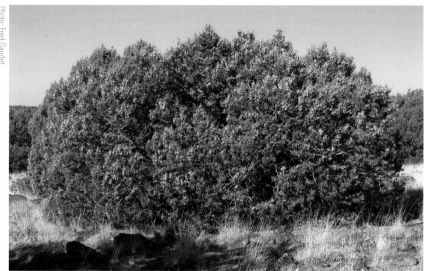

One-seeded junipers (*Juniperus monosperma*) dominate the landscape across Hardscrabble Mesa, and their sweet, pungent odor fills the air after each rainstorm.

The power-line trail crosses the headwaters of Rock Creek, where you might find a moderate flow of water. A calm grove of ponderosa pines makes for an inviting campsite. After 3 miles the trail veers a bit right (south) of the power-line corridor. In another 0.5 mile, avoid a dirt road that forks right (south-southwest); instead continue straight (southeast) for 50 yards to pass through a gate as you climb into a pleasant oak, juniper, and ponderosa forest.

Watch carefully where the road forks when you reach another power line. Follow carsonite posts onto the right (southeast) fork and continue on Trail 251. The road

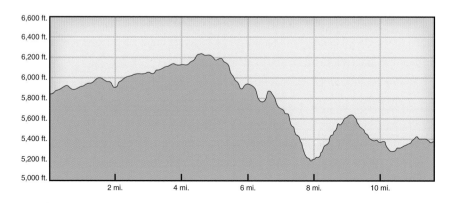

descends to the south and southeast for the next mile. Swing left (northeast) to pass East Tank. As you continue from this tank, look east-northeast for views of the flat top of the Mogollon Rim.

The road passes back under the power line and then dips into the drainage of Tank Gulch. Then it climbs steeply up a rocky roadbed to the southeast for 0.1 mile and then descends for another 0.1 mile. At this point, look on the left side of the road for cairns that mark a very faint singletrack trail descending to the northeast. Where signs indicate Trail 251 (which is the AZT), turn onto it and follow cairns through rocky terrain. The faint trail descends, occasionally steeply, with cairns marking most of the way, until you reach a sign for Oak Spring. The spring is a short distance behind the sign to the southeast—not on the canyon floor.

TURNAROUND NOTE: If you're day-hiking from the beginning of this passage and you haven't arranged a car shuttle, Oak Spring is a great spot to turn around and reverse your route.

Heading forward, the trail leaves Oak Spring to the north. Soon a sign indicates you're on Oak Spring Trail (Trail 16). Turn right (northeast), continue into Oak Spring Canyon, and reach the bottom of the canyon in 0.1 mile. Follow a steep climb, through many switchbacks, out of the canyon and into a pleasant forest of tall ponderosa pines. Pass by Bradshaw Tank and cross through the drainage below the tank, following cairns where the tread is obscure. Then pick up a clear singletrack continuing to the northeast.

When the trail meets Pine Creek (dry) at mile 10.9, turn right and walk downstream 100 yards, and then cross the creek to the east. Turn left (northeast) and follow a clear singletrack away from the creek. The trail soon curves to the right (east) and follows the south edge of a tributary of Pine Creek. The trail—now more of a road—bends to the right (south). In 0.1 mile, carsonite posts mark a left (east) turn off the road onto a singletrack.

Within earshot of AZ 87, pass through a gate, walk 70 yards, and cross the highway with care to pick up a clear trail on the other side. This trail descends from the highway and bends right (northeast). Within 100 yards, the trail turns back to the north to cross a stream marked by some cairns. Shortly after that, take the left (west-northwest) branch at a fork, and continue to the Pine Trailhead parking area and the end of Passage 26.

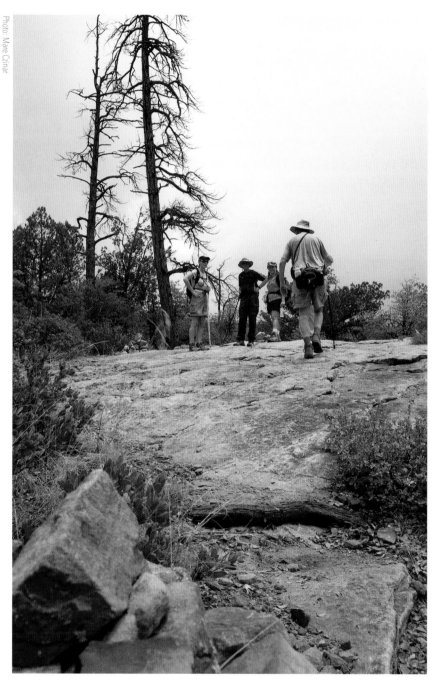

Photo: Mare Czinar

Starting from the Gateway Community of Pine, day-hikers can explore the dense forest of Passage 26.

Mountain Bike Notes

Most of this passage consists of intermediate riding over rocky terrain, with one very important exception. Only the most skilled riders will be able to negotiate the drop into and subsequent climb out of Oak Spring Canyon. This is a 2-mile stretch in the second half of the passage. Most riders will have to push their bikes through here. *For more information about mountain biking along the Arizona National Scenic Trail, visit* **aztrail.org.**

SOUTHERN ACCESS: Twin Buttes (FR 194)

From AZ 87, turn west into the town of Strawberry and continue west on Fossil Creek Road for 2.8 miles. Turn left (south) onto FR 428, continue for almost 1 mile, and then turn right onto FR 194. Follow FR 194 for 4.2 miles to AZT markers.

NORTHERN ACCESS: Pine Trailhead

If you want to hit the trail from here, please follow the trail description in reverse order. Drive south of Pine on AZ 87 for 0.6 mile, and turn left (east) to reach a large parking area and the trailhead.

PASSAGE 27

Highline

KEY INFO

LOCATION Pine Trailhead to Mogollon Rim

DISTANCE 19.3 miles one-way

DAY-TRIP OPTION Day-trippers could plan numerous loops and out-and-back options using forest trails and roads. Also see the turnaround note in the trail description.

SHUTTLE RECOMMENDATIONS Southern access point, Geronimo Trailhead (FR 440), and northern access point

DIFFICULTY Strenuous

LAND MANAGER Tonto National Forest, Payson Ranger District, **www.fs.usda.gov/tonto,** 928-474-7936

RECOMMENDED MONTHS March–November

GATEWAY COMMUNITIES See Pine and Strawberry (page 326).

GEOLOGY HIGHLIGHTS Not applicable

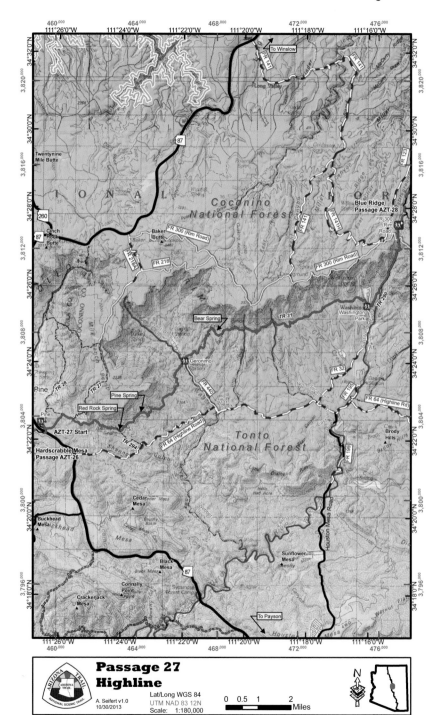

Passage 27
Highline

ARIZONA TRAIL
NATIONAL SCENIC TRAIL

A. Seifert v1.0
10/30/2013

Lat/Long WGS 84
UTM NAD 83 12N
Scale: 1:180,000

0   0.5   1   2
Miles

N

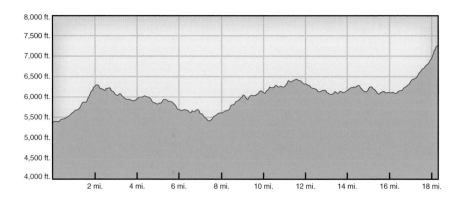

OVERVIEW

The first 17 miles of Passage 27 follows the Highline Trail, a National Recreation Trail that is visually stunning, historically significant, and brutally challenging. The AZT heads east from the Pine Trailhead, and once it reaches Washington Park Trailhead, it leaves the Highline Trail and makes a steep climb to the top of the magnificent Mogollon Rim. The Highline Trail dates back to the 19th century, when ranchers traveled back and forth on horseback to neighboring homesteads. The trail passes in and out of areas burned in the tragic 1990 Dude Fire, in which six firefighters died. It crosses numerous drainages and several springs as it traverses the steep sandstone slopes of the rim, with outstanding views to the south and great glimpses of the rim itself. There are many good locations for camping, and several creeks have flowing water most of the time, but they occasionally dry up. Its numerous access trails and evenly spaced trailheads (see Alternate Access, page 209) make this passage ideal for day-hiking.

As you leave the Pine Trailhead and make the mild climb out of the Pine area, the trail rambles about 6 miles through mostly arid forests. At 8.3 miles, you reach the popular Geronimo Trailhead with nice stands of pine and majestic fir trees, and a few good campsites nearby. Nearing the end of the passage and reaching the Washington Park Trailhead, you leave the Highline Trail and gain more than 1,000 feet on a 2-mile climb to General Springs, an area with plenty of great camping locations.

Because of the fires and ensuing monsoon rains, many portions of the Highline Trail have suffered extreme tread damage due to erosion. The entire trail is being studied for potential realignments.

ON THE TRAIL

From the Pine Trailhead and parking area, follow the signage for a short distance to access the AZT. Once you reach the junction with the AZT, head east and stay on the Highline Trail (Trail 31). You quickly pass trail junctions for Trail 28 and Trail 27 and reach a high vantage point on a ridge with distant landmarks to the south, including the Mazatzal Mountains and the craggy Four Peaks. The trail continues to roll across steep terrain until it reaches Red Rock Spring, where there is a place to camp a short distance to the left (northeast). About 70 yards beyond the spring, continue east on the Highline Trail as the Red Rock Trail (Trail 294) cuts right to descend to the Control Road in the valley floor.

TURNAROUND NOTE: If you're interested in a great day hike, consider leaving a car at Red Rock Trailhead for a 5-mile point-to-point adventure.

Next, you pass Pine Spring and cross through a number of drainages, eventually descending to an intersection with the old roadbed of Geronimo Trail. Turn right (east) and continue descending on the roadbed, which soon parallels a large stream. In 0.2 mile, follow the stream across an intersecting roadbed, turn right (east), and descend through a beautiful forest of very large ponderosa pines. Cross the two channels of Webber Creek to arrive at Geronimo Trailhead and the access road (FR 440).

After you leave Geronimo Trailhead, head northwest and, in about 0.5 mile, ignore a roadbed paralleling the trail on the left, and continue on the singletrack. Eventually you reach a trough of water from Bear Spring and a T-intersection that looks like a road. Turn right (south) and, where the road bends left, stay on singletrack to the east. The trail occasionally approaches steep, rocky walls of the rim, passing through thick patches of crimson-stemmed manzanita, alligator juniper, oak, and ponderosa pine. Pick your way across two broad sections of red slickrock, and then cross Bray Creek.

Soon afterward, you come to East Bray Creek, a section of trail that is being restored after years of erosion. Continue on to a crossing of North Sycamore Creek. The trail is somewhat faint on the other side of the creek; walk downstream about 20 yards and look for a faint tread heading east. The trail rambles through cool pine

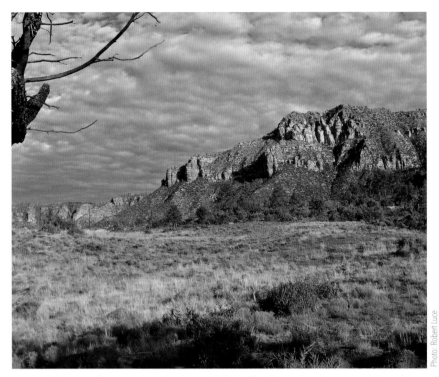

Photo: Robert Luce

Views of the Mogollon Rim, one of Arizona's defining landforms, can be enjoyed throughout most of Passage 27.

forests and across several more streams, and then it begins a steady descent through a series of switchbacks, terminating at a road junction.

Cross the road and stay to the left, noting the hiker sign that marks the continuation of the AZT on singletrack. Over the next 0.5 mile, the trail swings around the south side of a ridge before it turns back to the north, passes under a power line, and continues to the north-northeast. Follow the singletrack as it descends and crosses a small drainage before emerging from the trees just north of the Washington Park Trailhead.

The AZT leaves the Highline Trail here and heads north along the Colonel Devin Trail (Trail 290) on an old road. To reach the Washington Park Trailhead, turn right (southeast), and descend 50 yards to the parking area.

The AZT now parallels the headwaters of the East Verde River. A singletrack on the right (east) leaves the road you've been climbing. A sign indicating the Tunnel Trail (Trail 390) and the Colonel Devin Trail marks this intersection. Turn onto the single-track, which immediately crosses the stream and then curves left (north-northeast).

Shortly after the trail begins to climb steeply, you'll see a trail on the right that leads 0.25 mile to an uncompleted railroad tunnel, which was intended to carry ore from central Arizona mining towns through the Mogollon Rim to Flagstaff. To continue on the AZT, follow a switchback to the left (northwest). The trail crosses back over a drainage that is East Verde River, soon to arrive on top of the Mogollon Rim and the southern edge of the Colorado Plateau (7,200 feet). Continue north less than 0.1 mile to cross FR 300, near the historical marker for the Battle of Big Dry Wash, and then walk another 0.4 mile to the parking area at General Springs Cabin and the end of Passage 27.

Mountain Bike Notes

Short sections of this trail are fun on a bike, but you'll spend most of your time walking and pushing your bike. Mountain bikers consistently rate it their least favorite passage. *For more information about mountain biking along the Arizona National Scenic Trail, visit* **aztrail.org.**

SOUTHERN ACCESS: Pine Trailhead

Drive south of Pine on AZ 87 for 0.6 mile, and turn left (east) to reach a large parking area and the trailhead.

NORTHERN ACCESS: FR 300 Trailhead

If you want to hit the trail from here, please follow the trail description in reverse order. From the intersection of AZ 87 and AZ 260 north of Pine, drive east 2.6 miles on AZ 87, then turn right (south) toward FR 300. Go 0.1 mile and turn left onto FR 300. Avoid the frequent side roads, and drive 12 miles on FR 300 to a turnoff on the left (north), at a historical marker for the Battle of Big Dry Wash. Turn left and follow a power line 0.3 mile to General Springs Cabin. The road curves right, to a small parking area and the trailhead.

ALTERNATE ACCESS: Washington Park Trailhead

Drive south of Pine on AZ 87 for 2.2 miles and turn left (east) at a sign that says CONTROL ROAD (FR 64). Drive 9.3 miles and turn left on FR 32. Continue 3.3 miles, then turn right at a sign for Washington Park Trailhead. Make an immediate left turn and drive 1 mile to the large parking area at the trailhead. Follow the trail from the north side of the parking lot. In about 100 yards, you reach the AZT at the intersection of the Highline Trail (Trail 31) and the Colonel Devin Trail (Trail 290).

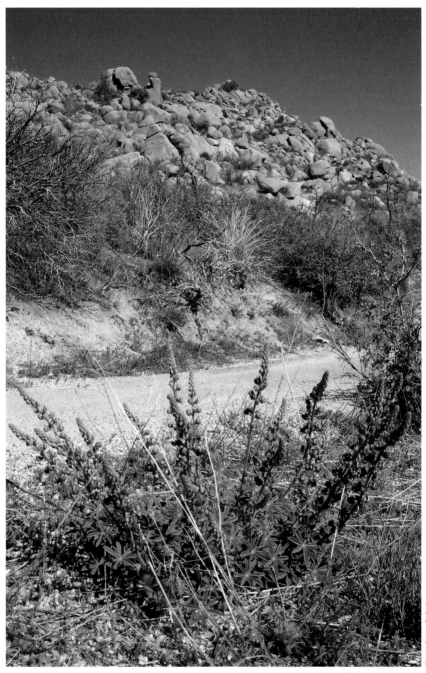

Photo: Sirena Dufault

Anyone traveling along the remote passages of the AZT's Central Section will be treated to unforgettable bursts of color and contrast during every season.

AZT North Section

Passages 28 through 43

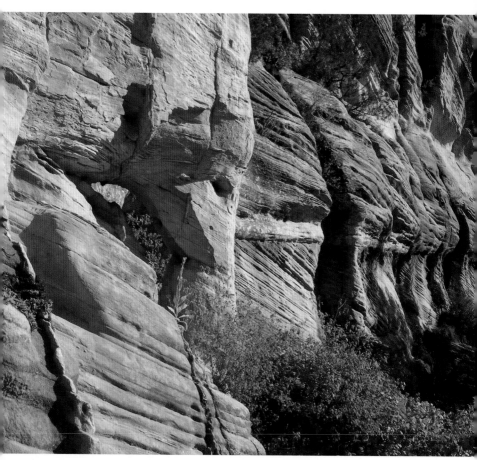

The wind-sculpted cliffs along Passage 31 are evidence of massive sand dunes that once covered this part of the planet.

Photo: Sirena Dufault

Blue Ridge

LOCATION Mogollon Rim to AZ 87

DISTANCE 16.1 miles one-way

DAY-TRIP OPTION See turnaround note in the trail description.

SHUTTLE RECOMMENDATIONS FR 123 (passage mile 5.3), FR 751 (passage mile 11.6)

DIFFICULTY Moderate

LAND MANAGER Coconino National Forest, Mogollon Rim Ranger District, **www.fs.usda.gov/coconino,** 928-477-2255

RECOMMENDED MONTHS April–November

GATEWAY COMMUNITY Not applicable

GEOLOGY HIGHLIGHTS Not applicable

OVERVIEW

This passage is mostly flat, with two notable exceptions. The first is the 500-foot-deep gorge carved by East Clear Creek, which flows into Blue Ridge Reservoir. The second is the steep drop from Blue Ridge to AZ 87. Neither is particularly difficult, and this passage as a whole is relatively easy. You'll cross pockets of pristine natural beauty, including the quiet sanctuary of General Springs Canyon, early in the passage. The

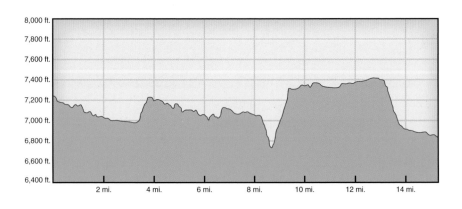

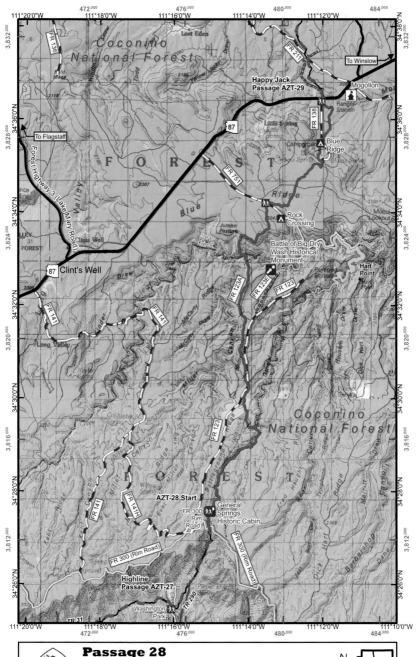

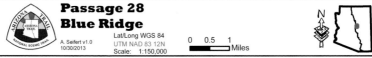

Passage 28
Blue Ridge

A. Seifert v1.0
10/30/2013

Lat/Long WGS 84
UTM NAD 83 12N
Scale: 1:150,000

0   0.5   1
Miles

N

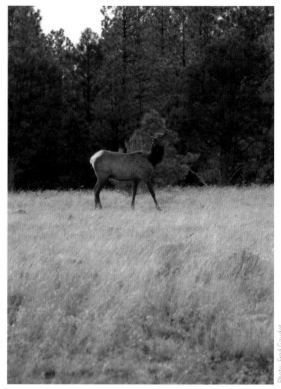

Trail adventures in northern Arizona are frequently shared with Roosevelt elk (*Cervus canadendis roosevelti*), and in autumn their unmistakable bugles can he heard throughout the forest.

Photo: Fred Gaudet

drop into East Clear Creek, which passes thick stands of pine and fir trees, is equally inspirational. Although roads bisect much of the passage, none are heavily traveled, and their presence does not spoil this quiet corner of the Mogollon Rim.

ON THE TRAIL

The trail exits the parking area to the left (west) of an elk fence, a structure designed to enhance stream habitat conditions for the endangered Little Colorado spinedace fish. Rock cairns and brown carsonite posts guide you through the forest along General Springs Canyon. The deeper you follow the winding trail into the canyon, the more beautiful it becomes.

At a trail fork, turn left (north) to climb out of the drainage. After a series of steep switchbacks, the Arizona National Scenic Trail (AZT) reaches level ground and turns sharply right (north) to join an old road. In 0.5 mile, the road bends left (west-northwest) and reaches a second dirt road at a T-intersection. Go straight across this road onto singletrack, as a carsonite post indicates. The trail immediately curves back to the right and crosses under power lines in 0.1 mile.

The AZT zigzags along, following cairns by the power line. It crosses dirt FR 123 and continues on the other side (northwest). For about the next 2 miles, the trail parallels FR 123. Follow the cairns and carsonite posts until you reach FR 123A, an old doubletrack. Turn left (northwest) and continue to a fork, where you should bear right (north-northeast).

Just northwest of where the road forks, stay left and find a stock tank with usually clear water right next to the road. If you have the time and energy to take it, explore the Battle of Big Dry Wash Historical Monument by taking the fork to the right.

Approximately 0.5 mile farther north, leave the road and continue straight ahead (north) on a singletrack. Go through a gate and immediately begin a steep descent into the canyon of East Clear Creek. This gate is as far as mountain bikes can reasonably ride (see Mountain Bike Notes, page 217). For hikers, a dense forest in the canyon offers respite from the heat of the plateau.

TURNAROUND NOTE: For day-trippers who haven't arranged a car shuttle, East Clear Creek is an excellent destination for the day. By the time you return to your vehicle at General Springs Historic Cabin, you'll have 18.4 miles under your boots, tires, or hooves.

To continue, cross the flat, gravelly bottom of the canyon. You may find water here, near the upper reaches of Blue Ridge Reservoir. Cross the canyon diagonally to your left (due west), and pick up a clear trail ascending the bank.

After climbing out of East Clear Creek Canyon, the trail levels abruptly on the plateau above the canyon, known as Blue Ridge. The trail heads almost due east, offering another nice view into East Clear Creek Canyon. At about 0.3 mile before Rock Crossing Campground, you come to a trail junction, where the AZT heads to the left (northeast). This trail lets the AZT traveler bypass the campground, which is closed most of the year. Signage indicates that the trail continuing east goes to Rock Crossing Campground.

During summer, when the campground is open, water and restrooms are available, and hikers and mountain bikers can stay in the campground for a fee. Horses are prohibited.

The AZT route around the campground goes northeast for about 0.5 mile, where it crosses FR 751. The trail heads east again, and in about 0.7 mile, you come to a doubletrack north of the campground. As you enjoy views of the vast expanse of flat pine forest stretching to the north, the trail bends right to head east-southeast. It curves back to the north to begin a rocky descent down the lush slopes of Blue Ridge.

Before you reach Blue Ridge Campground, you come to a trail route bypassing the campground for the same reasons and seasonal limitations as the Rock Crossing Campground. Follow the signs on an old doubletrack that heads left (north) to FR 138, and then turn right (south) on FR 138. In about 100 yards, the entrance to the campground is on the left and the AZT continues north, also on the left. During summer when it's open, Blue Ridge Campground has water.

Head north on a clear singletrack. The trail passes through enchanting stands of aspen before it reaches a road crossing. After the road crossing, there is a stock pond.

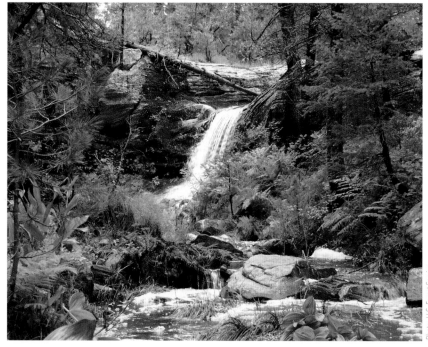

Photo: U.S. Forest Service

Once you reach Clear Creek along Passage 28, you'll understand why this is one of the most beloved waterways in Arizona.

The trail bends to the right to pass the pond and then continues north. Avoid a side trail on the left that heads west-northwest.

Trend northeast on a clear singletrack, then intersect a faint trail by a large cairn and a sign. Turn left (west) and follow cairns and carsonite posts to mile 16.1, where you'll find a parking area, an informal trailhead, and the end of Passage 28.

Mountain Bike Notes

Parts of this passage are rideable, but the dip into East Clear Creek is not. From mile 9.5 to the end, the riding is very difficult because of extremely rocky terrain. Only the most hardcore riders will enjoy this section. *For more information about mountain biking along the Arizona National Scenic Trail, visit* **aztrail.org.**

SOUTHERN ACCESS: FR 300 (Rim Road)

From the intersection of AZ 87 and AZ 260 north of Pine, drive east 2.6 miles on AZ 87, then turn right (south) toward FR 300. Go 0.1 mile and turn left onto FR 300. Avoid the frequent side roads, and drive 12 miles on FR 300 to a turnoff on the left (north) at a historical marker for the Battle of Big Dry Wash. This is where the AZT crosses FR 300. Turn left and follow a power line 0.3 mile to General Springs Historic Cabin. The road curves right to a small parking area and the trailhead.

NORTHERN ACCESS: AZ 87

From the intersection of AZ 87 and AZ 260 north of Pine, drive northeast 19.5 miles on AZ 87, and then turn right (south) on FR 138. (This turnoff is about 0.8 mile west of the Mogollon Rim Ranger Station on AZ 87.) Signs on the highway point to Moqui Campground. The trailhead is about 100 yards south on FR 138, on the left (east) side of the road.

Happy Jack

KEY INFO

LOCATION AZ 87 to Gooseberry Springs Trailhead

DISTANCE 30.7 miles one-way

DAY-TRIP OPTION See turnaround note in the trail description.

SHUTTLE RECOMMENDATIONS FR 93 (passage mile 8.6), FR 294 (passage mile 21.2)

DIFFICULTY Easy

LAND MANAGER Coconino National Forest, Mogollon Rim Ranger District, **www.fs.usda.gov/coconino,** 928-527-3600

RECOMMENDED MONTHS April–November

GATEWAY COMMUNITY See Mormon Lake (page 328).

GEOLOGY HIGHLIGHTS Not applicable

OVERVIEW

This passage traverses some attractive terrain, but much of it follows roads that are open to motorized vehicles. In the absence of natural barriers on the Mogollon Plateau, vehicles have thoroughly explored the area, and roads are more prevalent than trails. There are exceptions, including the first 5.1 miles of the south end of this passage where you'll enjoy singletrack through scenic canyons, although the route crosses and briefly follows roads at several points.

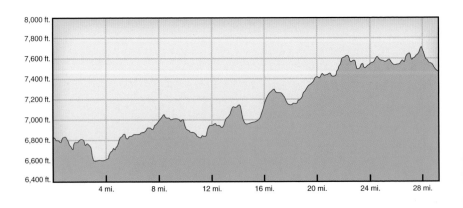

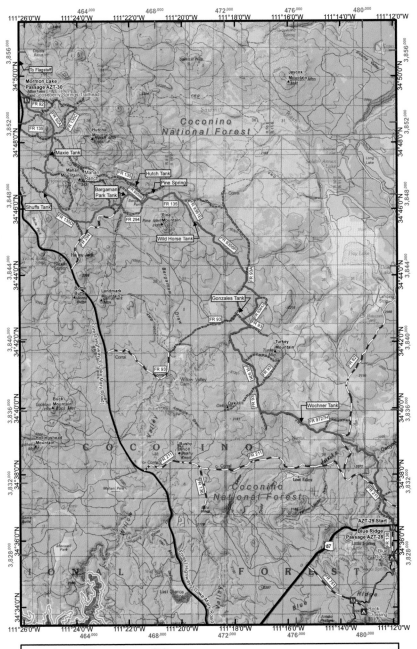

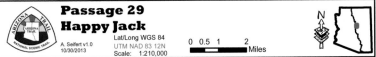

Passage 29
Happy Jack

Lat/Long WGS 84
UTM NAD 83 12N
Scale: 1:210,000

A. Seifert v1.0
10/30/2013

0 0.5 1   2
Miles

N

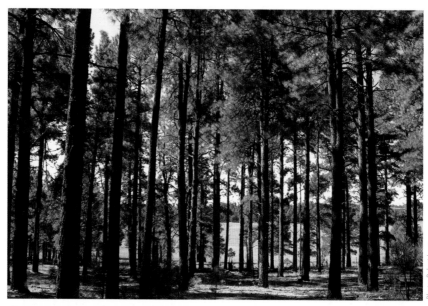

Photo: Robert Luce

The entire Colorado Plateau is dominated by ponderosa pine (*Pinus ponderosa*) forest, which provides a dense canopy and ample shade for AZT hikers, mountain bikers, and equestrians.

In 2012 the U.S. Forest Service completed a lengthy administrative process to develop a traffic-management plan for the forest, which will close many unnecessary roads to reduce impact on the forest. Many of the roads in this passage fall under this program, and much of the AZT will eventually be located on roads that have been converted to singletrack.

There are no guaranteed water sources, but stock tanks are plentiful, and Pine Spring is fairly reliable. You'll find good campsites all along this passage.

ON THE TRAIL

From the trailhead, travel 100 yards north on the dirt road to AZ 87, turn right (east) on the highway, go about 40 yards, and turn left (north) onto FR 138. Pass through a gate and continue along the road 0.1 mile to a sign indicating a singletrack on the right (northeast).

Cairns and brown carsonite posts show the way when the trail is faint. The AZT reaches a road and bends left to parallel it for 0.2 mile before crossing it to the northeast. The trail joins another road that forks immediately. Take the right fork and follow the road about 100 yards until it bends to the right. Leave the road on singletrack, continuing straight ahead (northeast).

The trail bends left (northwest) to descend into Jacks Canyon. In 0.2 mile, join a very faint old road in the bottom of the scenic canyon, follow it west approximately 1.2 miles, and exit the drainage bottom to the left (west). In another 0.7 mile along a wide level area, cross a high-quality dirt road, and continue northwest 0.6 mile to reach FR 9727H. Turn left (west) and follow this road, wending your way around chunks of lava rock, as you travel through pretty ponderosa forests.

Pass Wochner Tank, which appears as Waldroup Tank on the 1970 USGS *Turkey Mountain* topographic map, and in about a mile look to the left for an unnamed pond. You may find clear water here when Wochner Tank is dry or muddy.

TURNAROUND NOTE: If you're just out for the day, Wochner Tank (passage mile 6.8) or the unnamed pond (passage mile 7.7) makes a nice place to turn around and reverse your route.

Turn right (north) at a T-intersection with FR 93. Bear right (northeast) at a triangular intersection to stay on FR 93. Walk a little more than 0.1 mile to turn left (northwest) onto FR 93K. In about 2 miles, the trail veers right (east) and continues another 1 mile to rejoin FR 93. Turn left (north-northwest), continue 0.4 mile, and then turn right (northeast) on FR 9364J.

Gonzales Tank is about 0.25 mile northwest of the intersection of FR 93 and FR 9364J. Please be careful in this environmentally sensitive area. After 0.7 mile of climbing on FR 9364J, the road curves left (north) and then, in another 0.3 mile, curves back to the right (east). At this point, at the signed turn just past the gate, veer left (northwest) and follow the singletrack trail about 0.75 mile over a flat ridge before you descend to FR 93A.

Turn right (northeast) and walk a short distance to FR 9356P. Turn left (northwest) onto this road, and begin a steady climb. After topping out around 7,300 feet, this road descends to Wild Horse Tank. Join FR 9361E at the tank, follow it north for 1.6 miles to FR 135, and bear left (west).

Continue to a signed singletrack to the left, just before reaching a T-intersection with a road. If you want to get water at Pine Spring, turn right at the T-intersection and walk on this road for less than 0.1 mile to a second fork. Turn right and continue 0.2 mile to the spring. Pine Spring flows into a stock pond that provides the easiest access to the water; plus, it has some nice places to camp.

If you don't want to go to Pine Spring, follow the trail about 0.15 mile through the trees (note the steel AZT sign) south of the road just before the T-intersection with FR 294, until it crosses FR 294. The trail then follows FR 9356B northwest through a narrow gate strung between two large trees until it reaches a four-way junction of these rugged backcountry roads. Two steel-tower transmission lines loom ahead. Turn sharply left (south) at the junction, head through a gate and along FR 9255U a short distance. Just past the first steel tower, head west again on faint singletrack toward Bargaman Park Tank.

Pass Bargaman Park Tank and continue southwest to FR 135D. Turn right (northwest) for 1.9 miles on FR 135D to Shuffs Tank. Turn right (north), following signs and rock cairns to Maxie Tank.

Continue following the signs and heading north-northeast 0.6 mile to FR 135. Cross this road and follow FR 135C for 0.2 mile to FR 92A, which curves north-northwest around a low peak on the left. Descend slightly to an open park, and continue into the trees. The trail skirts a mound associated with the now-abandoned railroad and continues northerly along the railroad grade. You reach busy, graded dirt FR 92 and a steel AZT sign, which is the end of Passage 29.

Mountain Bike Notes

The broken basalt tread along this passage is anything but comfortable. Bring your full-suspension bike, and be prepared for a sore undercarriage. The worst stretch is the road from mile 5.7 to mile 8.6. *For more information about mountain biking along the Arizona National Scenic Trail, visit* **aztrail.org.**

SOUTHERN ACCESS: AZ 87

From the intersection of AZ 87 and AZ 260 north of Pine, drive northeast 19.5 miles on AZ 87, and then turn right (south) on FR 138. (This is about 0.8 mile west of the Blue Ridge Ranger Station on AZ 87.) Signs on the highway point to Moqui Campground. The trailhead is about 100 yards south on FR 138, on the left (east) side of the road.

NORTHERN ACCESS: Gooseberry Springs Trailhead

From the turnoff leading from Forest Highway 3 to Mormon Lake Village, continue south on FH 3 for approximately 5 miles, turn left onto a prominent road on the south side of an open meadow, and drive 0.25 mile to a sharp left turn in the road. The trailhead and a steel AZT sign are on your right. You can also reach this point from AZ 87 by driving north on FH 3.

Mormon Lake

KEY INFO

LOCATION Gooseberry Springs Trailhead to Marshall Lake Trailhead

DISTANCE 33.9 miles one-way

DAY-TRIP OPTION See turnaround note in the trail description.

SHUTTLE RECOMMENDATIONS FR 219 (passage mile 7.1), FR 240 (passage mile 12.5), FR 651 (passage mile 22.3)

DIFFICULTY Easy

LAND MANAGER Coconino National Forest, Flagstaff Ranger District, **www.fs.usda.gov/coconino,** 928-526-0866

RECOMMENDED MONTHS April–October

GATEWAY COMMUNITY See Mormon Lake (page 328).

GEOLOGY HIGHLIGHTS Not applicable

OVERVIEW

This easy, nearly 34-mile section crosses beautiful open meadows beside aspen and pine forests, with fine views of the San Francisco Peaks. Passage 30 appeals equally to hikers, mountain bikers, and equestrians, especially in late summer, when its sunflowers are in full bloom. Together, the passage's southern and northern maps, on the next page and 226, respectively, provide a comprehensive view of this popular route.

ON THE TRAIL

As shown on the southern map (next page), this passage begins at the Gooseberry Springs Trailhead, 0.25 mile east of paved Forest Highway 3 (Lake Mary Road), along FR 92 at the steel Arizona National Scenic Trail (AZT) sign. The trail proceeds north across the road onto singletrack through the meadow to the edge of the woods, turns left (northwest), and comes to Lake Mary Road in about 0.5 mile. The trail winds northwest toward Railroad Spring, about 3 miles south of Mormon Lake. Rock cairns and brown carsonite posts show the way. Occasionally you'll also see a wooden directional Forest Service sign.

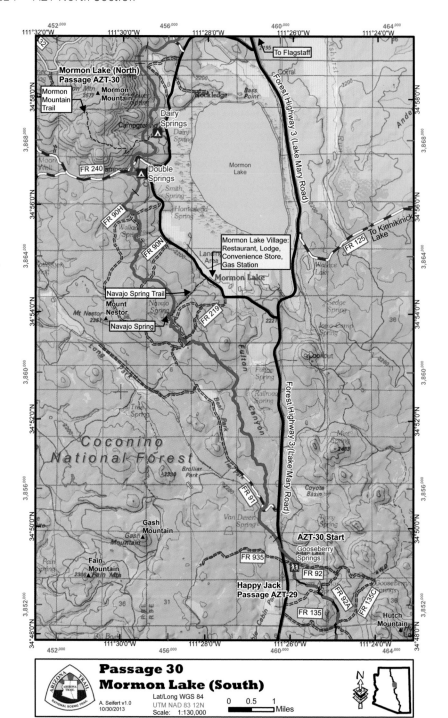

Passage 30
Mormon Lake (South)

Lat/Long WGS 84
A. Seifert v1.0
10/30/2013
UTM NAD 83 12N
Scale: 1:130,000

0   0.5   1
Miles

At mile 5.0 the route joins a road, and 1 mile later it exits left (northwest) back onto singletrack. It crosses a road at mile 6.5, goes through a gate at mile 6.8, and descends to FR 219. Shortly, the trail reaches its high point of the passage, and then descends to FR 219A, which it crosses at mile 7.7 and again at mile 7.9. This is the location of Navajo Spring (about 100 yards off the trail), a seasonal spring in a tranquil meadow.

TURNAROUND NOTE: At nearly 8 miles into the passage, Navajo Spring is a perfect destination for out-and-back hikers who haven't arranged a car shuttle. Mountain bikers will likely continue farther down the trail before turning around, and a variety of campgrounds found north of Navajo Spring make ideal places to refill bottles and reverse your route.

Moving on, at mile 7.9 the AZT reaches the junction with the Navajo Spring Trail, a 1-mile spur that leads directly into Mormon Lake Lodge. Only 1 mile from the AZT, the beautiful mountain community of Mormon Lake Village offers one of the best stops or staging areas anywhere along the entirety of the AZT's route. In addition to privately owned cabins and RV spaces, Mormon Lake Lodge offers cabin rentals, camping, RV parking, showers, and laundry facilities. Visitors can also enjoy the amenities of a bar, restaurant, store, and post office. Mormon Lake Lodge, a Forever Resort, has been a major partner with the Arizona Trail Association in providing the necessary resources to complete the Arizona National Scenic Trail around Mormon Lake. For more information, write to P.O. Box 3801, Mormon Lake, AZ 86038; call 928-354-2227; or visit **mormonlakelodge.com.**

From the Navajo Spring Trail junction, the AZT continues generally north through a healthy pine forest. It crosses FR 90N at mile 9 and joins a doubletrack at mile 10.5.

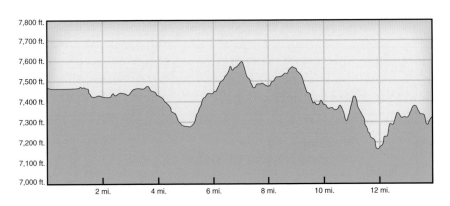

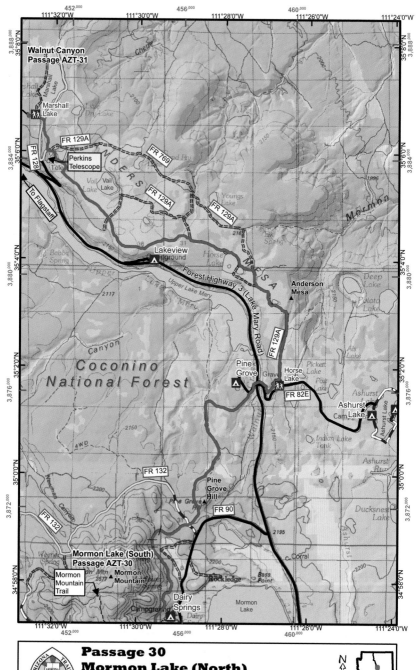

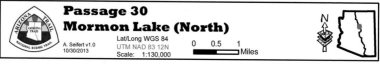

Passage 30
Mormon Lake (North)

A. Seifert v1.0
10/30/2013

Lat/Long WGS 84
UTM NAD 83 12N
Scale: 1:130,000

0   0.5   1
Miles

N

After 0.3 mile it becomes a singletrack again and crosses FR 90H and then FR 90B. At mile 11.7 the trail crosses the Lakeview Trail, and then the AZT descends to Double Springs Campground.

When the campground is open (usually late spring to early fall), it offers reliable water. The trail runs through the campground, climbs to the west, switchbacks east and then north, and crosses FR 240 at mile 13.1. After curving east and then west, the trail reaches a junction with the Mormon Mountain Trail, which connects to Dairy Springs Campground. Even when the campground is closed, a natural spring nearby offers a fairly reliable water source.

The northern passage map shows that you continue generally north, and the trail skirts some open areas staying on the edge of the woods. It passes through a series of gates, swings to the east, and then crosses FR 132 at mile 17.7. About 0.25 mile prior to this, the route joins an abandoned railroad bed that it follows for more than 3 miles before turning off of it at mile 20.9. After a short climb there is an easy descent to a crossing of FR 651—the access road for the Pine Grove Campground, which (similar to Double Springs) also has good water when it is open.

Just beyond this the trail crosses FH 3 and climbs steeply onto Anderson Mesa. It passes a short spur trail that connects to the Horse Lake Trailhead at mile 23.4 and then continues due north for several miles. Watch for intermittent views of the San Francisco Peaks from the doubletrack. Stay right at a road junction at mile 26, go through a fence, and then stay left at another road junction at mile 26.2. The trail curves around the mostly dry Horse Lake and heads east, finally leaving the road at mile 28.2.

The trail passes Lakeview Campground at mile 28.9, but as of this book's printing there is no access to the campground without climbing down a limestone bluff. The AZT crosses FR 129A at mile 30.7, then heads northwest across open country and crosses through two

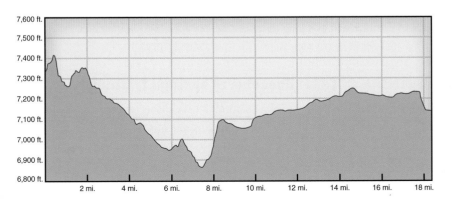

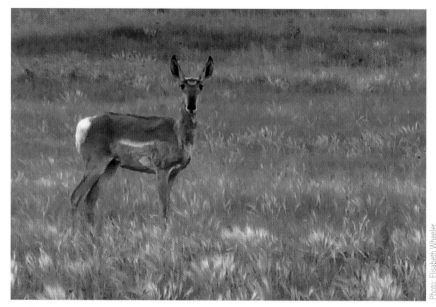

Photo: Elisabeth Wheeler

The lush meadows of Passage 30 provide abundant forage for northern Arizona wildlife.

gates in a game fence around Prime Lake. Equestrians must follow the fence around the lake. Shortly after crossing through the second gate the trail reaches the trailhead and small parking lot at the Lowell Observatory's Perkins Telescope site. The trail crosses an open meadow and then descends a wooded hillside to FR 128. Continue straight ahead (west) for 0.2 mile to the Marshall Lake Trailhead and the end of Passage 30.

Mountain Bike Notes

The entire passage provides excellent, easy-to-moderate singletrack riding. You can ride point-to-point by leaving a vehicle at one of the access points or do an out-and-back from either end as a long-distance ride. *For more information about mountain biking along the Arizona National Scenic Trail, visit* **aztrail.org.**

SOUTHERN ACCESS: Gooseberry Springs Trailhead

From the turnoff leading from FH 3 to Mormon Lake Village, continue south on FH 3 for approximately 5 miles. Turn left onto a prominent road (FR 92) on the south side of the open meadow, and drive 0.25 mile to a sharp left turn in the road; the trailhead and a steel AZT sign is on your right. You can also reach this point from AZ 87 by driving north on FH 3.

NORTHERN ACCESS: Marshall Lake

From Flagstaff, take the Lake Mary Road (FH 3) exit (339) off I-17 for 9 miles, and then turn left (east) onto FR 128 at the sign for Marshall Lake. As the paved road to the observatory makes a hard right, continue forward onto the graded gravel road 2.2 miles to the large Marshall Lake sign. Turn left and park beyond the AZT sign on the left. If you're coming from the south on Lake Mary Road, the Marshall Lake turnoff is 7.5 miles north of Pine Grove Campground.

PASSAGE 31

Walnut Canyon

KEY INFO

- **LOCATION** Marshall Lake to I-40
- **DISTANCE** 18.5 miles one-way
- **DAY-TRIP OPTION** See turnaround note in the trail description.
- **SHUTTLE RECOMMENDATION** FR 301 (passage mile 7.2) or Walnut Canyon Road (passage mile 16.1)
- **DIFFICULTY** Easy
- **LAND MANAGER** Coconino National Forest, Flagstaff Ranger District, **www.fs.usda.gov/coconino,** 928-527-3600
- **RECOMMENDED MONTHS** April–October
- **GATEWAY COMMUNITY** See Flagstaff (page 329).
- **GEOLOGY HIGHLIGHTS** Not applicable

OVERVIEW

This passage's peaceful traverse of Anderson Mesa from Marshall Lake and along Walnut Canyon belies its proximity to the city of Flagstaff. In the bottom of Sandy's Canyon, before the Arizona National Scenic Trail (AZT) ascends to the Fisher Point area, you will come to a junction. The left fork, a resupply route for thru-hikers, heads north into Flagstaff (see Passage 33, page 238). The right fork takes Passage 31 northeast and follows the edge of Walnut Canyon after passing Fisher Point (a popular destination for Flagstaff locals). The latter is also the equestrian bypass around Flagstaff.

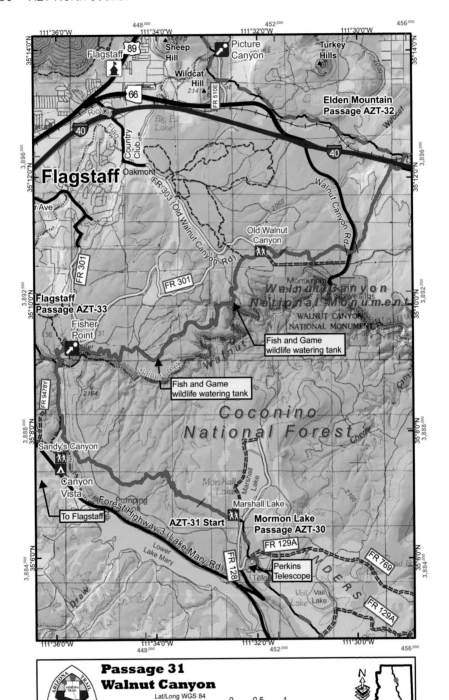

Passage 31
Walnut Canyon

Lat/Long WGS 84
A. Seifert v1.0
10/30/2013
UTM NAD 83 12N
Scale: 1:110,000

0   0.5   1
Miles

N

ON THE TRAIL

A large steel AZT sign marks the singletrack departure point from the trailhead that lies southwest of Marshall Lake (7,122 feet). The trail passes through a pleasant, flat woodland of ponderosa pine and oak. At mile 1.2, the trail begins a short descent into a canyon, and then it heads west and crosses a forest road to climb the other side of this small canyon. The AZT crosses FR 128B at mile 4.0 before it descends steeply into lower Walnut Canyon. In the bottom of the canyon at mile 5.5 is the intersection with Sandy's Canyon Trail; you can turn left to reach Canyon Vista Campground, or you can stay on the AZT and continue toward Fisher Point. The trail forks at mile 6.4. The left fork is Passage 33, the resupply route through Flagstaff. Passage 31 takes the right fork and ascends out of the canyon to Fisher Point.

TURNAROUND NOTE: A magical spot among the pines, Fisher Point makes for a pleasant destination if you're doing an out-and-back hike for the day.

To continue along the AZT, skirt the edge of the canyon and pass a trail junction with the FR 301 trailhead. At about mile 12.2 the trail makes a steep descent into and out of a branch of Walnut Canyon. A major Arizona Trail trailhead is located on FR 303, the Old Walnut Canyon Road. After you cross Old Walnut Canyon Road, the trail gradually transitions from a ponderosa pine forest to a piñon–juniper forest. The trail crosses the paved Walnut Canyon National Monument entry road and continues east before turning north to cross under the I-40 at Cosnino Road, where Passage 31 ends. An excursion along this passage wouldn't be complete without a side trip to Walnut

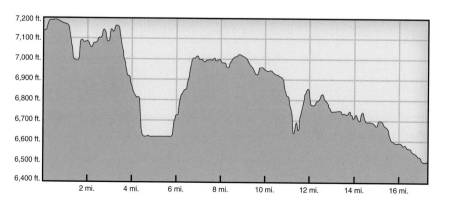

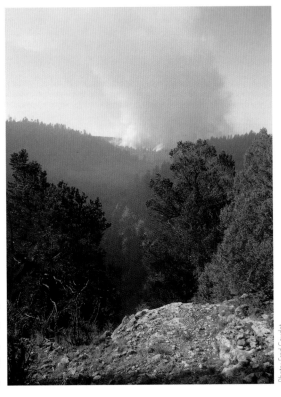

Fires are necessary to maintain the health of the pine forests of northern Arizona, and both controlled burns and wildfires are common.

Photo: Fred Gaudet

Canyon National Monument, where 25 cliff dwelling rooms of the Sinagua people are well preserved within their natural surroundings.

Mountain Bike Notes

Anderson Mesa is rocky but relatively level singletrack until you drop into Walnut Canyon. There are several climbs into and out of canyons where you might need to walk your bike. The northern half of the passage is smooth singletrack through the forest and along the rim of Walnut Canyon with one 250-foot descent into a branch of Walnut Canyon. *For more information about mountain biking along the Arizona National Scenic Trail, visit* **aztrail.org**.

SOUTHERN ACCESS: Marshall Lake

From Flagstaff, take the Lake Mary Road (FH 3) exit (339) off I-17 for 9 miles, and turn left (east) on FR 128 at the sign for Marshall Lake. Pass the observatory turnoff. At 2.2

miles, turn left before Marshall Lake (7,136 feet), and park at the AZT sign on the left. If you're coming from the south on Lake Mary Road, the Marshall Lake turnoff is 7.5 miles north of Pine Grove Campground.

ALTERNATE ACCESS: Old Walnut Canyon Trailhead

From Flagstaff, take I-40 east to Exit 205. Go south on the access road to Walnut Canyon Monument. Near the entrance is a junction with FR 303 and a sign to the AZT. Old Walnut Canyon Trailhead, which has room for horse trailers, is about 1.75 miles west on the left (south) side of FR 303.

ALTERNATE ACCESS: Forest Road 9478Y

Just north of Canyon Vista Campground, turn onto FR 9478Y and continue 0.25 mile to a parking area. From there it's a short walk to a trail marked ACCESS TO ARIZONA TRAIL.

NORTHERN ACCESS: I-40, Cosnino Road Exit

Heading east from Flagstaff, turn right off I-40 at Cosnino Road (Exit 207), and take the next right onto the frontage road (Old Route 66). There is no official parking area; however, there is space to park along the frontage road.

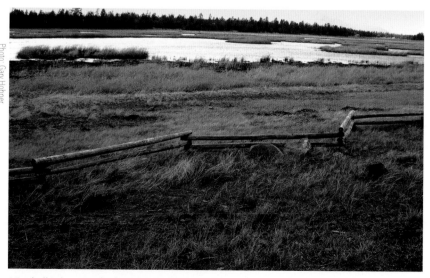

Photo: Gary Hohner

Marshall Lake, near the beginning of Passage 31

Elden Mountain

KEY INFO

LOCATION I-40 to Schultz Pass

DISTANCE 14 miles one-way

DAY-TRIP OPTION See turnaround note in the trail description.

SHUTTLE RECOMMENDATION AZ 89 (passage mile 7.0)

DIFFICULTY Moderate

LAND MANAGER Coconino National Forest, Flagstaff Ranger District, **www.fs.usda.gov/coconino**, 928-527-3600

RECOMMENDED MONTHS April–October

GATEWAY COMMUNITY Flagstaff

GEOLOGY HIGHLIGHTS See "Elden Mountain: A Volcano Unlike the Others" (page 344).

OVERVIEW

The first half of this passage skirts the Turkey Hills and crosses the Rio de Flag near Elden Pueblo. The second half is part of the Elden Mountain Trail System and follows the base of Little Elden Mountain on its way up to Schultz Pass. This passage is known as the equestrian bypass because it is used by horseback riders to avoid traveling through the city of Flagstaff. If you're in need of resupply or simply interested in seeing a little bit of Arizona's most famous mountain town, you may wish to use the Flagstaff passage (33) instead. But if you're more interested in maintaining the wilderness experience of

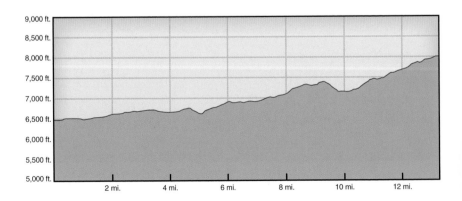

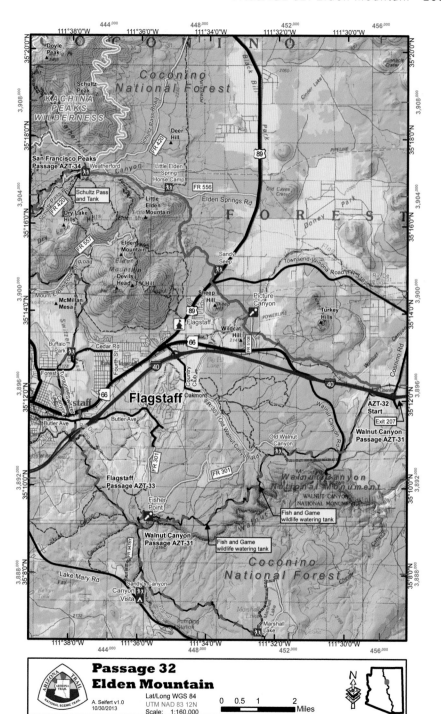

Passage 32
Elden Mountain

A. Seifert v1.0
10/30/2013

Lat/Long WGS 84
UTM NAD 83 12N
Scale: 1:160,000

0   0.5   1   2
Miles

N

the Arizona National Scenic Trail (AZT) than in playing around downtown Flagstaff, this is the passage for you.

ON THE TRAIL

Passage 32 begins near the Cosnino Road exit from I-40. From the trail underpass at the interstate, it is a short distance to the railroad tracks. Cross under the interstate and then make a sharp turn to the left (west). The route parallels the tracks and the interstate for several miles. Cross FR 510 at mile 3.3, and then the trail heads out into a large open area. Here, the passage offers nice views of Elden Mountain and the San Francisco Peaks. There are gates at miles 3.7 and 4.4. After crossing FR 510E, the trail contours around the side of Wildcat Hill and works its way up to the bridge over the Rio de Flag. Turn to the northwest, and gradually climb to US 89 at mile 7. Once under the highway, the trail turns right (north) and works its way over to the Sandy Seep Trail junction.

> **TURNAROUND NOTE:** If you're just out for the day and you haven't arranged a car shuttle, either the crossing under AZ 89 or the Sandy Seep Trail junction makes a great place to turn around and reverse your route for a 14-mile outing.

Turn left onto the Sandy Seep Trail and follow it for 1.4 miles up to the Little Elden Trail. Turn right at the T-intersection and follow this trail as it climbs up and around Little Elden Mountain. A right turn at the junction at mile 13.9 puts you on Schultz Pass Road and the end of the passage.

Mountain Bike Notes

The trail west of US 89 is part of the Dry Lake Hills–Elden Mountain Trail System, a popular system of trails for mountain biking in the Flagstaff area. The northern 6.5 miles of the trail climb gradually up to the mountain pass. *For more information about mountain biking along the Arizona National Scenic Trail, visit* **aztrail.org.**

SOUTHERN ACCESS: I-40 (Cosnino Road Exit)

Heading east from Flagstaff, turn right off I-40 at Cosnino Road (Exit 207) and take the next right onto the frontage road (Old Route 66). There is no official parking area; however, there is space to park along the frontage road.

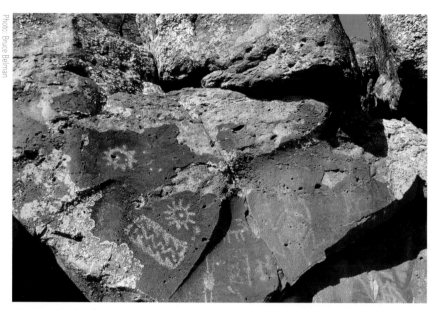

Photo: Bruce Belman

The petroglyphs of Picture Canyon exemplify the rich cultural history of northern Arizona.

ALTERNATE ACCESS: Sandy Seep Trailhead

Take US 89 north from the Flagstaff Mall, then turn left to the trailhead just after the US 89 intersection with Townsend–Winona Road.

ALTERNATE ACCESS: Little Elden Spring
Horse Camp and Trailhead

Take US 89 north of Flagstaff past the Silver Saddle Road stoplight. Turn left onto Elden Spring Road (FR 556), a gravel road, to the trailhead and horse camp.

NORTHERN ACCESS: Schultz Pass

From downtown Flagstaff, drive north on US 180 (North Fort Valley Road). After you pass the Sechrist School on your right, continue 1.5 miles and then turn right (north) where a sign indicates Schultz Pass Road (FR 420). Follow this paved road 0.7 mile through a right turn and a left turn. After the pavement ends, continue 4.5 miles to a parking area on the right (south) side of the road. Passage 32 connects to the Weatherford Trail and AZT Passage 34, on the north side of Schultz Pass Road just across from the parking lot.

Flagstaff (Resupply Route)

KEY INFO

LOCATION Fisher Point to Schultz Pass

DISTANCE 15.5 miles one-way

DAY-TRIP OPTION Not applicable

SHUTTLE RECOMMENDATION Buffalo Park (passage mile 7.2)

DIFFICULTY Moderate

LAND MANAGERS Coconino National Forest, Flagstaff Ranger District, **www.fs.usda.gov/coconino,** 928-527-3600; City of Flagstaff, **flagstaff.az.gov,** 928-213-2192

RECOMMENDED MONTHS April–October

GATEWAY COMMUNITY See Flagstaff (page 329).

GEOLOGY HIGHLIGHTS Not applicable

OVERVIEW

An urban route, Passage 33 takes you across the center of the city of Flagstaff, which offers diverse experiences from beginning to end. Long-distance-trail users can use this opportunity to resupply and revitalize in Arizona's most exciting mountain town. Great food, live entertainment, outdoor-gear suppliers, microbrews, a massage service, and much more can be found in downtown Flagstaff. The total mileage of the Arizona National Scenic Trail (AZT) does not include this route.

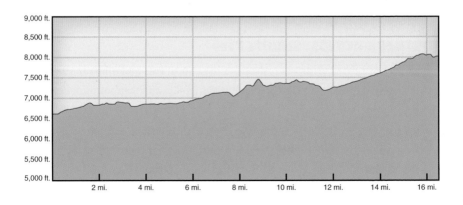

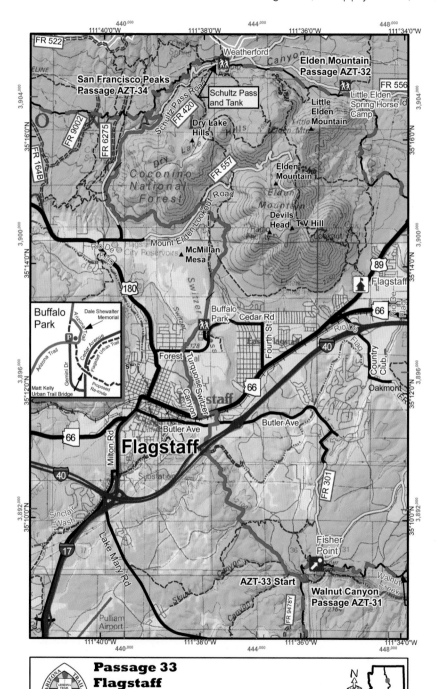

Passage 33
Flagstaff

A. Seifert v1.0
10/30/2013

Lat/Long WGS 84
UTM NAD 83 12N
Scale: 1:110,000

0   0.5   1
Miles

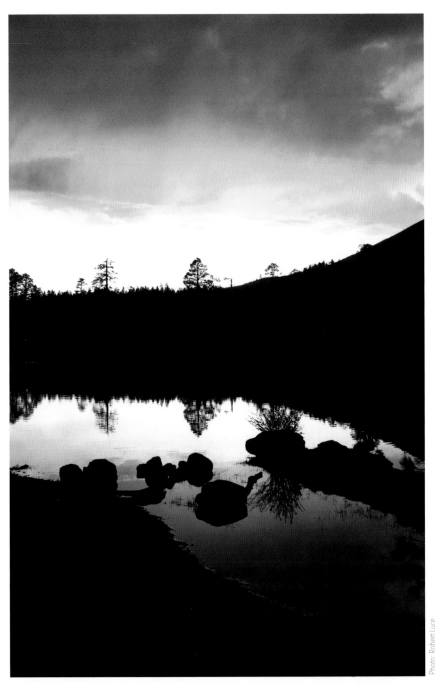

Sunset over Schultz Pass Tank, near the convergence of Passages 32, 33, and 34

The passage starts along the Fisher Point area trail system, passes through an underpass at one of the city's busiest intersections at Ponderosa Parkway (formerly Enterprise Road), and then climbs to McMillan Mesa on city streets and the Flagstaff Urban Trails System. Then the trail passes through beautiful Buffalo Park and enters the Dry Lake Hills trail system.

ON THE TRAIL

Passage 33 begins at a fork of Passage 31 about 0.5 mile southwest of Fisher Point. Passage 31 heads east towards Fisher Point, and Passage 33 heads north into Flagstaff. At 1 mile up the hill, turn right at the fence walk-through and continue north for 1.8 miles. Take the left fork at each of the next two major trail junctions. The trail drops down a steep hill and leads to an effluent pond just below I-40—don't even think about dipping your water bottles here.

From the bottom of the hill, follow the route around the east side of the pond, pass under I-40, and take the road to the right. You end up at the intersection of South Babbitt Drive and East Butler Avenue, between an Ace Hardware store and a Taco Bell. Additional chain restaurants and motels lie a short distance east at the I-40 and Ponderosa Parkway (formerly called Enterprise) interchange.

Turn right at East Butler Avenue and take the underpass at Ponderosa Parkway, north, to Route 66. Turn left at Route 66, then right onto Switzer Canyon Road. Turn right onto Turquoise Drive, which quickly bends to the north. Continue north on Turquoise Drive and look for the YMCA Family Center on the west side of the street, which is open to visiting members for showers. Continue north and cross Forest Avenue to the urban trail on the northeast corner, which leads you up the hill to Buffalo Park.

Flagstaff was the home of AZT founder Dale Shewalter, who in the 1970s envisioned a continuous path across Arizona and who launched the efforts leading to the 800-plus miles described in this guidebook. Buffalo Park is home to a commemorative sign and a memorial bench that honor the Shewalter Family. Trail users—especially those who've traveled 570-plus miles from the Mexican border—may wish to reflect a moment on the incredible contribution of this former schoolteacher. From the Buffalo Park parking lot, continue a short distance east around the large green water tank. Turn left on the McMillan Mesa Trail, which is a short loop off and back onto the AZT. The commemorative sign is on the right; Dale Shewalter passed away January 10, 2010, shortly before the AZT was completed.

From the Buffalo Park entrance, take the trail north to the national-forest boundary where it heads northwest around the foot of Elden Mountain and the Dry Lake Hills, escarpments that form the elevated horizon to the north and east. This is the Oldham Trail, which links with the Rocky Ridge Trail east of the Elden Lookout Road. Turn left on the Rocky Ridge Trail and begin a wide, climbing turn toward the Schultz Pass Trailhead. In 2.1 miles, at the Schultz Creek Trailhead, turn right onto the Schultz Creek Trail and continue northeast along the drainage approximately 3.9 miles, climbing toward the connector trail where Passage 33 crosses Schultz Pass Road and meets Passage 34.

Mountain Bike Notes

The portions of this route south and north of the city are some of the most popular mountain biking trails in town for commuters and recreational riders alike. The hills and elevation make these challenging for novice riders and out-of-towners. *For more information about mountain biking along the Arizona National Scenic Trail, visit* **aztrail.org.**

SOUTHERN ACCESS: Near Fisher Point

Fisher Point has no road access. The closest trail access is on Trail 106 from Canyon Vista Campground, 4 miles south of Flagstaff on Forest Highway 3.

ALTERNATE SOUTHERN ACCESS: Buffalo Park

From downtown Flagstaff, head north on North Fort Valley Road (US 180) to Forest Avenue. Turn right (east) on Forest Avenue and drive 1 mile to Gemini Drive. Turn left (north) on Gemini, which leads directly to Buffalo Park.

NORTHERN ACCESS: Schultz Pass

From downtown Flagstaff, drive north on US 180 (North Fort Valley Road). After you pass the Sechrist School on your right, continue 1.5 miles and then turn right (north) where a sign indicates Schultz Pass Road (FR 420). Follow this paved road 0.7 mile through a right turn and a left turn. After the pavement ends, continue about 3.9 miles to a small parking area on the left side of Schultz Pass Road. Passage 33, crosses Schultz Pass Road at this location and connects to Passage 34 on the north side of Schultz Pass Road.

San Francisco Peaks

KEY INFO

LOCATION Schultz Pass to Cedar Ranch

DISTANCE 36 miles one-way

DAY-TRIP OPTION See turnaround note in the trail description.

SHUTTLE RECOMMENDATIONS Snowbowl Road
(passage mile 7.4), FR 418 (passage mile 19.5), or FR 523 (passage mile 25.9)

DIFFICULTY Moderate

LAND MANAGER Coconino National Forest, Flagstaff Ranger District,
www.fs.usda.gov/coconino, 928-527-3600

RECOMMENDED MONTHS May–October

GATEWAY COMMUNITY See Flagstaff (page 329).

GEOLOGY HIGHLIGHTS See "The San Francisco Peaks' Violent Past"
(page 345).

OVERVIEW

This passage travels through beautiful pine, spruce, and aspen forests at high elevation—
briefly reaching 9,000 feet—and then transitions down to typical Arizona high-desert
terrain. It skirts the west side of the San Francisco Peaks, whose high point, Humphreys
Peak, is Arizona's tallest summit, at 12,633 feet. A culturally significant landform to all
of the seven Native American tribes who live nearby, the Peaks figure prominently into
myths and history alike. Although they are officially named the San Francisco Peaks,
a title given by early Spanish friars in honor of St. Francis of Assisi in 1629, they are
known as the Kachina Peaks among many native people and Flagstaff locals. Together,
the southern and northern maps for this passage, on the next page and page 246, respectively, provide a comprehensive view of this route, rich with biodiversity.

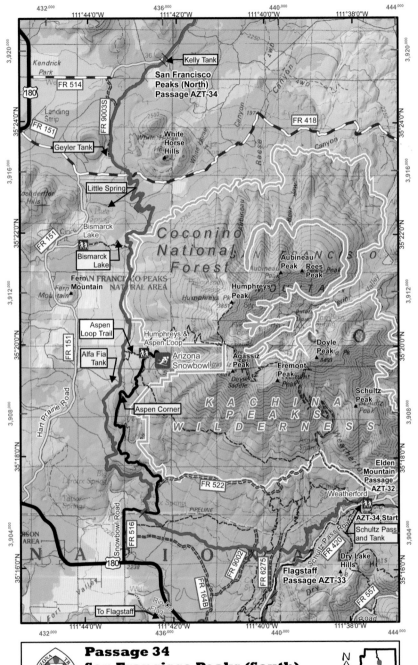

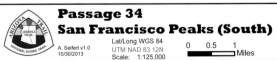

Passage 34
San Francisco Peaks (South)

A. Seifert v1.0
10/30/2013

Lat/Long WGS 84
UTM NAD 83 12N
Scale: 1:125,000

0   0.5   1
Miles

ON THE TRAIL

As the southern map for this passage (opposite) shows, this section begins at the Weatherford Trailhead on the north side of Schultz Pass Road. About 50 yards up the Weatherford Trail, the Arizona National Scenic Trail (AZT) immediately turns west and roughly follows the 7,500-foot elevation contour around the mountain. It crosses several old forest roads and passes through rolling ponderosa forest.

TURNAROUND NOTE: After 7.1 miles, the AZT crosses Snowbowl Road less than 1.5 miles from US 180. If you are day-hiking and need to reverse your route back to your vehicle, this landmark is a great turn-around location.

Continuing on, after the Snowbowl Road crossing, the trail then climbs 1,500 feet in elevation over the next 5 miles. It passes a junction with a spur trail that connects to the right about 0.25 mile to the Aspen Corner Trailhead, then continues on about 0.8 mile to the junction with the Aspen Loop Nature Trail, a link to the Arizona Snowbowl and Humphreys Trail. A side trip to the summit of this mighty peak is worth every step, but is a 14-mile round-trip from the Aspen Loop Nature Trail.

The AZT heads due north for about 2 miles across the upper reaches of Hart Prairie. In less than 0.5 mile, it reaches the Bismarck Lake Trail junction. The muddy puddle of a lake is about 300 yards northwest of the AZT and may or may not have water, depending on the season. Soon after the junction, the trail turns to the east around the northwest flank of Humphreys Peak and winds through a forest of giant firs and pines.

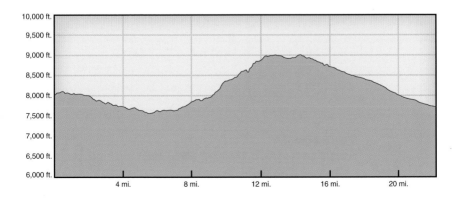

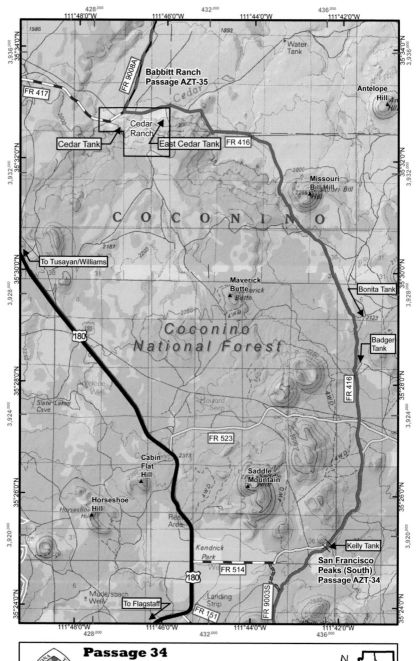

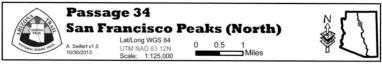

Passage 34
San Francisco Peaks (North)

Lat/Long WGS 84
UTM NAD 83 12N

A. Seifert v1.0
10/30/2013

Scale: 1:125,000

0   0.5   1
Miles

A little farther on, the trail begins working its way downhill in a northeastern direction. There are some large, gradual switchbacks, and the trail crosses an abandoned forest road. Little Spring, a reliable water source, is about 0.5 mile west of the trail on this road. The trail passes some more switchbacks on a gentle downhill grade to cross FR 418.

The trail crosses FR 418 to the northwest to pass around the southwestern flank of the White Horse Hills and begins a long sweeping turn to the north. About 1 mile north of FR 418, the trail joins FR 9003S, a fairly level doubletrack that continues north for about 0.7 mile, at which point the AZT becomes singletrack again. The trail heads northeast through open country with scattered trees, works its way around some private property, and then comes to a gate and Kelly Tank on FR 514. Kelly Tank has water during wet seasons, but getting water from the tank can be difficult because it has steep, muddy banks.

The northern map (opposite) picks up here, and you can see that just past Kelly Tank, the AZT crosses FR 514. The trail goes through a gate and continues northward, paralleling FR 514. The trail continues in a gradual downhill grade for about 2.8 miles where it crosses FR 523. One mile to the north you encounter Badger Tank, and another mile beyond is Bonita Tank; both hold water for just a short time after summer rains and winter snowmelt, but most of the time are dry and not considered reliable water sources. The AZT follows doubletrack for the remainder of the passage and proceeds northward on FR 416, turning slightly to the northwest. It levels out for a short distance and then goes downhill again as it passes Missouri Bill Hill on the right. About 1 mile past that hill, the trail turns to the west on FR 417 to the junction with FR 9008A and the end of Passage 34.

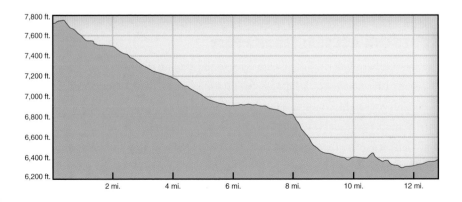

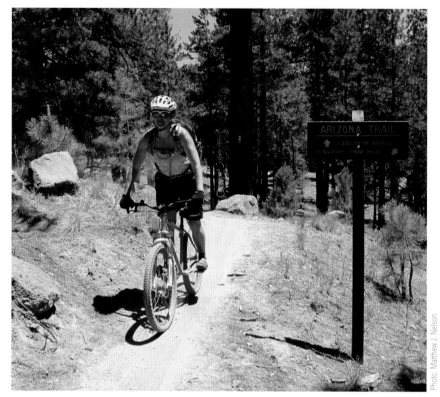

Photo: Matthew J. Nelson

With its expertly designed tread, breathtaking views, and proximity to Flagstaff, Passage 34 is a popular destination for mountain bikers.

Mountain Bike Notes

This entire passage is a world-class route for mountain biking. *For more information about mountain biking along the Arizona National Scenic Trail, visit* **aztrail.org.**

SOUTHERN ACCESS: Schultz Pass

For the southern half of this passage, refer to the map on page 244. From downtown Flagstaff, drive north on US 180 (North Fort Valley Road). After you pass the Sechrist School on your right, continue 1.5 miles and then turn right (north) where a sign indicates Schultz Pass Road (FR 420). Follow this paved road 0.7 mile through a right turn and a left turn. After the pavement ends, continue 5 miles to a parking area on the right (south) side of the road. Passage 34 starts on the Weatherford Trail, just across Schultz Pass Road from the parking area.

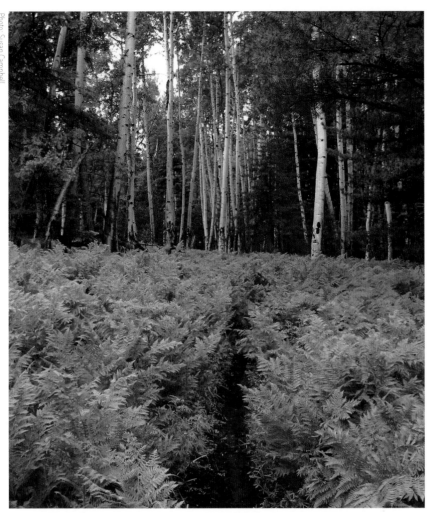

Along Passage 34, the AZT slices through spectacular fields of ferns and towering aspens.

NORTHERN ACCESS: **Cedar Ranch**

For the northern half of this passage, refer to the map on page 246. From Flagstaff drive
north on US 180 about 33.0 miles, and turn right (east) onto FR 417 near mile marker
248. (If you reach the Kaibab National Forest sign, you've gone too far by 0.4 mile.)
Continue 5.2 miles to a point just a short distance north of Cedar Ranch Headquarters,
where a side road (FR 9008A) leaves FR 417 to the left.

Babbitt Ranch

KEY INFO

LOCATION Cedar Ranch to Moqui Stage Station

DISTANCE 25.6 miles one-way

DAY-TRIP OPTION See turnaround note in the trail description.

SHUTTLE RECOMMENDATION Grandview Road (FR 301) (passage mile 18.5)

DIFFICULTY Easy

LAND MANAGERS Kaibab National Forest, Tusayan Ranger District, **www.fs.usda.gov/kaibab,** 928-638-2443; Arizona State Land Department, **azland.gov,** 602-542-4631; Babbitt Ranch, **babbittranches.com,** 928-774-6199

RECOMMENDED MONTHS April–June and September–November

GATEWAY COMMUNITY Not applicable

GEOLOGY HIGHLIGHTS Not applicable

OVERVIEW

Along this passage, the Arizona National Scenic Trail (AZT) follows ranch roads, but traffic is infrequent and the unique terrain is an integral part of the rich variety of landscapes along the entire Arizona Trail. As you look south toward the stunning San Francisco Peaks, try to imagine the scene 1 million years ago when lava spewed from an 18,000-foot supervolcano over thousands of miles.

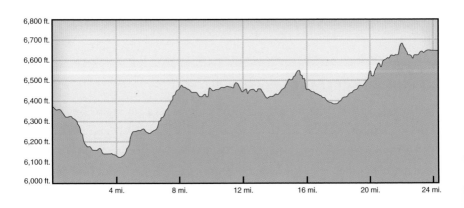

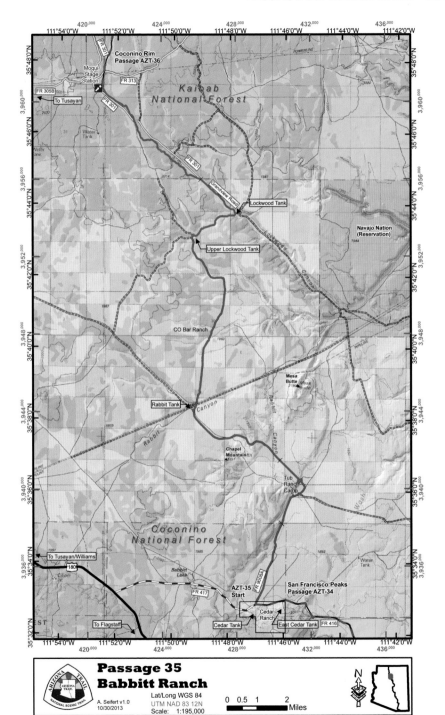

Passage 35
Babbitt Ranch

A. Seifert v1.0
10/30/2013

Lat/Long WGS 84
UTM NAD 83 12N
Scale: 1:195,000

0   0.5   1   2
Miles

N

The route is easy to follow because volunteers have done a good job marking the various road intersections with AZT-branded, four-by-four posts. The final 5 miles follow singletrack that is occasionally obscure but makes a nice diversion from the road.

Note that this passage crosses Arizona State Lands and a permit is required to camp outside the 15-foot trail corridor. This passage also crosses land owned by the Babbitts, one of the oldest and most well-respected ranching families in the state.

ON THE TRAIL

Head north-northeast on FR 9008A, as indicated by AZT signs. Walk through a sparsely vegetated landscape of juniper trees and rabbitbrush to a fork at mile 3.6. Stay on the main road, which breaks off to the right around Tub Ranch. Go through the gate—leaving it as you found it—and bear left and up the hill onto a beautiful high plateau at the first intersection. Take a moment to absorb the view, especially of the San Francisco Peaks to the south.

The road enters small hills dotted with trees. Cross a wash in 0.2 mile, bear left (southwest), and climb gradually. After some power lines come into view, you reach a fork. Bear right and continue 0.1 mile to another fork. Stay right again and continue straight ahead (north) to Rabbit Tank, which is 0.5 mile west of the trail.

TURNAROUND NOTE: If you're just out for the day and you haven't arranged a car shuttle, Rabbit Tank (passage mile 6.4) is a great place to turn around and reverse your route.

From the small dirt tank, cross under the buzzing power lines, follow a right fork to the north up a hill, and begin a long traverse of another broad, featureless plateau. After bearing north and finally northwest, you pass Upper Lockwood Tank. Follow the old road as it curves to the right around the tank, heading northeast along a tributary of Lockwood Canyon. You reach Lockwood Tank at a fence with two gates. Go straight through the gate in front of you, bear left, and continue through another distinctive gate to Grandview Road on the north side of the tank. Turn left and head northwest.

A cattle guard, a fence, and several signs mark your crossing into the Kaibab National Forest (the road you're following becomes FR 301). Cross the cattle guard and look to the left for a wooden sign for Kaibab National Forest. Behind this sign, head west on a faint singletrack. Look for several large rock cairns that mark the trail ahead. Aim for a lone juniper tree, and look for AZT signs to help guide your way.

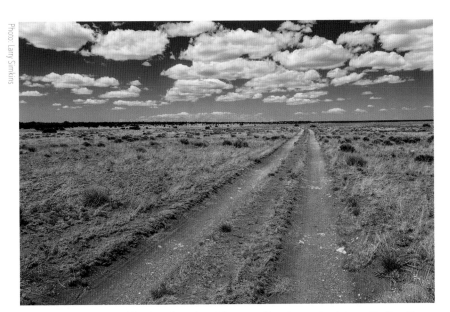

Passage 35 traverses Babbitt Ranch under wide-open skies that contrast dramatically with the dense pine forest to the south.

The trail improves as it reaches the trees and bends briefly to the left (southwest) before curving back to the northwest. Cross an old dirt road at a right angle. The trail winds and rolls through a dry piñon–juniper forest as it parallels FR 301 to the northwest, then becomes less distinct as it crosses FR 301. Follow the singletrack to the northwest on the other side.

The trail breaks out of the trees into a clearing and all but disappears. If you can't see the faint trail heading across the clearing, take a compass bearing of 330° and head for the opposite side. There you reach a fork in the trail that marks the end of Passage 35. The right fork is the continuation of the AZT into Passage 36. To reach the parking area at Moqui Stage Station, turn left (west) and continue 0.2 mile to a Forest Service sign marking the trailhead.

Mountain Bike Notes

This passage follows dirt ranch roads over its first 19 miles and then jumps onto a faint but pleasant singletrack. The entire passage offers fun riding, with views of surreal landscapes rarely seen on most rides. *For more information about mountain biking along the Arizona National Scenic Trail, visit* **aztrail.org.**

SOUTHERN ACCESS: Cedar Ranch

From Flagstaff, drive north on US 180 about 33 miles, and turn right (east) onto FR 417 near mile marker 248 (if you reach the Kaibab National Forest sign, you've gone too far by 0.4 mile). Continue 5.2 miles to a point just a short distance north of Cedar Ranch where a side road (FR 9008A) leaves FR 417 to the left. The passage begins here and follows FR 9008A north-northeast.

NORTHERN ACCESS: Moqui Stage Station

From the intersection of US 180 and AZ 64 in the town of Valle, go north on AZ 64 for 11 miles to FR 320 (mile marker 224). Turn right (east) onto FR 320 and drive 16 miles to an intersection with FR 301. Turn right (south) on FR 301 and drive 3.5 miles to the Moqui Stage Station. Park here, walk up a road that curves to the right (northeast), pass an old stone well in 50 yards, and follow singletrack east through the trees 0.1 mile to intersect the very distinct AZT. (To follow the AZT northbound, turn left toward Russell Tank.)

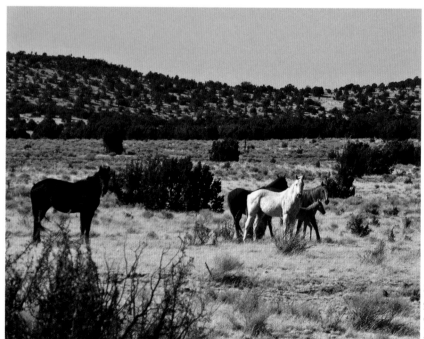

Horses outnumber humans along Passage 35.

Photo: Fred Gaudet

Coconino Rim

KEY INFO

LOCATION Moqui Stage Station to Grandview Lookout Tower

DISTANCE 19 miles one-way

DAY-TRIP OPTION See turnaround note in the trail description.

SHUTTLE RECOMMENDATION FR 310 (passage mile 8.8)

DIFFICULTY Easy

LAND MANAGER Kaibab National Forest, Tusayan Ranger District, **www.fs.usda.gov/kaibab,** 928-638-2443

RECOMMENDED MONTHS April–November

GATEWAY COMMUNITY See Tusayan and Grand Canyon Village (page 331).

GEOLOGY HIGHLIGHTS Not applicable

OVERVIEW

This passage offers a classic northern Arizona experience, with long stretches of beautiful ponderosa pine forest, prime elk habitat, and tantalizing views of the Grand Canyon. This relatively flat stretch has abundant campsites. While it has little fresh water, the frequent tanks and ponds may be promising. As you head northwest along the Coconino Rim, some of the drainages dropping to the northeast may contain water. However, you will find water only in the upper reaches of these valleys if the ground is saturated from winter snowmelt or recent rainfall. Carsonite posts bearing the Arizona National Scenic Trail (AZT) symbol frequently mark this trail.

ON THE TRAIL

The AZT descends to cross a dirt road 0.5 mile north of the intersection by Moqui Stage Station. Go straight across and continue north on a reclaimed doubletrack that meanders through ponderosa pines. As the road fades, pass through a gate into a fenced area and then continue on a faint doubletrack just west of north. Anderson Tank is just out of view on the right.

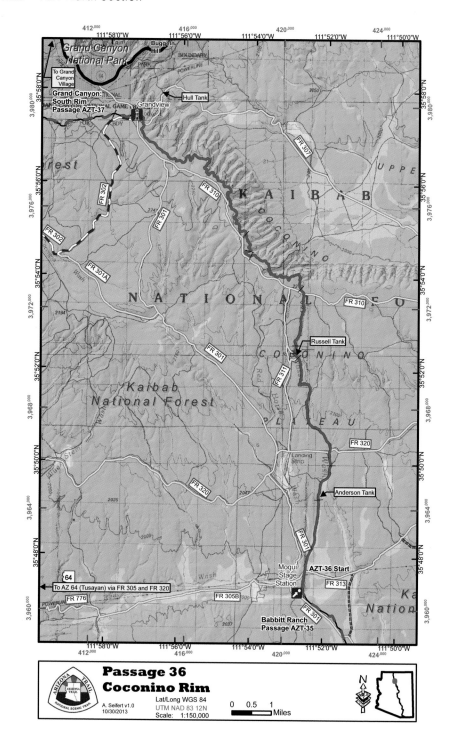

Passage 36
Coconino Rim

A. Seifert v1.0
10/30/2013

Lat/Long WGS 84
UTM NAD 83 12N
Scale: 1:150,000

0   0.5   1
Miles

N

In 1 mile, after you pass through another gate at mile 3.4, the road virtually disappears. Turn left and parallel the fence line due north: don't be tricked by the path that continues straight ahead to the northeast.

A faint doubletrack soon develops. When the fence ends, follow the doubletrack straight ahead, crossing FR 320. You pass a small, metal water tank at mile 4, after which the AZT follows Russell Wash through a deepening ponderosa forest. At this point, the trail veers left (west) out of the wash. The clear tread soon veers back to the right (north) and, after another 0.7 mile, passes through a modern gate near the large Russell Tank. At Russell Tank, there is a permanent toilet about 100 yards off the trail to the west.

TURNAROUND NOTE: For those who are just out for the day and haven't arranged a car shuttle, Russell Tank is an excellent spot to turn around and head south.

The AZT continues north and passes through another gate, crossing FR 310. After rambling through some oak-lined drainages, the trail trends west. Then the AZT breaks onto the edge of the Coconino Rim, offering far-ranging views to the north. After 1 mile, a trail sign indicates a bike bypass taking the left (westernmost) route. Hikers should stay right. Where the trail fades in about 0.1 mile, continue to a fence, turn back to the right, and follow a faint tread that switchbacks down the slope.

If you lose this elusive trail, make your way toward the bottom of the wash. The trail crosses the bottom 25 yards east of the fence and is much clearer as it climbs the north side for 0.2 mile to reach a road. Here, the bike bypass rejoins the main route, which

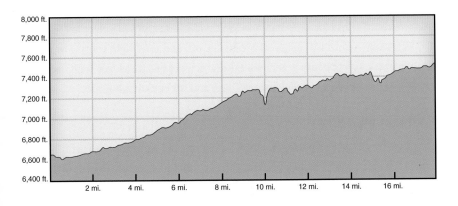

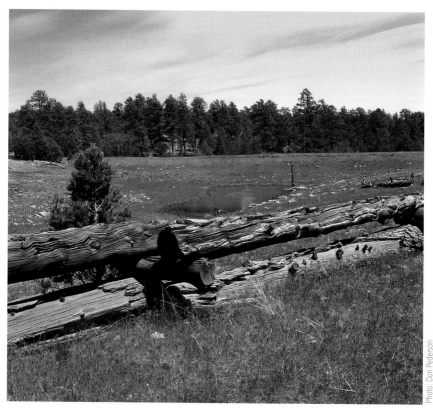

Photo: Dori Pederson

Cattle tanks may look and smell unpleasant, but they're among the most reliable water sources along Passage 36.

continues north on a singletrack. Over the next 3 miles, cross through several gates and minor washes, and get your first close-up views of the Grand Canyon to the north.

Toward the end of the passage, you begin to see interpretive signs explaining the effects of dwarf mistletoe on ponderosa pine populations. When you reach FR 307, turn left (west) onto this road, cross a cattle guard, and turn right (north) to rejoin the singletrack. A few steps farther, join the gravel tread of a developed loop trail, and follow it west to the Grandview Lookout Tower and the end of Passage 36.

Mountain Bike Notes

The entire length of this passage is open for riding, and for the most part it is easy going. One spot midway in the passage requires a short bike detour (signed) where the trail switchbacks down and up the steep walls of a drainage. Watch out for abundant prickly pear cactus and goathead thorns, a cyclist's nemesis. *For more information about mountain biking along the Arizona National Scenic Trail, visit* **aztrail.org.**

SOUTHERN ACCESS: Moqui Stage Station

From the intersection of US 180 and AZ 64 in the town of Valle, go north on AZ 64 for 11 miles to FR 320 (mile marker 224). Turn right (east) onto FR 320 and drive 16 miles to an intersection with FR 301. Turn right (south) on FR 301 and drive 3.5 miles to the Moqui Stage Station. Park here, walk up a road that curves to the right (northeast), pass an old stone well in 50 yards, and follow singletrack east through the trees 0.1 mile to intersect the very distinct AZT. (To follow the AZT northbound, turn left toward Russell Tank.)

NORTHERN ACCESS: Grandview Lookout Tower

Follow Grand Canyon National Park's Rim Drive (AZ 64) to its southernmost dip, about 11 miles east of Grand Canyon Village. From this junction, follow FR 310 (Coconino Rim Drive) 1.3 miles south to the trailhead.

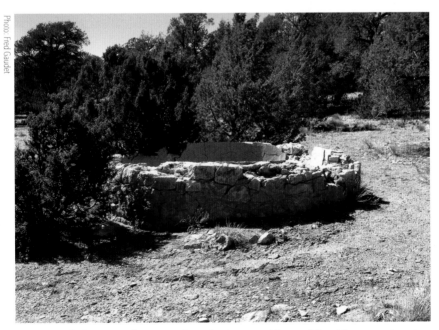

Photo: Fred Gaudet

Remnants of a historic well at Moqui Stage Station are evidence of the old stagecoach route from Flagstaff to Grand Canyon.

Grand Canyon: South Rim

KEY INFO

LOCATION Grandview Lookout Tower to South Kaibab Trailhead

DISTANCE 23.5 miles one-way

DAY-TRIP OPTION See turnaround note in trail description.

SHUTTLE RECOMMENDATION Tusayan Greenway Trailhead (passage mile 16.1)

DIFFICULTY Easy

LAND MANAGERS Kaibab National Forest, Tusayan Ranger District, **www.fs.usda.gov/kaibab,** 928-638-2443; Grand Canyon National Park, **nps.gov/grca,** 928-638-7888 for general visitor information

RECOMMENDED MONTHS April–November

GATEWAY COMMUNITY See Tusayan and Grand Canyon Village (page 331).

GEOLOGY HIGHLIGHTS See "The Grand Canyon: A Geological Masterpiece" (page 346).

OVERVIEW

Starting from the Grandview Lookout Tower, the Arizona National Scenic Trail (AZT) follows the Tusayan Bike Paths toward Tusayan and then enters Grand Canyon National Park. In the park it makes use of old doubletracks and bike paths toward Yaki Point and the South Kaibab Trailhead.

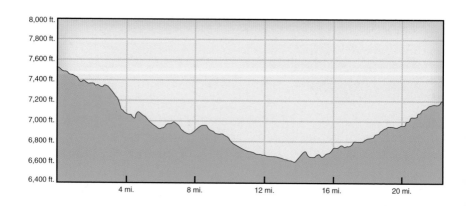

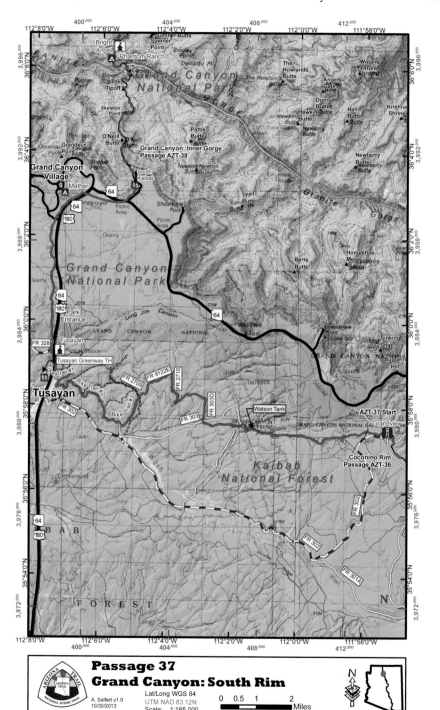

Passage 37
Grand Canyon: South Rim

Lat/Long WGS 84
UTM NAD 83 12N
Scale: 1:165,000

A. Seifert v1.0
10/30/2013

0   0.5   1   2
                                  Miles

ON THE TRAIL

Across FR 310, west of the Grandview Lookout Tower, is a parking lot that has a trail sign noting a bike trail and a distance of 16 miles to Tusayan. Passage 37 begins by heading west through open forest. It crosses a road at mile 1.3 and continues west.

Eventually the trail drops into an unnamed canyon and comes to Watson Tank at mile 4.4. Depending on the time of year, this tank might have water in it, but it's not reliable.

From the tank, the trail goes about 0.2 mile, turns right (north), and climbs up to FR 303. The route follows this road for about 1.7 miles to a junction with FR 303D at mile 6.2. Turn right (north) here and stay on this dirt road for about 0.5 mile, until it ends at mile 7.3.

TURNAROUND NOTE: Depending on the time of year and your endurance, turnaround spots for day-trippers may include Watson Tank (passage mile 4.4), FR 2709 (passage mile 10.3), or the town of Tusayan (passage mile 16.1).

Continuing north, the trail heads south about 0.5 mile and arrives at a gate and FR 2710B. Turn right (north) and follow this road to mile 8.7, a junction with FR 2710. Take FR 2710 north about 0.25 mile to FR 9122E, and turn left (southwest) on FR 9122E.

Follow FR 9122E until it reaches FR 2709 at mile 10.3. This road is also known as Bike Route #2 on the *Tusayan Bike Trail* map. Follow Bike Route #2 to Bike Route #1, which takes you very close to Tusayan and then turns to the north.

The bike trail crosses under the highway through a large concrete culvert and ends at AZ 64/US 180, 0.3 mile north of Tusayan. This point is 0.4 mile south of the Forest Service Tusayan Ranger Station.

There is a trail junction here at mile 16.1. Left (south) connects to the Tusayan Greenway Trailhead. The AZT heads north (right) here, paralleling the highway and crossing FR 328 at mile 16.5 and then an open area that was once the site of the old Moqui Lodge. Just beyond is an archway marking the entrance into Grand Canyon National Park.

The route is now on an old doubletrack that has been reconditioned into a bicycle and pedestrian trail. Follow this Greenway Trail to Mather Campground at mile 21.2, and then continue northeast along the well-marked path for another 2 miles. This path crosses paved roads, and although traffic is usually moving slowly, beware of drivers

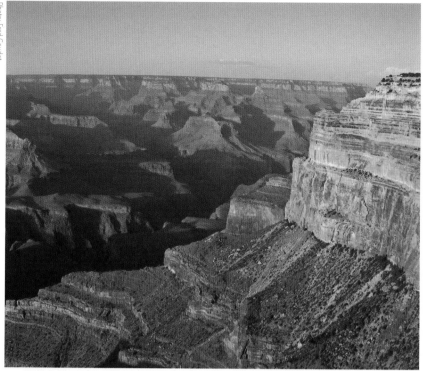

Watching the sun set over the Grand Canyon is an experience unlike any other.

from around the world who are likely to be distracted by one of the most spectacular natural wonders of the world outside their window. The Greenway Trail proceeds into the parking lot and the South Kaibab Trailhead, marking the end of Passage 37.

Mountain Bike Notes

This entire passage is excellent for mountain biking. Bike paths run through some beautifully forested areas with minimal elevation change. The route into the park allows a nearly car-free experience all the way to the South Rim of the Grand Canyon. *For more information about mountain biking along the Arizona National Scenic Trail, visit* **aztrail.org.**

SOUTHERN ACCESS: Grandview Lookout Tower

Follow Grand Canyon National Park's Rim Drive (AZ 64) to its southernmost dip, about 11 miles east of Grand Canyon Village. From this junction, follow FR 310 (Coconino Rim Drive) 1.3 miles south to the trailhead.

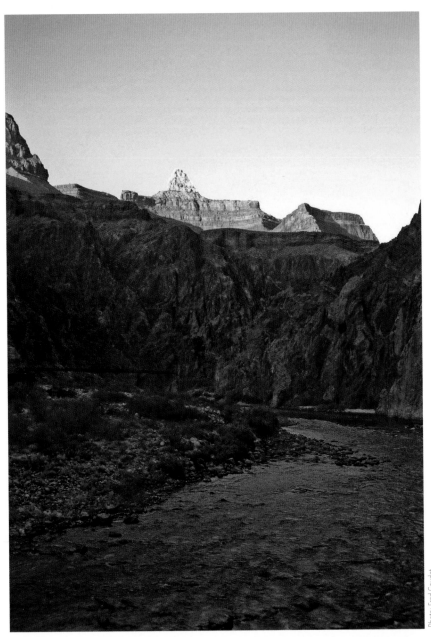

Photo: Fred Gaudet

The beauty and immensity of the Grand Canyon are best appreciated by hiking into its depths.

NORTHERN ACCESS: South Kaibab Trailhead

Take a shuttle from Grand Canyon Village, near the intersection of US 180 and AZ 64, because there is no overnight parking or camping at the trailhead. The park guide you'll receive at the entrance kiosk provides information, as do the park's visitor centers.

PASSAGE 38

Grand Canyon: Inner Gorge

KEY INFO

LOCATION South Kaibab Trailhead to North Kaibab Trailhead

DISTANCE 21.4 miles one-way

DAY-TRIP OPTION See turnaround note in the trail description.

SHUTTLE RECOMMENDATION Not applicable

DIFFICULTY Strenuous

LAND MANAGER Grand Canyon National Park, **nps.gov/grca,** 928-638-7888 for general visitor information

RECOMMENDED MONTHS April–June and September–mid-November

GATEWAY COMMUNITY Not applicable

GEOLOGY HIGHLIGHTS See "The Grand Canyon: A Geological Masterpiece" (page 346).

OVERVIEW

Through the high Kaibab Plateau in northern Arizona, the Colorado River has carved a canyon 277 miles long. It took approximately 6 million years to create this mile-deep canyon, and the result is a masterpiece of stone. Many people consider this passage the crown jewel of the Arizona National Scenic Trail (AZT). Nowhere else in the country does a few hours' walk take you through 2 billion years of geologic history. Photographs and words cannot capture the massive scale of the Grand Canyon. The relatively few individuals who physically traverse the canyon, feeling each foot of elevation loss and gain in their legs and lungs, are the only ones who can have a real sense of the grandeur of this place.

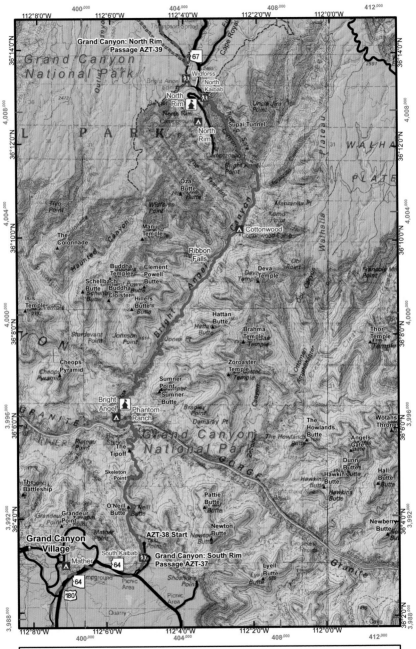

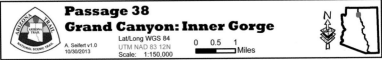

Passage 38
Grand Canyon: Inner Gorge

A. Seifert v1.0
10/30/2013

Lat/Long WGS 84
UTM NAD 83 12N
Scale: 1:150,000

0   0.5   1
Miles

N

For all its beauty, however, hiking into and back out of the Grand Canyon is a potentially life-threatening undertaking. Park Service literature and signs near trailheads warn about heat exhaustion and dehydration for good reason: more than 300 rescues are initiated each year, and most of the patients are fit young men who test themselves against the canyon and its rigorous environment. Running rim-to-rim has become increasingly popular, but endeavors like this are insane for anyone but the superfit ultrarunner who has thousands of difficult trail miles under his or her soles.

A desert climate prevails partway into the canyon, and temperatures exceeding 100 degrees are not uncommon. It's particularly demanding and dangerous to attempt to hike in and out of the canyon in one day. By all means, invest a minimum of two days and one night for a safe, fun traverse of the canyon. To experience the canyon more fully, spend two nights at the bottom—that way you'll get to see more than just the trail in front of your boots. The true beauty of the Grand Canyon can be found only when you sit in one place for a long, silent period of time.

To spend a night or two at the bottom of the Grand Canyon, you must plan well in advance. On the AZT, you may stay only at Bright Angel Campground or in a rental cabin at Phantom Ranch (near passage mile 7), and at Cottonwood Campground at mile 14.4. At the campgrounds, you will need all of the standard equipment, including the means to cook your own food. At Phantom Ranch, you can take a break from camping and enjoy a bed with sheets and blankets, a shower and towels, air conditioning, and even an outgoing telephone. Even if you're not staying there, you can sign up for the hearty meals at Phantom Ranch; reservations must be made well in advance.

The Grand Canyon National Park Backcountry Office accepts permit applications for inner-canyon campgrounds up to four months in advance—and you should submit

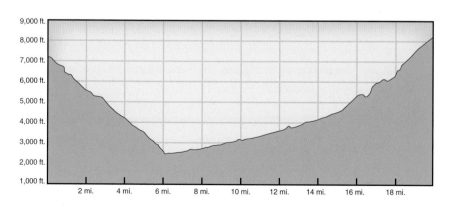

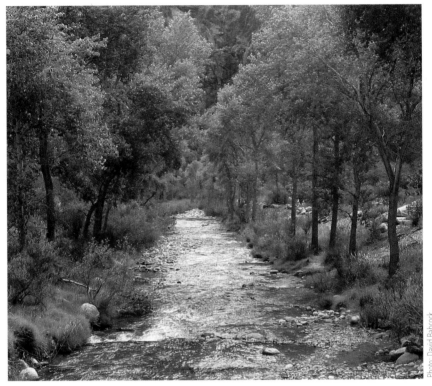

The AZT follows Bright Angel Creek through the Inner Gorge of the Grand Canyon.

an application by mail as early as possible. Walk-up permits are also possible, and the Backcountry Office handles accommodations for long-distance hikers, bikers, and equestrians traveling the entire length of the AZT. Xanterra Parks and Resorts takes reservations for Phantom Ranch up to 23 months in advance, and the rooms often fill very early. Due to sensitive resources, few developed sites, and worldwide popularity, camping in the Grand Canyon is closely managed. Rangers regularly patrol all areas of the canyon, and violations result in stiff fines and loss of future travel privileges inside this incredible national wonder.

ON THE TRAIL

The South Kaibab Trail is well marked, and although it is less popular than the Bright Angel Trail to the west, you're still likely to see quite a few people. If you encounter mule trains, stand to the inside of the trail and let them pass.

After leaving the trailhead, drop immediately along numerous switchbacks. The trail straightens somewhat and trends north-northwest, and then the sharp drops resume along Cedar Ridge. After passing under the prominent pinnacle of O'Neill Butte, the trail levels briefly on a stunning high plateau before plunging through countless painful switchbacks toward the sparsely vegetated Tonto Plateau below at Skeleton Point.

TURNAROUND NOTE: If you're day-hiking, don't try to descend beyond Skeleton Point (passage mile 3). The Grand Canyon is deceptively easy on the downhill and unbelievably challenging on the uphill. Most day-hikers reverse their route at Cedar Ridge (passage mile 1.5) or Skeleton Point. To go beyond these landmarks on a day trip is not only unrealistic but very dangerous.

On the plateau above the Colorado River, you reach the intersection with the Tonto Trail and continue straight to the north for the spectacular, winding descent into the Inner Gorge. On a geologic scale, you've now traveled 1.2 billion years back in time.

Just above the mighty Colorado River, you reach an intersection with the River Trail. Turn right (east), and continue through a tunnel and across the river on a suspension bridge. Follow the trail west (there are some Native American ruins about 0.1 mile past the bridge) and then north along Bright Angel Creek. Cross one of the two bridges to the west to access Bright Angel Campground.

Continuing north, pass the Ranger Station and bear right at a fork, and you'll arrive at Phantom Ranch. Continue to the canteen to purchase a cold beverage or basic resupply items.

Assuming you're well rested after a stay at Bright Angel Campground or the plush Phantom Ranch, head north along Bright Angel Creek. Pass the turnoff to the Clear Creek Trail, which offers a nice day hike for those taking a rest day in the Phantom Ranch area, and continue along this relatively easy stretch of trail toward Cottonwood Campground. The sound of Bright Angel Creek will provide a refreshing soundtrack every step of the way as thousands of vertical feet of chocolate-colored rocks rise around you.

For a spectacular side trip, head north across a bridge at passage mile 13.5 a short distance west of Cottonwood Campground. Ribbon Falls is among the many hidden wonders within Grand Canyon's Inner Gorge, and a walk through the canyon wouldn't be complete without standing in the cold spray of this otherworldly phenomenon.

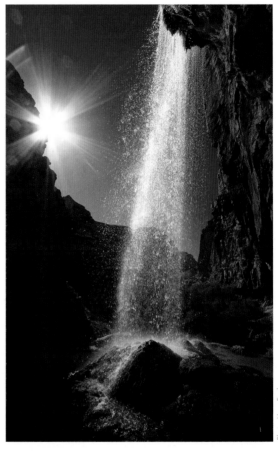

Ribbon Falls is one of the many natural wonders hidden deep within the Inner Gorge of the Grand Canyon.

Photo: Harry Ford

Beyond Cottonwood Campground, where bathrooms and water can be found, continue north and cross to the west side of Bright Angel Creek on a sturdy bridge. In another 0.1 mile, you'll find a rest house with shade and water. In a short distance, the trail begins climbing to the left (northwest) as it leaves Bright Angel Canyon. Follow Roaring Springs Canyon for the final climb to the North Rim. You'll see this side canyon's namesake falls, which do indeed roar. (Roaring Springs provides all the water for the facilities on both rims of the Grand Canyon.) Pass through Supai Tunnel, a small rest area with seasonal water and restrooms, and then continue another 2.1 miles to reach the North Kaibab Trailhead, and the end of Passage 38.

If you plan to visit the North Rim Lodge and other services at the North Rim, you can save about 0.6 mile by avoiding the main road and bearing left at a sign that says

GRAND LODGE 1.1 MILES. It's farther than that to the lodge, but in about 0.5 mile this path takes you to a general store, laundry facilities, and showers near a campground across the highway.

Mountain Bike Notes

Mountain bikes are prohibited on trails inside Grand Canyon National Park. The Arizona Trail Association (ATA) has a cooperative agreement with the park that allows long-distance bikepackers to carry their bikes through the canyon as long as their "wheels never touch dirt." You can also have your bike transported the 212 miles to the North Rim through **Trans Canyon Shuttle** (call 928-638-2820 or visit **trans-canyonshuttle.com**). This service is available May 15–October 15. *For more information about mountain biking along the Arizona National Scenic Trail, visit* **aztrail.org.**

SOUTHERN ACCESS: South Kaibab Trailhead

Take a shuttle from Grand Canyon Village, near the intersection of US 180 and AZ 64—there is no parking at the trailhead. For more information, inquire at the park's visitor centers.

NORTHERN ACCESS: North Kaibab Trailhead

The parking area is on the east side of AZ 67, 41 miles south of Jacob Lake and 2.3 miles north of Grand Canyon Lodge. The trailhead is at the south end of the parking lot.

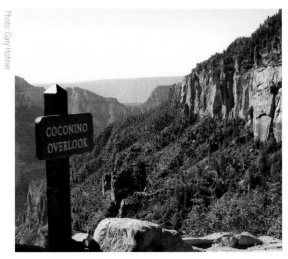

Looking back toward the South Rim after an arduous climb out of one of the world's deepest canyons

Grand Canyon: North Rim

KEY INFO

LOCATION North Kaibab Trailhead to Kaibab National Forest boundary

DISTANCE 12.6 miles one-way

DAY-TRIP OPTION See turnaround note in the trail description.

SHUTTLE RECOMMENDATION AZ 67 (passage mile 6.1)

DIFFICULTY Moderate

LAND MANAGER Grand Canyon National Park, **nps.gov/grca,** 928-638-7888 for general visitor information

RECOMMENDED MONTHS May–October

GATEWAY COMMUNITY See North Rim to Jacob Lake (page 332).

GEOLOGY HIGHLIGHTS See "The Grand Canyon: A Geological Masterpiece" (page 346).

OVERVIEW

This passage traverses the seldom-used northern side of Grand Canyon National Park as it heads through rolling, forested hills to the Kaibab National Forest. This section of the Arizona National Scenic Trail (AZT) follows graded dirt roads for 2 miles, but the majority of the route follows a primitive, remote utility corridor through lush forest. You're unlikely to see many other people along this passage.

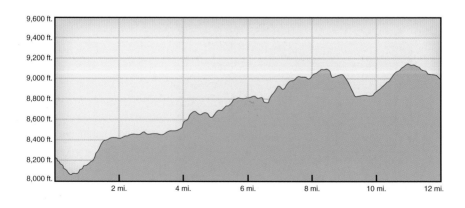

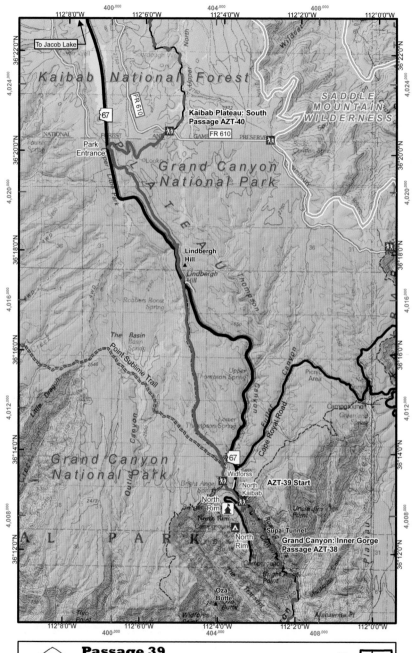

Passage 39
Grand Canyon: North Rim

Lat/Long WGS 84
UTM NAD 83 12N
Scale: 1:140,000

A. Seifert v1.0
10/30/2013

0   0.5   1
Miles

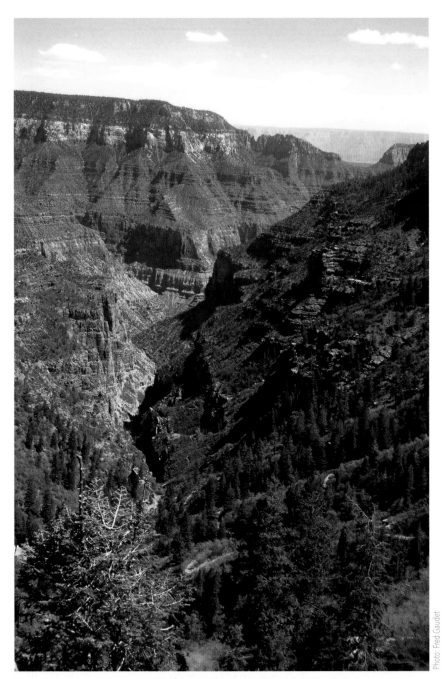

View into Roaring Springs Canyon from the North Rim, near the beginning of Passage 39

For equestrians, the park has a place for you to camp just north of the North Rim parking lot. Follow the road at the end of the parking lot, and head north, up a hill, and bear left as you travel up the road. Call the North Rim Ranger Station 928-638-7875) to check availability.

Just as it is for humans, conditioning is a big issue for horses traveling on the North Rim, which is at 8,800 feet in elevation: they feel the effects of the high altitude, too. Dehydration is also a concern; make sure you and your livestock consume enough water and calories during long hours on the trail.

ON THE TRAIL

From the parking lot, carefully cross the highway due west, pass a large metal AZT trailhead sign, and follow a well-defined trail down a drainage to a high-quality dirt road. Turn left (west), and follow the road past the parking lot for the Widforss Trail to a road junction. Bear left and follow the road 0.1 mile to a singletrack that departs on the right side. The trail soon joins a utility corridor. Stay on this corridor as it crosses several dirt roads. Many deer and turkeys that show little fear of humans inhabit this grassy area.

When the trail reaches AZ 67 at mile 6.1 (there is a paved parking area and picnic table as well as another large metal AZT sign), cross the highway carefully and follow a dirt road east for 60 yards.

TURNAROUND NOTE: If you're just out for the day, the trail crossing at AZ 67 (Lindbergh Hill) is a great place to turn around.

To continue along the AZT, turn left (north) onto a primitive road and continue along the utility corridor again. Where the utility corridor reaches a steep-sided drainage, the trail leaves the wide path to the right (east) onto a singletrack through the trees. The trail descends, crosses a drainage, and switchbacks back up the north slope, crossing the utility corridor several times.

Rejoin the utility corridor and reach this passage's second-highest point, where a steep descent begins. A flat stretch then takes you to where the trail leaves the utility corridor through the trees to the left, a few hundred yards southeast of the national park's north entrance station. If you stay on the utility corridor, you'll pass through the grounds of a small residence used by the National Park Service (NPS). Follow the trail to the parking lot just east of the entrance station, and then pick up Lookout Road going east around the back of the NPS residence.

Pass through a gate and follow Lookout Road along a gradual climb. At mile 11.2 you pass the highest point on the entire AZT, at 9,275 feet elevation. In another 0.3 mile, look for a well-signed junction of the AZT departing on the left (northeast). Notice the carvings on the large aspen trees on either side of the AZT at the junction. These arborglyphs mark the historic North Kaibab 101 Trail, used by early settlers and ranchers. In 0.7 mile, cross a fence marking the north boundary of the national park, the end of Passage 39. Ahead the trail crosses a long meadow to the north-northeast and heads to the FR 610 Trailhead.

Mountain Bike Notes

This passage is open to bikes, with mostly intermediate riding. The trail may be obscure in places, and you'll likely walk up some of the steeper grades given the high elevation along the Kaibab Plateau. *For more information about mountain biking along the Arizona National Scenic Trail, visit* **aztrail.org.**

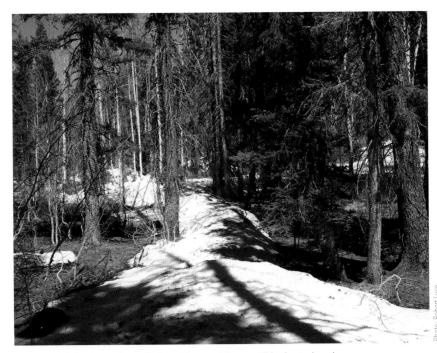

Photo: Robert Luce

Even in early summer, the trail along Passage 39 can still be buried under snow.

SOUTHERN ACCESS: **North Kaibab Trailhead**

The parking area is on the east side of AZ 67, 41 miles south of Jacob Lake and 2.3 miles north of Grand Canyon Lodge. The trailhead is at south end of the parking lot.

NORTHERN ACCESS: **Kaibab National Forest Boundary**

From Jacob Lake, drive south on AZ 67 for 26 miles, then turn left (east) onto FR 611 (4.5 miles north of the Grand Canyon National Park North Entrance Station and 1 mile south of Kaibab Lodge). Drive 1.1 miles and then turn right (east) onto FR 610. Wind south and then east 5.1 miles to the FR 610 Trailhead, on the south side of the road. The trailhead, which includes a permanent toilet, is located near where the AZT crosses FR 610, about 0.5 mile north of the boundary of Grand Canyon National Park.

PASSAGE 40

Kaibab Plateau: South

KEY INFO

LOCATION Kaibab National Forest boundary to Telephone Hill

DISTANCE 21.4 miles one-way

DAY-TRIP OPTION See turnaround note in the trail description.

SHUTTLE RECOMMENDATIONS East Rim View Trailhead (passage mile 7.8), FR 213 (passage mile 13.1)

DIFFICULTY Easy

LAND MANAGER Kaibab National Forest, North Kaibab Ranger District, **www.fs.usda.gov/kaibab,** 928-643-7395

RECOMMENDED MONTHS May–October

GATEWAY COMMUNITY See North Rim to Jacob Lake (page 332).

GEOLOGY HIGHLIGHTS Not applicable

OVERVIEW

As it follows the Kaibab Plateau Trail (Trail 101), this section of the Arizona National Scenic Trail (AZT) might just offer the easiest and most pleasant traveling along the entire 800-plus miles. It crosses a much overlooked and delightful area of northern

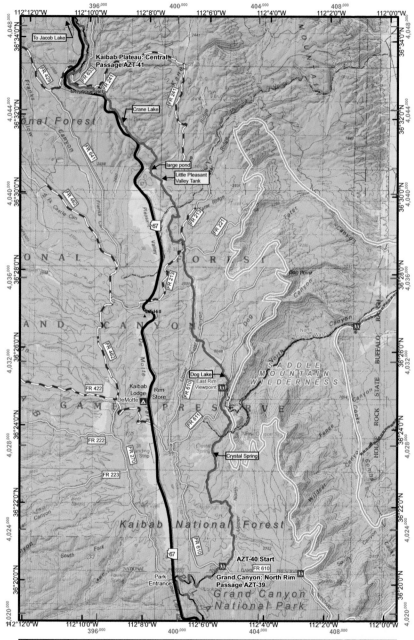

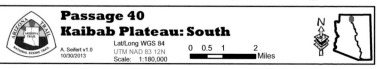

Passage 40
Kaibab Plateau: South

Lat/Long WGS 84
UTM NAD 83 12N
Scale: 1:180,000

A. Seifert v1.0
10/30/2013

0   0.5   1   2
Miles

N

Arizona, passing through an idyllic forest of spruce, pine, and aspen. For about a mile, the trail dodges in and out of stately trees along the East Rim of the Grand Canyon, offering breathtaking views of Marble Canyon to the east and the Vermilion Cliffs to the north, the final Arizona landmark before the canyon country of Utah. Another attraction: water is plentiful except in drought conditions. You can camp almost anywhere, as long as you're out of sight of the trail and roads.

ON THE TRAIL

Follow a singletrack northeast from the north boundary of Grand Canyon National Park across FR 610 and into Upper North Canyon Valley. The singletrack is marked by carsonite posts bearing the AZT symbol. After 1 mile, the trail follows an old road left (west-northwest) into an adjacent valley. In 0.1 mile, it joins another valley and turns back to the right (north) to meander through beautiful forests and sublime meadows. The AZT crosses FR 612 at mile 3.7.

At a sign indicating the Kaibab Plateau Trail (Trail 101), leave the road and turn right (north) onto a faint singletrack. In 200 feet, you pass a pond. After 2.3 miles, the trail leaves the valley by climbing a side drainage to the left (southwest). In 0.1 mile, the trail curves back to the right (north) to climb more steeply into a thick spruce–fir forest. Within the next mile, cross diagonally over two old roads and stay on the singletrack.

When you reach a jeep road, as indicated by carsonite posts, turn right (north). When the road forks in 0.7 mile, take the right fork, and continue on the double-track to a pond at Crystal Spring. From here follow the singletrack to the northeast as the trail approaches the North Canyon Rim. A gradual descent ends, Trail 4 proceeds

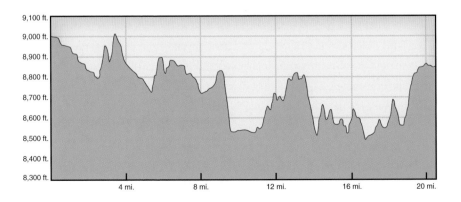

straight ahead about 0.6 mile over the edge of the rim and drops about 450 feet in elevation to North Canyon Spring, the most reliable water source on or near this passage.

The AZT turns to the north at the junction with Trail 4 and climbs through giant, old-growth ponderosa pines. The trail levels along the East Rim, with awesome views east into the Saddle Mountain Wilderness. Soon you can see Marble Canyon, upstream from the Grand Canyon. Far to the north lie the majestic Vermilion Cliffs.

The trail winds along the rim and reaches the vehicle-accessible East Rim Viewpoint Trailhead at 8,822 feet. With restroom facilities and good photography and napping possibilities, East Rim Viewpoint makes for a fine rest stop; however, camping is prohibited within 0.25 mile.

TURNAROUND NOTE: For day-hikers without a car shuttle, the East Rim View Trailhead is a prime destination; you can easily spend a few hours here before reversing your route. By the time you return to the beginning of the passage, you'll have traveled nearly 15 unforgettable miles.

Back on the AZT, join a dirt road for a brief distance, staying near the rim, and then follow a singletrack that goes around the right (east) side of a camping area. Avoid Trail #7, which descends off the rim, and stay on the very clear singletrack as it ambles along the rim to the north.

As you leave the East Rim Viewpoint, the trail widens into a road and passes a campsite on the left. Pick up a singletrack that takes off to the left by a carsonite post. Go about 40 yards, cross FR 611 at a right angle, and continue on a doubletrack to the west-northwest. Soon you pass a scenic pond called Dog Lake. About 0.5 mile past Dog Lake, follow a doubletrack northwest through a long meadow for 0.6 mile. When you reenter the trees, the AZT leaves the road to the left on a singletrack. The trail crosses two old roads and then begins a major descent through a series of switchbacks to reach the peaceful valley called Upper Tater Canyon.

Turn right (north) onto an old doubletrack and walk along the narrow, flat meadow. Watch for a carsonite AZT sign, and be careful to avoid a faint doubletrack that climbs out of the valley to the left. Near the north end of the valley, the road you're following curves to the left. Look for carsonite posts marking a singletrack that branches off to the right. Follow it for 0.1 mile, and then turn right onto a doubletrack that climbs northwest away from the meadow. Cross a fence and an adjacent road at a right angle, and then follow a singletrack on the other side.

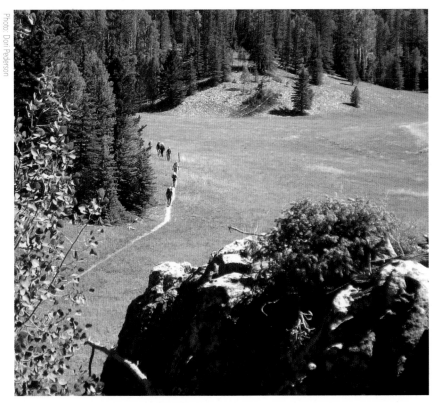

During summer and autumn, the AZT along Passage 40 is simply divine.

The trail winds through the forest, passing a murky pond. Cross a well-graded dirt road (FR 221). Continue on a singletrack, cross another road in 0.2 mile, and pick up a doubletrack trending just east of north, which quickly bends west before returning to a north-northwest direction. In 0.5 mile, follow a singletrack that leaves the right side of the road and curves northwest through a pleasant grove of aspen trees. Soon you see AZ 67 in sprawling Pleasant Valley to the west.

In less than 1 mile, the doubletrack fades to a singletrack that is occasionally obscure. It descends to a broad, grassy extension of Pleasant Valley and then climbs an old jeep road to the northwest. As the trail regains the trees, follow a left fork less than 100 yards to a singletrack that continues straight ahead to the northwest. Brown carsonite posts clearly mark the route.

Roll through the forest and meadows, entering a very large meadow 15 miles from the start of the passage. As the trail fades, follow a faint doubletrack to the left (west) along the north edge of the meadow, passing Little Pleasant Valley Tank. Descend to another meadow, and follow a singletrack to the right (north) past a large pond. The AZT climbs and then descends to parallel AZ 67, passing through an old corral before reaching Crane Lake in the middle of another large meadow. Crane Lake has seasonal water. Passage 40 ends at mile 21.4 about 2.75 miles beyond Crane Lake after a steep climb to the top of Telephone Hill at FR 241.

Mountain Bike Notes

With singletrack almost the entire way, this passage offers one of the best moderate rides along the AZT, passing through evergreen forests and peaceful meadows, with far-reaching views from the East Rim. Although it's a long way from anywhere, this passage should be a destination for mountain bikers everywhere. *For more information about mountain biking along the Arizona National Scenic Trail, visit* **aztrail.org.**

SOUTHERN ACCESS: Kaibab National Forest Boundary

From Jacob Lake, drive south on AZ 67 for 26 miles and turn left (east) onto FR 611 (4.5 miles north of the Grand Canyon National Park North Entrance Station and 1 mile

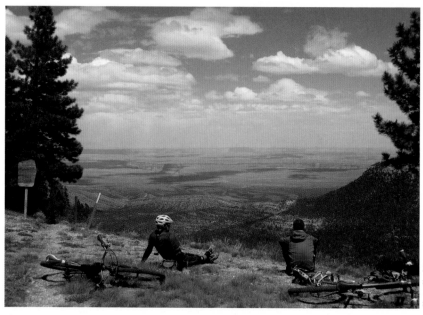

The East Rim Viewpoint along Passage 40 beckons trail travelers to stop and soak up the scenery.

Photo: Chad Brown

south of Kaibab Lodge). Drive 1.1 miles, and turn right (east) onto FR 610. Wind south and then east 5.1 miles to the FR 610 Trailhead on the south side of the road. The trailhead includes a permanent toilet and is located near where the AZT crosses FR 610 and about 0.5 mile north of the boundary of Grand Canyon National Park.

ALTERNATE SOUTHERN ACCESS: East Rim Viewpoint Trailhead

From Jacob Lake, head south on AZ 67 for 26.5 miles (0.7 mile beyond DeMotte Campground) and turn left (east) on FR 611. Follow FR 611 for 4 miles to the East Rim Viewpoint Trailhead.

NORTHERN ACCESS: Telephone Hill

About 13.5 miles south of Jacob Lake on AZ 67, look for a sign pointing to FR 429 on the west side. Do not turn right onto FR 429, but instead turn left (east) onto FR 241. In 0.1 mile, the AZT crosses the road, but there is no parking here. Continue another 0.1 mile to a little campsite on the left, where you may find a place to park.

PASSAGE 41

Kaibab Plateau: Central

KEY INFO

LOCATION Telephone Hill to US 89A

DISTANCE 17.2 miles one-way

DAY-TRIP OPTION See turnaround note in the trail description.

SHUTTLE RECOMMENDATION Murray Lake (FR 205) Trailhead (passage mile 8.6)

DIFFICULTY Easy

LAND MANAGER Kaibab National Forest, North Kaibab Ranger District, **www.fs.usda.gov/kaibab,** 928-643-7395

RECOMMENDED MONTHS April–October

GATEWAY COMMUNITIES See North Rim to Jacob Lake (page 332) and Page (page 334).

GEOLOGY HIGHLIGHTS Not applicable

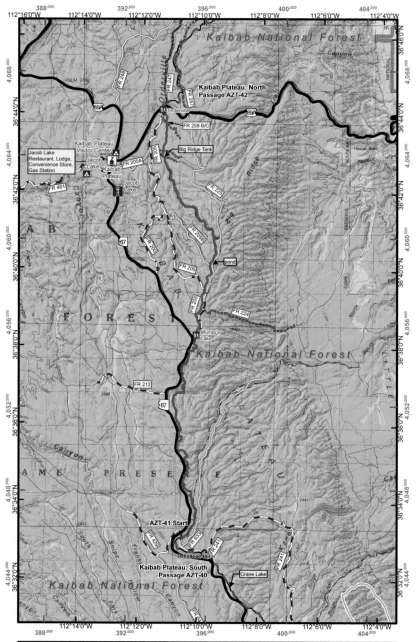

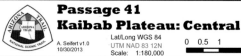

Passage 41
Kaibab Plateau: Central

Lat/Long WGS 84
UTM NAD 83 12N
Scale: 1:180,000

A. Seifert v1.0
10/30/2013

0   0.5   1   2
Miles

ARIZONA TRAIL
NATIONAL SCENIC TRAIL

OVERVIEW

The first half of Passage 41 crosses an area burned by the 2006 Warm Fire. The ponderosa pine forest was totally incinerated, but new growth of aspen trees and many species of grasses, shrubs, and flowers are beginning the natural restoration process. The AZT was reopened to users on August 15, 2011, after several years of clearing a corridor of dead timber and restoration of the trail by the U.S. Forest Service.

Beyond the burn area, the pleasant hiking and mountain biking experience of the Kaibab Plateau Trail (Trail 101) continues. As the trail gradually descends, the spruce trees of the previous passage give way to stands of ponderosa pine, and the land is noticeably drier. You're unlikely to encounter any free-flowing water. The trail crosses many dirt roads in this passage, but they are not busy. Hunting is popular here in the fall; consult the U.S. Forest Service for information about hunting seasons.

ON THE TRAIL

From the top of Telephone Hill at 8,848 feet, the AZT departs northbound, parallel to AZ 67, on a renovated logging skid road that has been converted into singletrack. It passes through the burn area of the 2006 Warm Fire; dead timber has been cleared back about 100 yards on either side of the trail.

At mile 5.5 the trail turns to the right (east) and drops steeply into a wooded canyon largely spared from the fire. The trail bends left (northwest) to climb out of the canyon. After a high point, it crosses a jeep road and makes a rolling descent on an old road to the northwest. Evidence of the Warm Fire fades, and the AZT crosses FR 205 at the Murray's Lake Trailhead near a parking lot and a toilet, and continues northward (see Turnaround Note, next page).

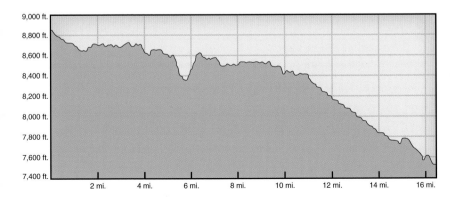

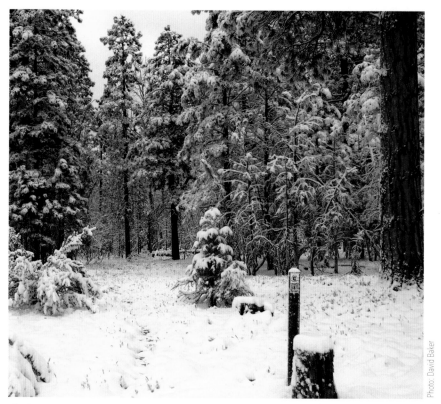

The high elevation and extreme climate of the Kaibab Plateau typically keep the trail blanketed with snow from November through May.

TURNAROUND NOTE: Day-hikers who haven't arranged a car shuttle should consider the Murray's Lake/FR 205 Trailhead their turnaround spot. Although it's tempting to continue heading north, the trailhead is 8.6 miles into the passage.

Following carsonite posts, the singletrack continues northward parallel to FR 205. It soon crosses two obscure forest roads and then rolls over flat, open forest terrain. The AZT crosses FR 205 when this road turns to the northwest and continues on to cross FR 205B. At mile 11.3 the trail passes a water-collection facility for wildlife, with a large storage tank on the right and a pond that may have seasonal water. The trail turns to the left and descends to an abandoned gas pipeline road in the bottom of the drainage. Follow the drainage downslope for the next 3 miles to pass a gravel pit and continue on a wide, old roadbed to the northwest.

The next seasonal water source, at mile 15.5, is Big Ridge Tank (7,738 feet). At the far side of the tank, the AZT follows a singletrack to the right (north-northwest). After crossing a dirt road, the trail proceeds northeast across a ridge. At an intersection marked by a sign for FR 258B/C, it turns left (north) and continues 0.2 mile on the road to a sign that marks a singletrack climbing away from the road to the right (north). Follow this trail 0.5 mile to reach the parking lot and Orderville Trailhead at the end of Passage 41. At the trailhead is a permanent toilet and a large wooden sign marking the first segment of the AZT, dedicated in 1988.

Mountain Bike Notes

This passage's cycling is mostly easy, with a clear trail and just a few steep climbs and descents. It's another one of the destination trails for mountain bikers visiting northern Arizona. *For more information about mountain biking along the Arizona National Scenic Trail, visit* aztrail.org.

SOUTHERN ACCESS: Telephone Hill

About 13.5 miles south of Jacob Lake on AZ 67, look for a sign pointing to FR 429 on the west side. Do not turn right onto FR 429, but instead turn left (east) onto FR 241. In 0.1 mile, the AZT crosses the road, but there is no parking here. Continue another 0.1 mile to a little campsite on the left, where you may be able to park.

NORTHERN ACCESS: Orderville Trailhead

From Jacob Lake, head east on US 89A for 2.2 miles, and then turn right (south) on FR 205. The trailhead is on the left after 0.1 mile.

Kaibab Plateau: North

KEY INFO

LOCATION US 89A to Winter Road

DISTANCE 17 miles

DAY-TRIP OPTION There are no obvious intermediate destinations along this passage, so day-trippers without a car shuttle should reverse their route based on individual endurance. The trail gradually loses elevation from start to finish, with a dramatic descent occurring after passage mile 7.2. Before your energy levels are halfway drained, remember that it's all uphill back to US 89A.

SHUTTLE RECOMMENDATION FR 248 (passage mile 11.6)

DIFFICULTY Moderate

LAND MANAGER Kaibab National Forest, North Kaibab Ranger District, **www.fs.usda.gov/kaibab,** 928-643-7395

RECOMMENDED MONTHS April–October

GATEWAY COMMUNITIES See North Rim to Jacob Lake (page 332) and Page (page 334).

GEOLOGY HIGHLIGHTS Not applicable

OVERVIEW

The Arizona National Scenic Trail's (AZT's) final major ecosystem change occurs on this route. The trail begins in a ponderosa pine forest and descends into high desert

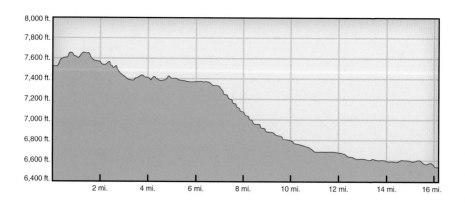

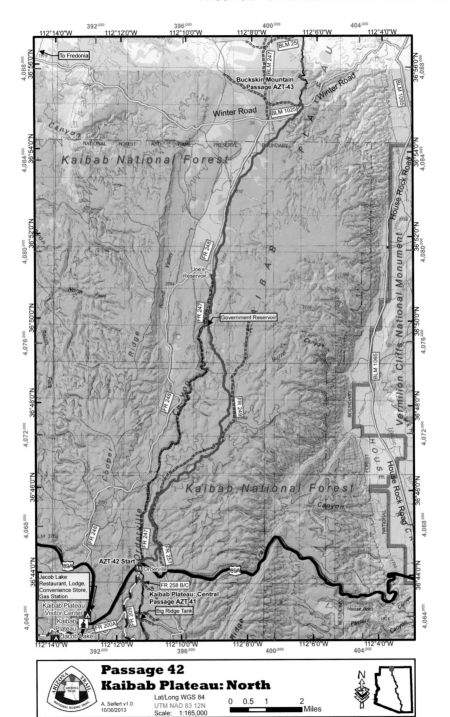

Passage 42
Kaibab Plateau: North

A. Seifert v1.0
10/30/2013

Lat/Long WGS 84
UTM NAD 83 12N
Scale: 1:165,000

0   0.5   1   2
━━━━━━━━━━━━ Miles

N

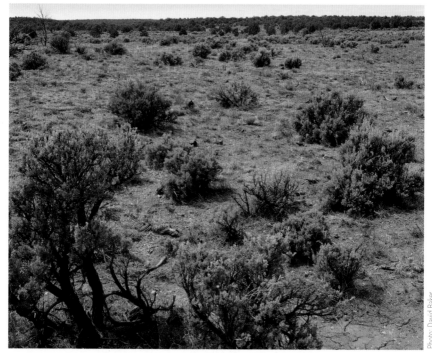

Descending from the Kaibab Plateau to the Great Basin Conifer Woodland, the landscape is soon covered with red dirt and big sagebrush (*Artemisia tridentata*).

populated with sagebrush, juniper trees, and creeping prickly pear. The trail is frequently faint, but cairns and signs for Trail 101 mark the route.

ON THE TRAIL

From the parking area at 7,523 feet, follow the dirt road north 50 yards to the paved highway. Bear diagonally right, and carefully cross the highway to a dirt road on the other side. Look for a sign on the right that says KAIBAB PLATEAU TRAIL #101. Follow a singletrack into the trees behind the sign, trending slightly east of north. After 0.2 mile, turn right at a barbed-wire fence and follow the fence line for 20 yards. Then curve left to follow a bend in the fence. In the next 0.5 mile the AZT winds its way along or near the fence. The trail is easy to follow as it makes its way to a ravine. The trail trends north, crossing FR 249 at a right angle. Follow signs for Trail 101.

Continue northward, staying above Orderville Canyon (to the west) and keeping dirt FR 249 to the east. The trail veers right (northeast) to cross at a right angle. After you cross another road at mile 4, the trail becomes invisible, but cairns show the way. The route parallels Orderville Canyon, which remains on your left (west). Stay away from the frequent doubletracks that try to lure you away to the east. Look for cairns to assist you.

Cross FR 249 about 5.5 miles from the start of this passage, and continue due north through a burn area, following cairns. The AZT continues to trend between northeast and northwest, occasionally crossing dirt roads. The trail descends into a shallow ravine, which it follows through ponderosa pines. The ravine ends abruptly at a gigantic clearing covered with sagebrush. Government Reservoir is across FR 247 about 500 yards but rarely has water.

The route is obvious, as a clear swath has been cut through the sage, heading north along the far right (east) side of this open area. Where the sagebrush ends, it becomes harder to follow the trail. Just keep the piñon and juniper trees close on your right, and follow denuded ground that indicates a trail. You come to an intersection with the Navajo Trail, which leads 0.25 mile west to Joe's Reservoir.

The trail winds through a pleasant high-desert forest of juniper and small pines for the next mile and then enters another large field of sage and promptly disappears. Look for an obscure swath through the sagebrush slightly west of north. Cross a faint road at a right angle and reenter the trees. In 1 mile, the forest gives way to a gothic landscape

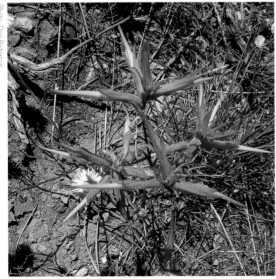

Photo: Dori Pederson

Indian paintbrush (*Castilleja linariifolia*) is a familiar flower along Passage 42.

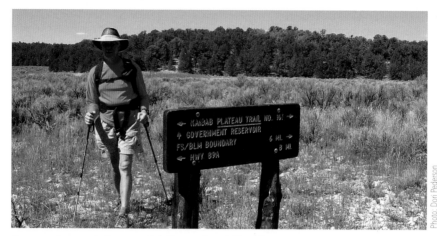

From south to north, Passage 42 follows a downhill grade toward the Utah border.

of dead trees where the trail disappears again. Continue in the same direction to reach the other side.

In 0.5 mile, you cross another large field of sage, but there is an obvious trail corridor. The AZT crosses a doubletrack and a sturdy barbed-wire fence. In 0.2 mile, after another road-and-fence encounter, a trail lined with logs and debris winds to the northeast. You reach Winter Road, or BLM Road 1025 at 6,531 feet and the end of Passage 42. There is a decent campsite about 250 yards west of Winter Road.

Mountain Bike Notes

The riding on this passage is mostly easy. Downed timber and soft ground present the toughest obstacles. *For more information about mountain biking along the Arizona National Scenic Trail, visit* **aztrail.org.**

SOUTHERN ACCESS: Orderville Trailhead

From Jacob Lake, head east on US 89A for 2.2 miles, and then turn right (south) on FR 205. The trailhead is on the left after 0.1 mile.

NORTHERN ACCESS: Winter Road

From US 89A, at House Rock Road, 13.7 miles east of Jacob Lake, turn north on House Rock Road for 15.6 miles to Winter Road (BLM Road 1025). Turn left (west) on Winter Road for 3.7 miles to the AZT, where a large metal AZT sign indicates the trailhead.

Buckskin Mountain

KEY INFO

LOCATION Winter Road to Utah border

DISTANCE 10.8 miles one-way

DAY-TRIP OPTION See turnaround note in the trail description.

SHUTTLE RECOMMENDATION BLM 14 (passage mile 6.7)

DIFFICULTY Easy

LAND MANAGER Bureau of Land Management, Arizona Strip Field Office, **blm.gov/az/st/en/fo/arizona_strip_field.html**, 602-417-9200

RECOMMENDED MONTHS March–November

GATEWAY COMMUNITIES See Page (page 334) and Fredonia, Arizona, and Kanab, Utah (page 335).

GEOLOGY HIGHLIGHTS Not applicable

OVERVIEW

The Arizona National Scenic Trail (AZT) ends in the north much like it began in the south: in the middle of nowhere. This is entirely appropriate, of course, because getting to the middle of nowhere defines the AZT experience. This spectacularly beautiful final passage along the eastern flank of Buckskin Mountain marks a return to the high-desert ecosystem of small cacti, colorful shrubs, and hardy piñon and juniper trees. You'll enjoy sweeping views of Utah to the north and the brightly colored Vermilion Cliffs to the east. The trail along most of this passage is clear and easy to follow.

ON THE TRAIL

From Winter Road at 6,531 feet, at a large steel AZT trailhead sign, follow a clear singletrack northwest through a pleasant juniper–piñon forest, rolling in and out of washes and crossing the occasional dusty road. Then begin a gradual descent to a shallow valley. The trail is sometimes obscure here, but cairns occasionally mark the way. The trail becomes clearer after crossing a faint road. After crossing a primitive road (BLM 14), the trail bends right to trend east-northeast.

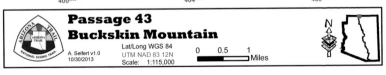

Passage 43
Buckskin Mountain

A. Seifert v1.0
10/30/2013

Lat/Long WGS 84
UTM NAD 83 12N
Scale: 1:115,000

0   0.5   1
Miles

N

TURNAROUND NOTE: Because this is among the shortest of the AZT's 43 passages, many people attempt it in a single push, especially if they're able to arrange a car shuttle. But day-hikers who want to get a taste of this passage or who prefer to cover the out-and-back distance with a shorter mileage commitment could ideally turn around at passage mile 6.7, where the trail meets the faint BLM Road 14.

Continuing along an eastern path the AZT begins its long descent toward Utah by joining the drainage of North Larkum Canyon. The trail dances in and out of this canyon until it exits on the left (north) and climbs gradually to the adjoining ridge. Straight ahead, you can see the dramatic Vermilion Cliffs.

At 8.5 miles from your starting point, the trail descends via switchbacks to the northeast and Coyote Valley comes into view. You reach the bottom of the switchbacks after 1.5 miles. Continue northeast across the sagebrush-covered valley to a low, rocky ridge. The trail descends the other side of this ridge to a parking lot marked by ramadas, picnic tables, restrooms (without water), and an informational kiosk at the trailhead at 4,992 feet. This staging area marks the end of the AZT, but perhaps the beginning of many wanderings into the wildlands of southern Utah, including Coyote Buttes and Paria Canyon.

Mountain Bike Notes

The excellent mountain biking of the Kaibab Plateau continues here, with mostly intermediate riding and the occasional technical section. A northbound ride is decidedly

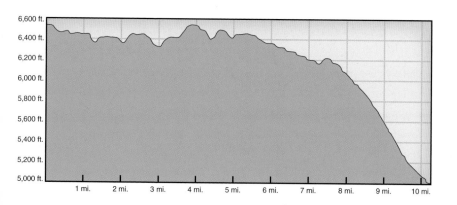

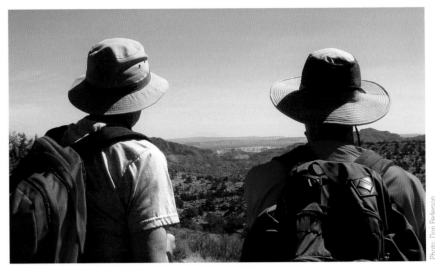

Photo: Dori Pederson

Although the AZT ends at the border of Utah, unlimited adventures await within the canyon country to the north.

easier than heading south because of the elevation loss. *For more information about mountain biking along the Arizona National Scenic Trail, visit* **aztrail.org.**

SOUTHERN ACCESS: Winter Road

From US 89A, at House Rock Road, 13.7 miles east of Jacob Lake, turn north on House Rock Road for 15.6 miles to Winter Road (BLM Road 1025). Turn left (west) on Winter Road for 3.7 miles to the AZT, where a large metal AZT sign marks the trailhead.

NORTHERN ACCESS: Stateline Trailhead

It may help to set your odometer to zero in Page, Arizona. From Page, head west on AZ 98 for 2.5 miles to US 89, and turn right (north). At mile 6.4, you pass Wahweap Marina, which offers camping. Cross the state line at mile 13. At mile 38 from Page, just after mile marker 25, you pass through a roadcut, and the highway begins a big, sweeping curve to the right. At the end of the guardrail on the left, turn left (south) onto a dirt road. This is 0.2 mile south of mile marker 26 (from Kanab, this turnoff is about 36 miles "south" according to signs—actually geographically east—on US 89).

Follow the dirt road for 10 miles, and then turn right (west) onto a well-graded dirt road. Continue 0.2 mile to a parking area, restrooms, and several campsites. The trailhead is on the left as you drive in. Park in designated spots only.

GATEWAY COMMUNITIES
(South to North)

TOWNS AND CITIES ALONG the Arizona National Scenic Trail (AZT) welcome hikers, cyclists, and equestrians. Trail users will find a wide variety of services in some communities, and a limited selection in others. Thus, categories of resources—such as Internet Venues, Lodging, or Feed and Tack—do not appear in all of the following listings (which are current as of this book's publication). Regardless of the array of services, all 32 Gateway Communities extend an invitation for you to relax and resupply—and to come again.

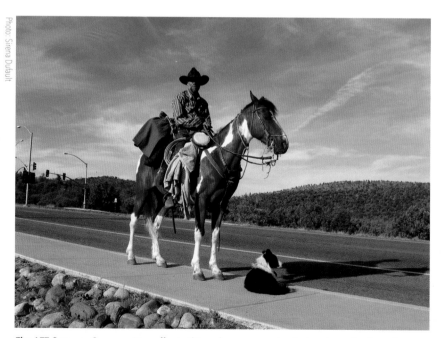

The AZT Gateway Communities offer trail travelers an opportunity to relax, refresh, and resupply before they head back out onto the trail.

GUIDE to
GATEWAY COMMUNITIES and GEOLOGY SITES

PASSAGE	GATEWAY COMMUNITY(IES)	GEOLOGY SITE
SOUTH SECTION		
1. Huachuca Mountains (page 50)	Sierra Vista (page 303)	Not applicable
2. Canelo Hills: East (page 58)	Not applicable	Not applicable
3. Canelo Hills: West (page 63)	Patagonia (page 305)	Not applicable
4. Temporal Gulch (page 69)	Patagonia (page 305) Sonoita (page 306)	Not applicable
5. Santa Rita Mountains (page 75)	Sonoita (page 306)	Not applicable
6. Las Colinas (page 81)	Not applicable	Not applicable
7. Las Cienegas (page 86)	Sonoita (page 306) Vail (page 308)	Not applicable
8. Rincon Valley (page 91)	Vail (page 308)	"The Karst of Colossal Cave" (page 338)
9. Rincon Mountains (page 96)	Tucson (page 310)	"The Mighty Santa Catalina and Rincon Mountains" (page 339)
10. Redington Pass (page 103)	Tucson (page 310)	"The Mighty Santa Catalina and Rincon Mountains" (page 339)
11. Santa Catalina Mountains (page 109)	Tucson (page 310) Summerhaven (page 312)	"The Mighty Santa Catalina and Rincon Mountains" (page 339)
12. Oracle Ridge (page 116)	Summerhaven (page 312) Oracle (page 314) San Manuel (page 317)	"The Mighty Santa Catalina and Rincon Mountains" (page 339)

GUIDE to
GATEWAY COMMUNITIES and GEOLOGY SITES

PASSAGE	GATEWAY COMMUNITY(IES)	GEOLOGY SITE
13. Oracle (page 122)	Oracle (page 314) Mammoth (page 315) San Manuel (page 317)	"The Mighty Santa Catalina and Rincon Mountains" (page 339)
14. Black Hills (page 127)	Central Copper Corridor: Dudleyville, Winkelman, Hayden, Kearny, and Kelvin and Riverside (page 318)	Not applicable
15. Tortilla Mountains (page 132)	Central Copper Corridor: Dudleyville, Winkelman, Hayden, Kearny, and Kelvin and Riverside (page 318) Florence (page 321)	Not applicable
CENTRAL SECTION		
16. Gila River Canyons (page 140)	Central Copper Corridor: Dudleyville, Winkelman, Hayden, Kearny, and Kelvin and Riverside (page 318) Florence (page 321)	"Supervolcanoes of the Superstition Mountains" (page 341)
17. Alamo Canyon (page 146)	Globe (page 319) Florence (page 321) Superior (page 322)	"Supervolcanoes of the Superstition Mountains" (page 341)
18. Reavis Canyon (page 152)	Globe (page 319) Superior (page 322)	"Supervolcanoes of the Superstition Mountains" (page 341)
19. Superstition Wilderness (page 158)	Globe (page 319) Roosevelt and Tonto Basin (page 323)	"Supervolcanoes of the Superstition Mountains" (page 341)
20. Four Peaks (page 165)	Roosevelt and Tonto Basin (page 323)	"Amazing Mazatzals" (page 342)
21. Pine Mountain (page 171)	Roosevelt and Tonto Basin (page 323)	"Amazing Mazatzals" (page 342)

GUIDE to
GATEWAY COMMUNITIES and GEOLOGY SITES

PASSAGE	GATEWAY COMMUNITY(IES)	GEOLOGY SITE
CENTRAL SECTION (*continued*)		
22. Saddle Mountain (page 176)	Not applicable	"Amazing Mazatzals" (page 342)
23. Mazatzal Divide (page 182)	Payson (page 325)	"Amazing Mazatzals" (page 342)
24. Red Hills (page 188)	Payson (page 325)	"Amazing Mazatzals" (page 342)
25. Whiterock Mesa (page 193)	Payson (page 325)	Not applicable
26. Hardscrabble Mesa (page 199)	Payson (page 325) Pine and Strawberry (page 326)	Not applicable
27. Highline (page 204)	Pine and Strawberry (page 326)	Not applicable
NORTH SECTION		
28. Blue Ridge (page 212)	Not applicable	Not applicable
29. Happy Jack (page 218)	Mormon Lake (page 328)	Not applicable
30. Mormon Lake (page 223)	Mormon Lake (page 328)	Not applicable
31. Walnut Canyon (page 229)	Flagstaff (page 329)	Not applicable
32. Elden Mountain (page 234)	Flagstaff (page 329)	"Elden Mountain: A Volcano Unlike the Others" (page 344)
33. Flagstaff (Resupply Route) (page 238)	Flagstaff (page 329)	Not applicable

GUIDE to
GATEWAY COMMUNITIES and GEOLOGY SITES

PASSAGE	GATEWAY COMMUNITY(IES)	GEOLOGY SITE
34. San Francisco Peaks (page 243)	Flagstaff (page 329)	"The San Francisco Peaks' Violent Past" (page 345)
35. Babbitt Ranch (page 250)	Not applicable	Not applicable
36. Coconino Rim (page 255)	Tusayan and Grand Canyon Village (page 331)	Not applicable
37. Grand Canyon: South Rim (page 260)	Tusayan and Grand Canyon Village (page 331)	"The Grand Canyon: A Geological Masterpiece" (page 346)
38. Grand Canyon: Inner Gorge (page 265)	Not applicable	"The Grand Canyon: A Geological Masterpiece" (page 346)
39. Grand Canyon: North Rim (page 272)	North Rim to Jacob Lake (page 332)	"The Grand Canyon: A Geological Masterpiece" (page 346)
40. Kaibab Plateau: South (page 277)	North Rim to Jacob Lake (page 332)	Not applicable
41. Kaibab Plateau: Central (page 283)	North Rim to Jacob Lake (page 332) Page (page 334)	Not applicable
42. Kaibab Plateau: North (page 288)	North Rim to Jacob Lake (page 332) Page (page 334)	Not applicable
43. Buckskin Mountain (page 293)	Page (page 334) Fredonia, AZ, and Kanab, UT (page 335)	Not applicable

MAP of
GATEWAY COMMUNITIES

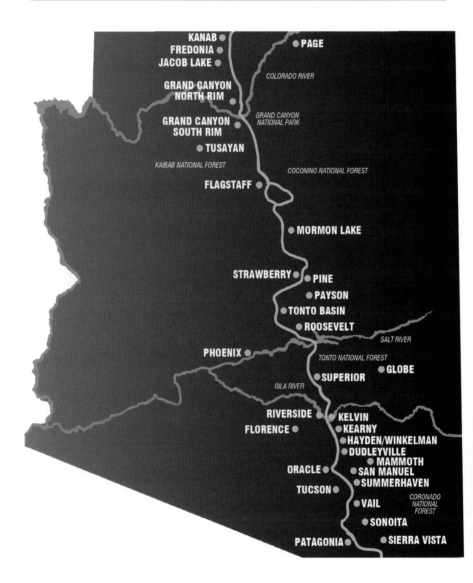

Map: Wide World of Maps / Arizona Trail Association

SIERRA VISTA

GATEWAY TO PASSAGE 1: Huachuca Mountains

OVERVIEW

Sierra Vista started out in 1877 as Camp Huachuca, established to protect settlers from attacks by Chiricahua Apache. The gateway to the southern terminus of the Arizona National Scenic Trail (AZT), Sierra Vista offers many services in locations throughout the town.

ELEVATION 4,633 feet

POPULATION 46,109

POST OFFICE 2300 East Fry Boulevard, 85635, 520-458-2540

INTERNET VENUES Sierra Vista City Library, 2600 East Tacoma Street, 520-458-4225

Groceries

Safeway, 2190 East Fry Boulevard, 520-459-4204

Sierra Vista Natural Foods Cooperative, 96 South Carmichael Avenue, 520-335-6676, **sierravistamarket.com**

Cafés and Restaurants

Gelato Java Stop, 1100 South AZ 92, 520-559-1614

Golden Dragon, 2151 AZ 92, 520-458-7575

La Casita, 465 East Fry Boulevard, 520-458-2376

Pizzeria Mimosa, 4755 East Neapolitan Way, Hereford, 520-378-0022, **pizzamimosa.com**

Lodging and Camping

Garden Place Suites, 100 North Garden Avenue, 520-439-3300, **gardenplacesuites.com**

Sierra Suites Hotel, 391 East Fry Boulevard, 520-459-4221, **sierravistasuites.com**

Bike Shops

M & M Cycling, 1301 East Fry Boulevard, 520-458-1316, **mandmcycling.com**

Sun 'n Spokes, 156 East Fry Boulevard, 520-458-0685, **sunnspokes.com**

Feed and Tack

Ramsey Canyon Feed & Pet, 4107 East Glenn Road, 520-378-9474

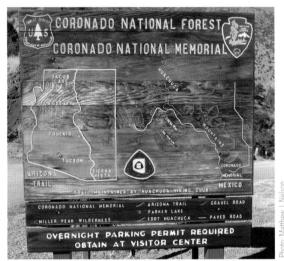

Photo: Matthew J. Nelson

The southern terminus of the AZT is just 10 miles southwest of the Gateway Community of Sierra Vista.

Other Services

Laundry: Several options are available along Fry Boulevard.

Massage: Bodyworks Therapeutic Massage, 3514 Kings Court Drive, 520-452-1776, bodyworksmassage.net

Shuttles

Arizona Sunshine Tours offers shuttles between Tucson International Airport and the AZT trailhead in Coronado National Memorial. Call 520-803-6713 or visit **arizonasunshinetours.com.**

Arizona World Shuttle Express will pick you up at the Tucson International Airport and take you to Sierra Vista and then to the Coronado National Memorial Visitor's Center near Montezuma Pass. Call 520-458-3330, 24 hours in advance.

Area Attractions

Coronado National Memorial, 4101 West Montezuma Canyon Road, Hereford, 520-366-5515: This national memorial at the Arizona National Scenic Trail's southern terminus commemorates the Francisco Vásquez de Coronado Expedition of 1540–1542.

Ramsey Canyon Nature Preserve, 27 East Ramsey Canyon Road, 520-378-2785, **tinyurl.com/ramseycanyonnp:** Ramsey Canyon, in the Huachuca Mountains within the Upper San Pedro River Basin, is renowned for its outstanding scenic beauty and the diversity of its plant and animal life, including 15 species of hummingbirds.

San Pedro Riparian National Conservation Area, 1763 Paseo San Luis, 520-439-6400: Located 6 miles east of Sierra Vista, this natural wonder contains 40 miles of protected riparian area along the San Pedro River. It also provides invaluable habitat for 250 species of migratory birds and contains archaeological sites representing human occupation from 13,000 years ago.

PATAGONIA

GATEWAY TO PASSAGE 3: Canelo Hills: West
and **PASSAGE 4:** Temporal Gulch

OVERVIEW

Native Americans, Spaniards, Mexicans, ranchers, miners, and Jesuit priests have all inhabited this land over the past 500 years. Now Patagonia is a tourist destination and naturalist's playground. Visit in mid-April for Patagonia Trail Day.

ELEVATION 4,055 feet
POPULATION 913
POST OFFICE 100 North Taylor Lane, 85624, 800-275-8777
INTERNET VENUES **Patagonia Public Library,** 346 Duquesne Avenue,
520-304-2010

Groceries

Patagonia Market, 292 Naugle Avenue, 520-394-2962

Red Mountain Foods, 347 McKeown Avenue, 520-394-2786

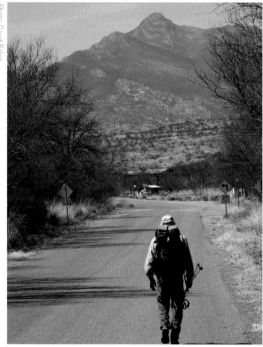

Photo: David Baker

Walking along Harshaw Road
(Passage 4) toward the
community of Patagonia

Cafés and Restaurants

Gathering Grounds, 319 McKeown Avenue, 520-394-2009, **patagoniasbuzz.com**

Mercedes Restaurant, 330 Naugle Avenue, 520-394-2331

Velvet Elvis, 292 Naugle Avenue, 520-394-2102, **velvetelvispizza.com**

Wild Horse Restaurant, 309 McKeown Avenue, 520-394-2344

Lodging and Camping

Stage Stop Inn, 303 McKeown Avenue, 520-394-2211, **stagestophotelpatagonia.com:** The Stage Stop Inn stands on the actual site of the Patagonia Stage Stop on the old Butterfield Trail. Relax in the comfy chairs by the fireplace, and grab a bite to eat at the Wild Horse Restaurant. Ask for the AZT discount.

In addition, many unique B&Bs, *casitas* (small houses), guest ranches, and rooms are available for rent in the Patagonia area. Visit **patagoniaaz.com** for more information on rates.

Other Services

Patagonia Area Business Association Visitors Center, 317 McKeown Avenue, 85624, 520-394-9186. On-site are **Mariposa Books and More (maripo@theriver.com)** and **Patagon Bike Rental** (520-604-0258, **patagonbikerental.com**). They accept packages for trail users.

Area Attractions

The Nature Conservancy's Patagonia-Sonoita Creek Preserve, 150 Blue Heaven Road, 520-394-2400, **tinyurl.com/pscpreserve:** The preserve is one of the best-known and most popular destinations for birding in the Southwest. The riparian area along Sonoita Creek contains some of the richest habitat remaining in southern Arizona. More than 300 species migrate, nest, and live in this critical habitat.

Patagonia Lake State Park, 400 Patagonia Lake Road, 520-287-6965: Hiking trails, rental boats, a campground, a day-use area, and picnic ramadas await you in the park, which also offers beach access and regularly scheduled birding tours on foot and by pontoon boat.

SONOITA

GATEWAY TO PASSAGE 4: Temporal Gulch, **PASSAGE 5:** Santa Rita Mountains, and **PASSAGE 7:** Las Cienegas

OVERVIEW

Sonoita is home to Arizona's Wine Country, in the rolling grasslands and oak forests at the junction of AZ 82 and 83 east of the Santa Rita Mountains. The Sonoita Valley used

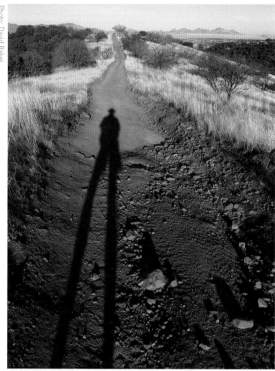

In the heart of Arizona's wine country, the town of Sonoita offers AZT users great food and basic trail necessities.

to be known for its cattle ranches and then for its contributions to the movie industry (*Oklahoma!* was filmed nearby).

ELEVATION 4,987 feet
POPULATION 1,000
POST OFFICE 3166 AZ 83, Suite 1, 85637, 520-455-5500
INTERNET VENUES **Sonoita Community Library,** 3147 AZ 83, 520-455-5517

Groceries

Sonoita Mercantile Country Store, 3235 AZ 82, 520-455-5788:
Has a gas station and ATM.

Sonoita Mini Market, 3160 AZ 82, 520-455-5613

Cafés and Restaurants

The Café, 3280 AZ 82, 520-455-5044, **cafesonoita.com**

The Steak Out Restaurant & Saloon, 3200 South Sonoita Highway, 520-455-5205, **azsteakout.com**

Tia Nita's Cantina, 3119 AZ 83, 520-455-0500

Lodging and Camping

Crown C Ranch, 139 Crown C Ranch Road, 520-455-5739, **crowncranch.com:** Single rooms and guest house. A ranch house is also available, accommodating groups of up to 18.

Sonoita Inn, 3243 AZ 82, 520-455-5935, **sonoita inn.com:** Rustic accommodations in the rolling grasslands of Sonoita.

Feed and Tack

Sonoita Feed, 3254 AZ 82, 520-455-5544

Massage Therapy

Cynthia Carlisi, 520-394-2104, **canyonwmn@theriver.com**

Area Attractions

Empire Ranch, AZ 83 at milepost 40, 520-439-6400: The Empire Ranch House is a 22-room adobe-and-wood-frame building that dates to 1870 and is listed on the National Register of Historic Places. Tours of the ranch are available, and miles of trails pass through towering cottonwoods along the flowing cienega.

Sonoita Wine Trail: Take a break from the Arizona Trail to hop on the Sonoita Wine Trail, which visits vineyards between Sonoita and Elgin. A map is available at **arizonawine.org/sonoitaWineTrail.html.**

Parker Canyon, 520-455-5847, **parkercanyonlake.com:** A beautiful 130-acre lake located in the high, cool, rolling hills of southern Arizona. Amenities include a mercantile and marina store, restrooms, drinking water, boat ramp, fishing pier, lakeside trail, and a 65-space campground with restrooms, picnic tables, and grills.

VAIL

GATEWAY TO PASSAGE 7: Las Cienegas
and **PASSAGE 8:** Rincon Valley

OVERVIEW

Originally a Southern Pacific railroad town, Vail is a growing community east of Tucson in the foothills of the Rincon Mountains. This "town between the tracks" is also home to Colossal Cave Mountain Park and the Gabe Zimmerman Memorial Trailhead.

ELEVATION 3,235 feet
POPULATION 10,208
POST OFFICE 13190 East Colossal Cave Road, 85641. (**Colossal Cave Mountain Park,** 16721 East Old Spanish Trail, Tucson, AZ 85641, also accepts packages.)

Groceries

Quik Mart, 13142 East Colossal Cave Road, 520-762-1009

Cafés and Restaurants

Dairy Queen, 13160 East Colossal Cave Road, 520-762-0343

Hot Rods Restaurant, Bar and Lounge, 10500 East Old Vail Road, 520-202-0987

La Posta Quemada Ranch in Colossal Cave Mountain Park: Follow the sign on the AZT for the spur trail with a knife and fork on it a quarter-mile west.

Montgomery's Grill and Saloon, 13190 East Colossal Cave Road, 520-762-0081

Nico's Taco Shop, 13303 East Colossal Cave Road, 520-762-8888

Valeria's Comida Mexicana, 11800 East Old Vail Road (no public phone number)

Bike Shops

Ben's Bikes, 7431 South Houghton Road, 520-574-2453: Full-service shop near the trail.

Area Attractions

Colossal Cave, 16721 East Old Spanish Trail, 520-647-7275, **colossalcave.com:** Cave tours are just a short distance from the Arizona Trail. The trail goes through Colossal Cave Mountain Park, but to see the cave itself requires a detour of 2 miles. Take the spur trail to La Posta Quemada Ranch and continue north on Colossal Cave Road.

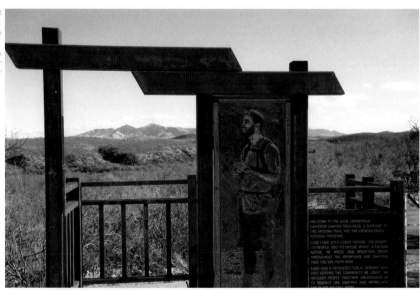

From the Gabe Zimmerman Trailhead at the northern end of Passage 7, the town of Vail is not far away.

Gabe Zimmerman Memorial Trailhead, Marsh Station Road: From I-10, Exit 281, loop exit to Marsh Station Road. Travel northeast on Marsh Station Road approximately 3 miles. Zimmerman, a 30-year-old aide to then–U.S. Representative Gabrielle Giffords, was killed along with five others in the January 8, 2011, Tucson shootings that injured Giffords and a dozen others. This trailhead and interpretive trail celebrates his life and love of the outdoors and Arizona Trail.

TUCSON

GATEWAY TO PASSAGE 9: Rincon Mountains, **PASSAGE 10:** Redington Pass, and **PASSAGE 11:** Santa Catalina Mountains

OVERVIEW

"The Old Pueblo," as Tucson is known, has a rich history stretching back to Archaic times. It is surrounded by mountain ranges that offer year-round outdoor recreation. All trail amenities are accessible from either Redington Road or Molino Basin. Services listed here are proximal to the AZT, but if you head into midtown or downtown, the possibilities for food, drink, and much more are unlimited.

ELEVATION 2,389 feet
POPULATION 525,796
POST OFFICE 8987 East Tanque Verde Road, 85749, 520-749-4845
INTERNET VENUES Kirk Bear Canyon Library, 8959 East Tanque Verde Road, 520-594-5275

Groceries

Safeway, 9125 East Tanque Verde Road, 520-760-6087

Cafés and Restaurants

The nearest intersection for restaurants is Catalina Highway and Tanque Verde Road.

Fortunato's Italian Deli, 9100 East Tanque Verde Road, 520-795-3354, **fortunatosdeli.com**

Le Buzz, 9121 East Tanque Verde Road, #125, 520-749-3903, **lebuzzcaffe.com**

Renee's Organic Oven, 7065 East Tanque Verde Road, 520-886-0484, **reneesorganicoven.com**

Lodging and Camping

Comfort Suites at Sabino Canyon, 7007 East Tanque Verde Road, 520-298-2300, **tucsoncs.com:** 13 miles from Molino Basin and 25 miles from Redington Road.

Ramada Inn and Suites, 6944 East Tanque Verde Road, 520-886-9595

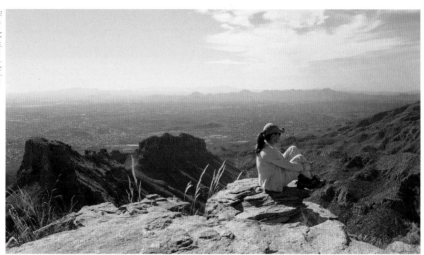

The big city of Tucson is quite a contrast to the remote valleys and mountains of Passages 10 and 11, but it's easily accessible from Redington Road and General Hitchcock Highway.

Bike and Other Outdoors Shops

Fleet Feet Sports Tucson, 7301 East Tanque Verde Road, 520-886-7800: Locally owned running, walking, and fitness specialty store.

Pro Bike, 6540 East Tanque Verde Road, 520-722-2453, **probiketucson.com**

Sabino Cycles, 7045 East Tanque Verde Road, 520-885-3666, **sabinocycles.com**

Summit Hut, 5045 East Speedway Boulevard, 520-325-1554; 7745 North Oracle Road, 520-888-1000; **summithut.com:** Local outdoor outfitter with a friendly and knowledgeable staff. Founder Dave Baker thru-hiked the AZT in 2008.

REI, 160 West Wetmore Road, 520-887-1938

Feed and Tack

Tanque Verde Hay Feed & Supply, 11050 East Tanque Verde Road, 520-749-0211

Tucson Feed & Pet Supply, 7878 East Tanque Verde Road, 520-731-8738, **thepetclub.net**

Other Services

Wayne Blankenship, LMT, 520-907-0412, **wayneblankenship@hotmail.com:** Discounts for trail users.

Angie Edge, LMT, 520-579-5980, **edge.angie@gmail.com**

Tanque Verde Chiropractic Clinic, 9100 East Tanque Verde Road, 520-749-2929, **tanqueverdechiropractic.com**

Area Attractions

Arizona-Sonora Desert Museum, 2021 North Kinney Road, 520-883-2702, **desert museum.org:** A world-renowned zoo, natural history museum, and botanical garden, all in one place! The museum offers interpretive displays of living animals and plants native to the Sonoran Desert. It's on the other side of town from the trail, but worth a visit if you have some time to explore Tucson.

Fourth Avenue and Congress Street: Fourth Avenue is Tucson's area for bars, clubs, and live music. Nearby is the historic **Hotel Congress,** established in 1919 and the location of the capture of John Dillinger in 1934.

SUMMERHAVEN

GATEWAY TO PASSAGE 11: Santa Catalina Mountains
and **PASSAGE 12:** Oracle Ridge

OVERVIEW

This small but important Gateway Community gives Arizona National Scenic Trail (AZT) users a chance to stop and refuel during their traverse of the Santa Catalina Mountains north of Tucson. Located at 8,200 feet, it has been rebuilt in the wake of the devastating Aspen Fire of 2003.

ELEVATION 8,200 feet
POPULATION 40
POST OFFICE 12984 North Sabino Canyon Road, Mt. Lemmon, 85619,
520-576-1427
INTERNET VENUES **Sawmill Run Restaurant** (see below) offers free Wi-Fi.

Groceries

Mt. Lemmon General Store & Gift Shop, 12856 North Sabino Canyon Parkway, 520-576-1468: Will hold packages for trail users.

Cafés and Restaurants

Iron Door Restaurant, 10300 East Ski Run Road, 520-576-1400: At Ski Valley, 1 mile northeast of Summerhaven

Mt. Lemmon Cookie Cabin, 12781 North Sabino Canyon Parkway, 520-576-1010

Sawmill Run Restaurant, 12976 North Sabino Canyon Parkway, 520-576-9147, sawmillrun.com

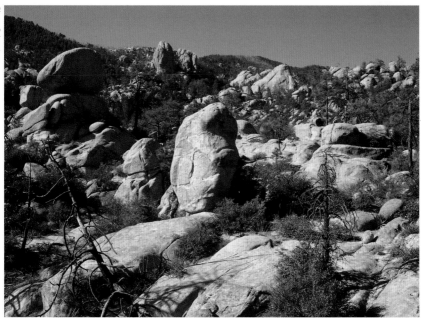

Photo: Robert Luce

The small community of Summerhaven provides immediate access to the Wilderness of Rocks, near the summit of the Santa Catalina Mountains.

Lodging and Camping

The Moose Cabin on Mt. Lemmon, 520-429-4232, **mtlemmoncabin.com:** Two-night minimum.

Mt. Lemmon Cabins, 520-576-1455, **mtlemmoncabins.com**

Other Services

Mount Lemmon Community Center, 12949 North Sabino Canyon Parkway, 520-877-6000: Facility has public restrooms with water.

Area Attractions

Mount Lemmon Ski Valley, 10300 East Ski Run Road, 520-576-1321, **skithelemmon .com:** One mile away from Summerhaven is the southernmost ski resort in the United States. When the conditions allow, ski 21 runs in winter, or get on the ski lift for a scenic ride to the top of the mountain in summer.

Santa Catalina Mountain trail system: An endless network of trails allows for all sorts of possibilities for loop- and shuttle-trail adventures. Check **www.fs.usda.gov /coronado** for maps and information.

ORACLE

GATEWAY TO PASSAGE 12: Oracle Ridge
and **PASSAGE 13:** Oracle

OVERVIEW

Oracle has had many incarnations: a gold-mining town, a haven for people suffering from tuberculosis, a Hollywood filming location, an artists' retreat, and a retirement community. The town is nestled in the foothills of the northern portion of the Santa Catalina Mountains.

ELEVATION 4,524 feet
POPULATION 3,563
POST OFFICE 905 East American Avenue, 85623, 520-896-2641
INTERNET VENUES **Oracle Public Library,** 565 East American Avenue, 520-896-2121

Groceries

Oracle Market, 760 East American Avenue, 520-896-2232

Cafés and Restaurants

Casa Rivera's, 1975 West American Avenue, 520-896-3747

De Marco's Pizza and Italian Food, 1885 West American Avenue, 520-896-9627

Oracle Inn Steakhouse, 305 East American Avenue, 520-896-3333, **oracleinn.com**

The Oracle Patio Cafe, 270 East American Avenue, 520-896-7615, **oraclepatiocafe.com**

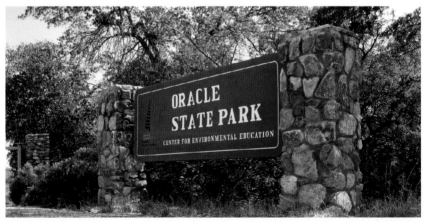

Photo: Terri Gay

The AZT travels through Oracle State Park and very close to the artistic, eclectic, and adorable town of Oracle.

Lodging and Camping

Chalet Village Motel, 1245 West American Avenue, 520-896-9171: A stay in the charming A-frame rooms in the center of Oracle will recharge you for the trail ahead. The motel accepts packages and shuttles hikers.

El Rancho Robles Guest Ranch, 1170 North Rancho Robles Road, 520-896-7651, **elranchorobles.com:** This restored dude ranch offers rooms and casitas among the oaks and boulders.

High Jinks Ranch Bed and Breakfast, highjinksranch.net: This site started out as Buffalo Bill Cody's 1912 gold claim and ranch, and is listed on the National Register of Historic Places. Contact **laurel@highjinksranch.net** to check on the availability of guest accommodations. It is located along the trail.

Peppersauce Campground, Coronado National Forest, Santa Catalina Ranger District, 520-749-8700, 6 miles southeast of Oracle on Forest Road 38 (40 miles northeast of Tucson): $10 per night, per vehicle.

Massage Therapy

Sanctuary Massage Studios, 1995 West American Avenue, 520-896-6539, **ramonassanctuary@gmail.com**

Area Attractions

Biosphere 2, 32540 South Biosphere Road, 520-838-6200, **b2science.org:** The Biosphere 2 facility serves as a center for research, outreach, teaching, and lifelong learning about earth, its living systems, and its place in the universe. From 1991 to 1993, eight researchers lived inside the biosphere and were required to get everything they needed from the closed system. Tours are available.

Oracle State Park, 3820 Wildlife Drive, 520-896-2425, **azstateparks.com:** Oracle State Park is a 4,000-acre wildlife refuge located on the northern foothills of the Santa Catalina Mountains north of Tucson. The park offers 15 miles of interconnecting loop trails through oak-grassland overlooking the San Pedro River Valley and has limited hours.

MAMMOTH

GATEWAY TO PASSAGE 13: Oracle

OVERVIEW

A small town perched between the San Pedro River and the Santa Catalina Mountains, Mammoth was founded in 1872 as Mammoth Camp, to serve the nearby Mammoth Mine. It later became a bedroom community for those working the massive San Manuel Mine, which closed in 2003. While few services exist in this rural Copper Corridor locale, the Mexican food is widely considered the best in this part of Arizona. Other

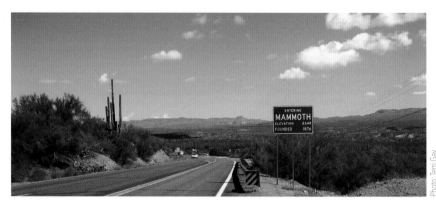

Photo: Terri Gay

Mammoth is one of many small towns within the Copper Corridor that welcome AZT travelers to its restaurants, markets, and shops.

attributes include Mammoth's epic views of the Galiuro Mountains and access to Aravaipa Canyon Wilderness.

ELEVATION 2,359 feet
POPULATION 1,457
POST OFFICE 230 South Main Street, 85618, 520-487-2861: Monday–Friday 8:30 a.m.–4:30 p.m.
INTERNET VENUES **Mammoth Public Library,** inside Mammoth Town Hall, 125 Clark Street, 520-487-2026: Free Wi-Fi.

Groceries

Circle K, 307 AZ 77, 520-487-2621

Corker's One Stop 732 AZ 77, 520-487-2411

Cafés and Restaurants

La Casita, 400 AZ 77, 520-487-9980

Las Michoacanas, 337 AZ 77, 520-487-2380

77 Drive In, 102 North AZ 77, 520-487-2783

Lodging

Foster's Lodge, 712 North AZ 77, 520-487-1904, **fosterslodge.com:** Outdoor pool, views of the Galiuro Mountains, and Wi-Fi.

Area Attractions

Aravaipa Canyon Wilderness: A perennial stream slices through a stunning canyon filled with myriad birds, wildlife, and lush riparian vegetation. A permit is required to visit; see **tinyurl.com/aravaipa** for details.

SAN MANUEL

GATEWAY TO PASSAGE 12: Oracle Ridge
and **PASSAGE 13:** Oracle

OVERVIEW

This former copper-mining town along the San Pedro River now attracts retirees. It hosts a tremendous panoramic viewshed.

ELEVATION 3,500 feet
POPULATION 3,551
POST OFFICE 430 South Avenue A, 85631, 520-385-9341
INTERNET VENUES San Manuel Library, 108 West Fifth Avenue, 520-385-4470

Groceries

Minit Market, 400 Avenue A, 520-385-2813

Cafés and Restaurants

La Casita Restaurant, 570 South Avenue A, 520-385-3025

Mel's Drive-In, 1034 West Third Avenue, 520-385-4212

San Pedro Valley Pizza Co., 326 South Alta Vista, 520-385-2041

Lodging and Camping

San Manuel Lodge, 666 West Eighth Avenue, 520-385-4340

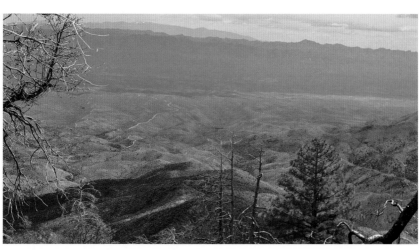

Photo: Sue and Mark Johnson

Nestled within the San Pedro River Valley is the Gateway Community of San Manuel.

CENTRAL COPPER CORRIDOR:
DUDLEYVILLE, WINKELMAN, HAYDEN, KEARNY, and KELVIN and RIVERSIDE

GATEWAY TO PASSAGE 14: Black Hills, **PASSAGE 15:** Tortilla Mountains, and **PASSAGE 16:** Gila River Canyons

OVERVIEW

The Copper Corridor extends from Oracle to Superior. It has a unique copper-mining history and culture, as well as abundant scenic and natural attractions, such as the San Pedro and Gila Rivers and numerous mountain ranges. The town of Kearny, the largest of the Copper Corridor communities in the region, was named after mid-1800s frontier general Stephen Kearny. At the base of the Pinal Mountains, the town was established in 1954 to accommodate nearby mine operations. There are no services or community resources in Dudleyville or Kelvin and Riverside.

ELEVATION Kelvin and Riverside: 1,808 feet; Hayden: 2,044 feet

POPULATION Dudleyville: 959; Hayden: 656; Kearny: 1,991; Kelvin and Riverside: few; Winkelman: 351

POST OFFICES 154 Park Lane, Hayden, 85135, 520-356-7042
388 Alden Road, Kearny, 85137, 520-363-5621
301 Giffin Avenue, Winkelman, 85192, 800-275-8777

INTERNET VENUES Arthur E. Pomeroy Library, 912-A Tilbury Drive, Kearny, 520-363-5861
Hayden Library, 175 Fifth Street, Hayden, 520-356-7031

Groceries

Giorsetti Grocery Store, 307 Giffin Avenue, Winkelman, 520-356-7221

IGA Foodliner, 345 Alden Road, Kearny, 520-363-5595

Cafés and Restaurants

Buzzy's Drive-In, 111 Tilbury Drive, Kearny, 520-363-7371

Cosmic Coffee Co., 334 Alden Road, Kearny, 520-363-9986

Maria's Restaurant, 640 Morris Road, Hayden, 520-356-6807

Old Time Pizza & Deli, 370 Alden Road, Kearny, 520-363-5523

Lodging and Camping

Free campground, near 13-acre Kearny Lake on the south end of town

General Kearny Inn, 301 Alden Road, Kearny, 520-363-5505

GLOBE

GATEWAY TO PASSAGE 17: Alamo Canyon, **PASSAGE 18:** Reavis Canyon, and **PASSAGE 19:** Superstition Wilderness

OVERVIEW

A mining town, Globe's past is laced with many historic events, such as murders, stagecoach robberies, outlaws, lynchings, and Apache raids. The majority of services are in downtown Globe, but the neighboring town of Miami offers some additional services.

ELEVATION 3,510 feet
POPULATION 7,532
POST OFFICE 101 South Hill Street, 85501, 800-275-8777
INTERNET VENUES Globe Public Library, 339 South Broad Street, 85501, 928-425-6111
Miami Memorial Library, 1052 Adonis Avenue, 85501, 928-473-2621

Groceries

There are two large grocery stores and a **Walmart** near the intersection of Highway 60 and Highway 188:

Fry's Food, 2115 US Highway 60, #200, 928-425-3276

Safeway, 4567 East US Highway 60, Miami, 520-425-7667

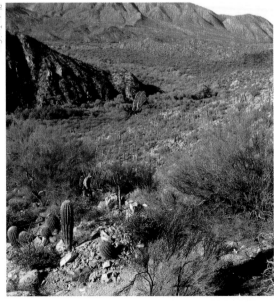

Photo: Terri Gay

Just a short distance from popular Passages 15 and 16 are many small towns within the Central Copper Corridor.

Cafés and Restaurants

The Globe–Miami area boasts so many great Mexican restaurants that it's hard to decide which one is the best. Choose from among these:

De Marcos's Restaurant, 1103 North Broad Street, 928-402-9232

Chalo's Casa Reynoso, 902 East Ash Street, 928-425-0515, chalosglobe.com

Guayo's on the Trail, 14239 Arizona 188, 928-425-9969

La Casita Café, 470 North Broad Street, 928-425-8462

Vida e Caffe, 157 West Cedar Street, Suite B, 928-425-2246

Lodging and Camping

America's Best Value Inn, 2370 East US Highway 60, 928-425-7151: Free Wi-Fi and breakfast.

Motel 6 Globe Hotel, 1699 East Ash Street, 928-425-5741: Pool, hot tub, and free Wi-Fi.

Other Services

Laundry: Wash 'n' Fluff Coin Laundry, 1324 North Broad Street, 928-425-3579

Massage: Adobe Ranch Wellness Spa, 138 South Broad Street, 928-425-3632

Showers: Globe Gym, 201 North Ash Street, 928-425-9304

Area Attractions

Besh-Ba-Gowah Museum, 1324 South Jesse Hayes Road, 928-425-0320: Salado archaeological site and botanical gardens and the largest collection of Salado pottery in the world.

Pinal Mountains, Globe Ranger District, 7680 South Six Shooter Canyon Road, 928-402-6200: The Pinal Mountains near Globe offer many options for camping, hiking, biking, and horseback riding. There is an unpaved road up to Pinal Peak's 7,848-foot summit.

FLORENCE

GATEWAY TO PASSAGE 15: Tortilla Mountains,
PASSAGE 16: Gila River Canyons, and **PASSAGE 17:** Alamo Canyon

OVERVIEW

One of Arizona's oldest towns, Florence was founded in 1866 and became the Pinal County seat of government in 1875. There are more than 140 historic buildings in

Florence, many of which are constructed of adobe brick. The district contains a mix of architectural styles from early territorial times through the post–World War II building boom.

ELEVATION 1,490 feet
POPULATION 25,536
POST OFFICE 501 North Main Street, 85132, 520-868-5651
INTERNET VENUES **Florence Community Library,** 1000 South Willow Street, 520-868-8311

Groceries

Pinal Food Market, 90 North Main Street, 520-868-5703

Safeway, 3325 North Hunt Highway, 520-723-0179

Cafés and Restaurants

L & B Inn, 695 South Main Street, 520-868-9981, **lbinn.com**

Mt. Athos Restaurant & Café, 444 South Pinal Parkway, 520-868-0735, **mountathoscafe.com**

Lodging and Camping

Holiday Inn Express Hotel & Suites, 240 West AZ 287, 520-868-9900

The Inn at Rancho Sonora, 9198 North AZ 79, 520-868-8000, **ranchosonora.com:** Courtyard rooms with Continental breakfast; pool and spa; casitas; RV park.

Feed and Tack

Western Feed & Supply, 255 South Main Street, 520-868-4141

Other Services

Laundry: Florence Coin-Op Laundry, 320 North Main Street

Massage: Essence of Life Massage Therapy, 26837 North Aladdin Road, 520-414-1589, **essenceoflife.massagetherapy.com**

Area Attractions

Casa Grande Ruins National Monument, 1100 West Ruins Drive, 520-723-3172: A Hohokam farming community and "Great House" are preserved at Casa Grande Ruins. One of the largest prehistoric structures ever built in North America, it was abandoned in 1450. The visitor center has a collection of artifacts from the site. The monument is 9 miles west of Florence.

SUPERIOR

GATEWAY TO PASSAGE 17: Alamo Canyon
and **PASSAGE 18:** Reavis Canyon

OVERVIEW

Set in an area with a rich mining history and cultural significance, Superior sits between the impressive mass of Picketpost Mountain and the cliffs of Apache Leap. Superior was the first Gateway Community to construct a connector trail to link the community to the AZT. See next page for more information about the Legends of Superior Trail (LOST).

ELEVATION 2,888 feet
POPULATION 2,896
POST OFFICE 25 North High School Avenue, 85173, 520-689-5790
INTERNET VENUES **Superior Public Library,** 99 Kellner Avenue,
   520-689-2327

Groceries

Circle K, 831 South Western Avenue, 520-689-5404

Family Dollar, 580 West US Highway 60, 520-689-5480

Save Money Market, 420 West Main Street, 520-689-2265

Superior Farmers Market, 798 West US Highway 60, 520-689-5845

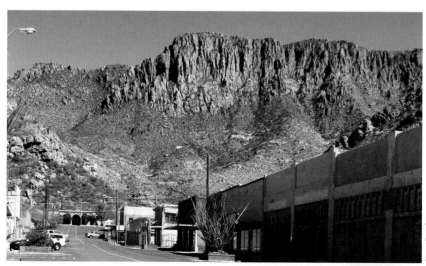

Hike from the AZT along the LOST to the town of Superior, a historic mining town well known for its natural resources.

Cafés and Restaurants

Buckboard City Café, 1111 West US Highway 60, 520-689-5800: Home to the World's Smallest Museum (see below).

Edwardo's Pizzaria, 701 Belmont Avenue, 520-689-2628

Jade Grill, 639 US Highway 60, 520-689-2885, **jadegrillasianbbq.com**

Los Hermanos, 835 West US Highway 60, 520-689-5465

Lodging and Camping

Copper Mountain Motel, 577 West Kiser Street, 520-689-2886: Friendly staff will accept packages. Wi-Fi in rooms, laundry facilities.

Area Attractions

Boyce Thompson Arboretum, 37615 US Highway 60, 520-689-2811, **arboretum .ag.arizona.edu:** Founded in the 1920s, Arizona's oldest and largest botanical garden is a great place to visit if you want to learn more about the many strange and wonderful plants of the world's deserts.

Legends of Superior Trail (LOST): The LOST connects the Arizona National Scenic Trail (AZT) to the town of Superior via a 6-mile interpretive trail. The trail goes through historic Pinal City, abandoned in 1891.

Queen Creek and Devil's Canyon: Some of central Arizona's greatest rock climbing can be found along the rhyolite cliffs near Superior. Devil's Canyon is a world-class canyoneering destination, featuring Arizona's largest natural plunge pools.

World's Smallest Museum, 1111 West US Highway 60, **worldssmallestmuseum.com:** Discover what wonders await at this curiosity next to the Buckboard City Café.

ROOSEVELT and TONTO BASIN

GATEWAY TO PASSAGE 19: Superstition Wilderness,
PASSAGE 20: Four Peaks, and **PASSAGE 21:** Pine Mountain

OVERVIEW

Facilities in Roosevelt are limited to the visitors center and marina. For more options, the town of Tonto Basin lies 17 miles north on AZ 188. The original town of Roosevelt was created to provide housing for workers during the construction of the Theodore Roosevelt Dam, which opened in 1911. After the dam was created, the town of Roosevelt was moved to higher ground and the old buildings were submerged.

ELEVATION 2,200 feet
POPULATION 1,424 (Tonto Basin)

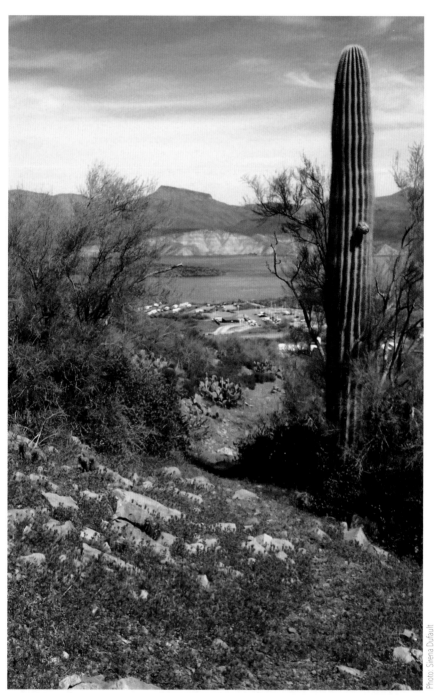

The Roosevelt Lake Visitors Center and Marina, as seen from Passage 20

Photo: Sirena Dufault

POST OFFICE The **Roosevelt Lake Visitors Center,** 28085 North AZ 188, 85545, accepts packages. The **Roosevelt Post Office** is 11 miles south of the marina: 9998 Main Street, 85545, 928-467-2215.

INTERNET VENUES Tonto Basin Public Library, 415 Old AZ 188, 928-479-2355, 25 miles north of the Roosevelt Lake Visitors Center

Groceries

Tonto Basin Marketplace, 45994 North AZ 188, 928-479-2000

Cafés and Restaurants

Big Daddy's Pizza, 100 Salado Trail, 928-479-3223

Butcher Hook Restaurant, AZ 188, milepost 259, 928-479-2712, butcherhook.com

Roosevelt Lake Marina, 28085 AZ 188, 602-912-1664

Lodging and Camping

Punkin Center Lodge, 249 Old AZ 188, 928-479-2229, punkincenteraz.com: This motel with attached bar and grill offers patio seating with views of the Tonto Basin.

Tonto Basin Inn, milepost 260 on AZ 188, 928-479-2891, tontobasininn.com

Area Attractions

Roosevelt Lake, 28085 AZ 188, 602-912-1664: Roosevelt Lake boasts the largest lake in central Arizona, consisting of 112 miles of shoreline and coves. Campgrounds are located all along AZ 188.

Tonto National Monument, 26260 North AZ 188, Suite 2, 928-467-2241: Salado cliff dwellings from the 13th to 15th centuries only 2.5 miles south on AZ 188 from the Roosevelt Visitors Center. On-site museum and tours are available.

PAYSON

GATEWAY TO PASSAGE 24: Red Hills, **PASSAGE 25:** Whiterock Mesa and **PASSAGE 26:** Hardscrabble Mesa

OVERVIEW

East of the Mazatzal Wilderness, Payson offers trail users a wide range of services.

ELEVATION 5,000 feet
POPULATION 15,301
POST OFFICE 100 West Frontier Street, 85541, 928-474-2972
INTERNET VENUES Payson Public Library, 328 North McLane Road, 928-474-9260

Groceries

Bashas', 142 AZ 260, 928-474-4495

Safeway, 401 AZ 260, 928-472-8208

VITA-MART, 516 South Beeline Highway, 928-474-4101

Cafés and Restaurants

Ayothaya Thai Café, 404 East AZ 260, 928-474-1112

Beeline Café, 815 South Beeline Highway, 928-474-9960: cash only

El Rancho Restaurant, 200 South Beeline Highway, 928-474-3111

Gerard's Italian Bistro, 512 North Beeline Highway, 928-468-6500

Lodging and Camping

America's Best Value Inn, 811 South Beeline Highway, 928-474-2283

LF Ranch, 928-970-3543, **lfranch.com:** Offers bunkhouse or camping options, picket lines for equines, and meals with advance reservations.

Majestic Mountain Inn, 602 AZ 260, 800-408-2442, **majesticmountaininn.com**

Outdoor Shops

Bicycle Adventurers, 201 West Main Street, Suite B, 928-474-2308

Massage Therapy

A Simple Touch, 805 East AZ 260, 928-978-4787, **asimpletouch.info**

Area Attractions

Rim Country Museum and Zane Grey Cabin, 700 Green Valley Parkway, 928-474-3483, **rimcountrymuseums.com:** Contains exhibits about Tonto Apache, pioneers, ranchers and miners, and the towns of Payson, Strawberry, and Pine. Also features a replica of writer Zane Grey's cabin, which burned down in the Dude Fire of 1990.

PINE and STRAWBERRY

GATEWAY TO PASSAGE 26: Hardscrabble Mesa
and **PASSAGE 27:** Highline

OVERVIEW

Tucked beneath the Mogollon Rim, these twin communities have lots to offer.

ELEVATION 5,448 feet (Pine); 5,883 feet (Strawberry)
POPULATION 1,963 (Pine); 961 (Strawberry)
POST OFFICE 3847 North AZ 87, Pine, 85544-9997
INTERNET VENUES Pine Public Library, 6124 North Randall Place, Pine, 928-476-3678

Groceries

Ponderosa Market, 6112 Hardscrabble Mesa Road, Pine, 928-476-3590

Cafés and Restaurants

HB's Place, 3854 North AZ 87, Pine, 928-476-4475

Pine Deli, 6240 Hardscrabble Mesa Road, Pine, 928-476-3536

That Brewery & Pub, 3270 North AZ 87, milepost 267, Pine, 928-476-3349, **thatbrewery.com:** Accepts packages and helps with shuttles. Brewers of Arizona Trail Ale, specially crafted for thirsty trail users.

Sidewinders Saloon, 6112 West Hardscrabble Mesa Road, Pine, 928-476-6434

Lodging and Camping

Pine Creek Cabins, 3901 AZ 87, Pine, 928-970-9511

The Ranch at Fossil Creek, 10379 West Fossil Creek Road, 928-476-5178, **ranchatfossilcreek.com:** A working goat and llama ranch offering homemade delicacies such as goat's milk fudge and cheese. Let a llama carry your gear on the trail. Yurt camping available

Strawberry Lodge, 8039 West Fossil Creek Road, Strawberry, 928-476-3333

That Cabin at That Brewery & Pub, 3270 North AZ 87, milepost 267, Pine, 928-476-3349, **thatbrewery.com:** Stay at That Cabin and ask for the trail-user discount.

Massage Therapy

A Touch from Heaven Massage, Pine, 928-476-3900

Area Attractions

Fossil Springs Wilderness, 928-527-3600, **tinyurl.com/fossilsprings:** This 11,550-acre wilderness contains one of the most diverse riparian areas in Arizona. More than 30 species of trees and shrubs and more than 100 species of birds have been observed here, and the stream seems to appear out of nowhere, gushing 20,000 gallons a minute out of a series of springs at the bottom of a 1,600-foot deep canyon.

Tonto Natural Bridge State Park, 928-476-4202, **azstateparks.com:** Believed to be the largest natural travertine bridge in the world, it stands 183 feet high over a 400-foot long tunnel that measures 150 feet at its widest point.

MORMON LAKE

GATEWAY TO PASSAGE 29: Happy Jack and **PASSAGE 30:** Mormon Lake

OVERVIEW

The name commemorates the Mormon settlers who operated dairy farms in the area. Mormon Lake, when full, is Arizona's largest natural lake. Sometimes the lake dries up and becomes a marsh. It's one of those Arizona idiosyncrasies, like rivers that sometimes have no water in them.

ELEVATION 7,100 feet
POPULATION The sign at Mormon Lake Village says 50 TO 5,000, a number that fluctuates depending on the season.
POST OFFICE 1 Mormon Lake Road, 86038, 928-779-2371
INTERNET VENUES None

Groceries

Mormon Lake Lodge Country Store, 928-354-2227, **mormonlakelodge.com**

Cafés and Restaurants

Mormon Lake Lodge Steakhouse & Saloon, 928-354-2227, **mormonlakelodge.com:** The saloon has entertainment on the weekends.

Lodging and Camping

Mormon Lake Lodge, 1991 Mormon Lake Road, 928-354-2227, **mormonlakelodge .com:** Duplex motel-style units, cabins, RV sites, and tent camping.

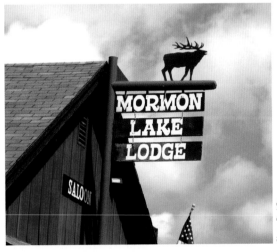

Mormon Lake Lodge, a popular destination for day-trippers to begin adventures on the AZT, is a necessity for long-distance trail travelers.

Photo: Terri Gay

Area Attractions

High Mountain Stables, 928-354-2359, **highmountainstablesaz.com:** Offers trail rides May–September, overnight campouts, wagon rides, surrey rides, and a free petting zoo.

Mountain bike rentals, Mormon Lake Lodge, 928-354-2227, **mormonlakelodge.com**

FLAGSTAFF

GATEWAY TO PASSAGE 31: Walnut Canyon,
PASSAGE 32: Elden Mountain, **PASSAGE 33:** Flagstaff,
and **PASSAGE 34:** San Francisco Peaks

OVERVIEW

The laid-back mountain town of Flagstaff is a favorite among AZT users, and has become one of the greatest trail towns in the Southwest. It was also the home of Dale Shewalter, "Father of the Arizona National Scenic Trail," and he is commemorated with an AZT sign and a bench in Buffalo Park. Flagstaff has a great bus system for getting around town and has all the amenities a trail user needs.

ELEVATION 6,910 feet
POPULATION 65,870
POST OFFICE 2400 North Postal Boulevard, 86004, 928-714-9302 (on the bus route)
INTERNET VENUES Flagstaff Public Library, 300 West Aspen Avenue, 928-779-7670

Groceries

Flagstaff has all the big grocery stores, but Fry's is the closest to the trail.

Fry's, Route 66 and Switzer Canyon Drive, 928-774-2719

New Frontiers Natural Marketplace, 320 South Cambridge Lane, 928-774-5747, **newfrontiersmarket.com**

Cafés and Restaurants

Alpha & Omega Greek Restaurant, 1580 East Route 66, 928-774-4337, **alphaomegagreekfood.squarespace.com**

Flagstaff Brewing Company, 16 East Route 66, 928-773-1442, **flagbrew.com**

Late for the Train, 22 East Birch Avenue, 928-779-5975, **lateforthetrain.com**

Macy's European Coffeehouse, 14 Beaver Street, 928-774-2243, **macyscoffee.net**

Pato Thai Cuisine, 104 North San Francisco Street, 928-213-1825, **patothai.com**

Lodging and Camping

Best Western Pony Soldier Inn and Suites, 3030 East Route 66, 928-526-2388: Indoor pool, jacuzzi, and free Wi-Fi.

DuBeau Hostel, 19 West Phoenix Avenue, 928-774-6731: This hostel has dorm rooms and private rooms and offers free breakfast and Wi-Fi. Both DuBeau and Grand Canyon Hostel are centrally located within one block of each other in quaint downtown Flagstaff, where you'll find everything within walking distance of the town square.

Grand Canyon Hostel, 19 South San Francisco Street, 928-779-9421

Bike and Other Outdoors Shops

Flagstaff has more bike shops per capita than any other city in Arizona.

Absolute Bikes, 202 East Route 66, 928-779-5969, **absolutebikes.net**

Cosmic Cycles, 612 North Humphreys Street, 928-779-1092, **cosmiccycles.com**

Flagstaff Bicycle Revolution, 3 Mikes Pike, 928-774-3042, **flagbikerev.com**

Flagstaff also has the largest selection of outdoors stores on the trail.

Aspen Sports, 15 North San Francisco Street, 928-779-1935, **flagstaffsportinggoods.com**

Peace Surplus, 14 West Route 66, 928-779-4521, **peacesurplus.com**

Feed and Tack

Olsen's Grain Inc., 2250 North Steve's Boulevard, 928-522-0568, **olsensgrain.com**

Other Services

Laundry: White Flag Coin-Op Laundry, 16 South Beaver Street, 928-774-7614

Massage: Bending Willow Massage, 928-606-7493: Discounts for trail users; **Stay Tuned Therapeutics,** 403 West Birch Avenue, 928-699-1999, **staytuned-az.com.**

Showers: YMCA Family Center, 1001 North Turquoise Drive, 928-556-9622

Area Attractions

Walnut Canyon National Monument, 3 Walnut Canyon Road, 928-526-3367, **nps.gov/waca:** See millions of years of geologic history and amazing Sinagua cliff dwellings at this popular monument, a short distance from Passage 33.

TUSAYAN and GRAND CANYON VILLAGE

GATEWAY TO PASSAGE 36: Coconino Rim and
PASSAGE 37: Grand Canyon: South Rim

OVERVIEW

The town of Tusayan is just south of the Grand Canyon National Park entrance. Most facilities in the Grand Canyon are 2.5 miles from the South Kaibab Trailhead.

ELEVATION 6,612 feet

POPULATION 558

POST OFFICES 100 Mather Business Center, Grand Canyon Village, 86023, 928-638-2512

Tusayan General Store, 236 AZ 64, Tusayan, 86023, 800-275-8777

INTERNET VENUES Grand Canyon Community Library, 208 Navajo Street, 928-638-2718: Eight public computers available for a small fee per half-hour; free 24-hour Wi-Fi, accessible outside.

Holiday Inn Express, AZ 64 in Tusayan, 928-638-3000: Nonguests are welcome to use the free Wi-Fi in its lobby, which is open 24 hours a day.

Groceries

Grand Canyon General Store, 100 Mather Business Center, 928-638-2262

Tusayan General Store, 236 AZ 64, 928-638-2854

Cafés and Restaurants

In Tusayan, try these eateries:

The Big E Steakhouse, 395 AZ 64, 928-638-0333, bigesteakhouse.com

We Cook Pizza & Pasta, 605 AZ 64, 928-638-2278, wecookpizzaandpasta.com

In Grand Canyon Village, options include the following (928-638-2631, **grandcanyon lodges.com**): the **Arizona Room,** just east of Bright Angel Lodge, for steaks, ribs, and fish; **Bright Angel Restaurant,** in Bright Angel Lodge; **Canyon Cafe,** in Yavapai Lodge; the **Delicatessen at the Marketplace,** in front of the general store; the **El Tovar Dining Room,** in the El Tovar Hotel; and **Maswik Cafeteria,** in Maswik Lodge.

Lodging and Camping

Tusayan is lined with hotels for a variety of budgets.

Best Western Premier Grand Canyon Squire Inn, 74 AZ 64, 928-638-2681, grandcanyonsquire.com: Hot breakfast, spa and sauna, free Wi-Fi.

The Grand Hotel, 149 AZ 64, 928-638-3333, grandcanyongrandhotel.com: If you're looking for an upscale place to stay in Tusayan, The Grand can't be beat.

Red Feather Lodge, 300 AZ 64, 928-638-2414, redfeatherlodge.com

The South Rim of the Grand Canyon offers a variety of lodging as well, from the modestly priced **Maswik** and **Bright Angel Lodges** to the opulent **El Tovar Hotel** (reservations for all three: 928-638-2631, grandcanyonlodges.com). In Grand Canyon Village is **Mather Campground:** 877-444-6777, recreation.gov.

Other Services

Bike Rental: Bright Angel Bicycles, 10 South Entrance Road, 928-638-3055, bikegrandcanyon.com: Rent a bike or take a guided tour to explore the scenic overlooks and forested greenways of Grand Canyon National Park.

Guided Tours: All-Star Grand Canyon Tours, 800-940-0445, allstargrandcanyontours.com: Offers custom private trips in Grand Canyon National Park and shuttle service.

Laundry and Showers: In Tusayan, the **Best Western Premier Grand Canyon Squire Inn** (74 AZ 64, 928-638-2681) lets hikers use its coin-operated laundry facilities. In Grand Canyon Village, laundry and shower facilities are available next to **Mather Campground** (see above); hours vary seasonally.

Area Attractions

Grand Canyon National Park, of course!

NORTH RIM to JACOB LAKE

GATEWAY TO PASSAGE 39: Grand Canyon, North Rim,
PASSAGE 40: Kaibab Plateau: South,
PASSAGE 41: Kaibab Plateau: Central,
and **PASSAGE 42:** Kaibab Plateau: North

OVERVIEW

Many of the services in this area are seasonal from May until October, depending upon when the roads close for winter. Call for details before you visit.

Jacob Lake is named for Jacob Hamblin, Mormon pioneer and explorer. This small lake sustained Mormon settlers as they traveled along the Honeymoon Trail on their way to get married at the temple in St. George, Utah. Known as the Arizona Strip, this part of the state is geographically separated from the rest of Arizona by the Grand Canyon.

ELEVATION 7,920 feet
POPULATION Few
POST OFFICE 85 North Main Street, North Rim, 86052
INTERNET VENUES Wi-Fi available at the camper store near North Rim Campground

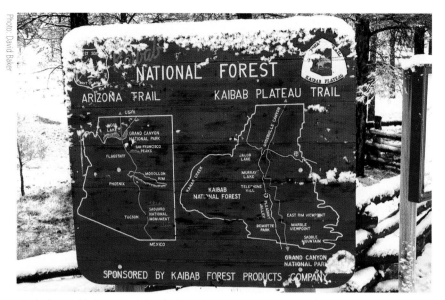

The lodge and bakery at Jacob Lake have saved many AZT travelers from the extreme elements of the Kaibab Plateau.

Groceries

North Rim Country Store, milepost 605, AZ 67, 928-638-2383, **northrimcountry store.com;** accepts packages. Six miles north of park entrance.

Grand Canyon Lodge at the North Rim (see below) also has a small general store with limited resupply items.

Cafés and Restaurants

Grand Canyon Lodge at the North Rim has a dining room, deli, coffee shop, and saloon. **Kaibab Lodge** and **Jacob Lake Inn** (see below) both have full restaurants.

Lodging and Camping

DeMotte Campground, 877-444-6777, **recreation.gov:** This Kaibab National Forest campground, 18 miles north of the rim on AZ 67, is open May 15–October 30.

Grand Canyon Lodge at the North Rim, 877-386-4383, **grandcanyonlodgenorth .com:** This is the only lodging inside the park on the North Rim. It offers cabins and hotel rooms and is open May 15–October 15.

Jacob Lake Inn, junction of AZ 89A and AZ 67, 928-643-7232, **jacoblake.com:** Built in 1929, Jacob Lake Inn has cabins, rooms, a restaurant, a small store with resupply items, and a bakery that shouldn't be missed. The inn, open year-round, offers discounts and shuttle services to trail users and accepts packages.

Kaibab Camper Village, 928-643-7804, **kaibabcampervillage.com:** One mile southwest of Jacob Lake on AZ 67, this facility offers tent and RV sites, laundry, and hot showers. Open May 12–October 15.

Kaibab Lodge, AZ 67, HC 64, Box 30, 86022, 928-638-2389, **kaibablodge.com:** Located 18 miles from the North Rim on Highway 67, the Kaibab Lodge has cabins, a restaurant, and a cozy fireplace you can relax in front of after a day on the trail. Open May 15–November 2.

North Rim Campground requires a reservation; call 877-444-6777 or visit **recreation .gov.** The campground is open May 15–October 15, with walk-in sites available until November 30 (facilities on the North Rim close on October 15).

Area Attractions

Allen's Trail Rides, 435-644-8150, **allensoutfittersandtrailrides.com, j.allen.guides@gmail.com:** 1-hour, 2-hour, half-day, full-day, and longer trips. Call to make reservations.

Kaibab Plateau: Miles of scenic trails and dirt roads crisscross the Kaibab Plateau, allowing for hiking, biking, horseback riding, and camping. Contact the Kaibab Plateau Visitor Center at 928-643-7298.

PAGE

GATEWAY TO PASSAGE 41: Kaibab Plateau: Central,
PASSAGE 42: Kaibab Plateau: North, and
PASSAGE 43: Buckskin Mountain

OVERVIEW

The city of Page was established in 1957 to house workers building the Glen Canyon Dam on the Colorado River. The main attraction in Page is Lake Powell, but the area hosts a number of great hiking, biking, and equestrian trails, as well as cultural experiences on the nearby Navajo Nation.

ELEVATION 4,118 feet
POPULATION 7,252
POST OFFICE 44 Sixth Avenue, 86040, 928-645-2571
INTERNET VENUES Page Library, 479 South Lake Powell Boulevard, 928-645-4270

Groceries

Safeway, 650 Elm Street, 928-645-8155

Walmart Supercenter, 1017 Industrial Road, 928-645-2622

Cafés and Restaurants

Asian Cuisine Indian and Thai Food, 107 Lake Powell Boulevard, 928-645-0094

Beans Gourmet Coffee House, 644 North Navajo Drive, 928-645-6858

Fiesta Mexicana, 125 South Lake Powell Boulevard, 928-645-4082

Slackers, 635 Elm Street, 928-645-5267, **slackersqualitygrub.com**

Lodging and Camping

Lake Powell Motel, 750 South Navajo Drive, 928-645-3919: These one- and two-bedroom suites on the "street of little motels" include a living room and kitchen.

Page Boy Motel, 150 North Lake Powell Boulevard, 928-645-2416: Free breakfast and Wi-Fi and a swimming pool.

Page-Lake Powell Campground, 849 South Coppermine Road, 928-645-3374, **pagecampground.com:** RV and tent sites, laundry, pool, hot tub, and free Wi-Fi.

Other Services

Laundry: Sunbeam Laundry, 112 South Lake Powell Boulevard, 928-645-6834

Massage: Adams Chiropractic Clinic, 635 Elm Street, #9, 928-645-8864

Area Attractions

Plan a couple of extra days in this remote corner of Arizona to take advantage of the many recreational opportunities in the area.

Antelope Canyon: One of the most famous and photographed slot canyons in the Southwest, **Upper Antelope Canyon** requires a guided tour, while **Lower Antelope Canyon** can be self-guided. Both lie within the Navajo Nation, which charges an entrance fee. More information: **navajonationparks.org/htm/antelopecanyon.htm.**

Colorado River: Normally, float trips on the Colorado require anywhere from 10 days to 3 weeks, but **Colorado River Discovery** offers half-day float trips and full-day paddle trips along the calm section between Glen Canyon Dam and Lee's Ferry. Floating along the sandstone walls of Glen Canyon is mesmerizing. Details: 888-522-6644, **raftthecanyon.com.**

Lake Powell: This narrow, 186-mile-long body of water is set amid the deep canyons, rocky outcrops, and spectacular scenery of the Glen Canyon National Recreation Area. Formed by Glen Canyon Dam, activities include kayaking, swimming, fishing, scuba diving, snorkeling, water skiing, hiking, and sightseeing. Kayaking is an amazing way to explore the sinuous shoreline and slot canyons of Lake Powell, and **Hidden Canyon Kayak** offers half-day, full-day, and multiday trip options as well as gear rentals. Details: 928-660-1836, **hiddencanyonkayak.com.**

FREDONIA, ARIZONA, and KANAB, UTAH

GATEWAY TO PASSAGE 43: Buckskin Mountain

OVERVIEW

The tiny town of Fredonia is Arizona's northernmost city and offers little in the way of services. Kanab, just over the border in Utah, has all the facilities trail users need. Known as "Little Hollywood" because of its rich movie history, it's also popular with outdoor enthusiasts visiting nearby attractions such as Zion and Bryce National Parks.

ELEVATION Fredonia: 4,671 feet; Kanab: 4,970 feet
POPULATION Fredonia: 1,314; Kanab: 4,391
POST OFFICES 85 North Main Street, Fredonia, 86022, 928-643-7122
39 South Main Street, Kanab, 84741, 435-644-2760
INTERNET VENUES Fredonia Public Library, 130 North Main Street,
Fredonia, 928-643-7137
Kanab Public Library, 374 North Main Street, Kanab, 435-644-2394

Groceries

Glazier's Family Market, 264 South 100 East, Kanab, 435-644-5029,
glaziersfamilymarket.com

Honey's Jubilee, 260 East 300 South, Kanab, 435-644-5877, **honeysfoods.com**

Cafés and Restaurants

Escobar's Mexican Restaurant, 373 East 300 South, Kanab, 435-644-3739

Houston's Trails End, 32 East Center Street, Kanab, 435-644-2488

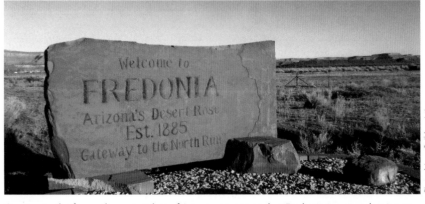

Welcome to
FREDONIA
Arizona's Desert Rose
Est. 1885
Gateway to the North Rim

Photo: Arizona Trail Association

Services in the far northern stretches of Arizona are sparse, but Fredonia is as good as it gets.

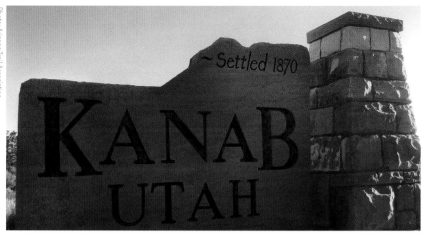

Just a bit farther north, Kanab has most everything a trail user might need.

Laid Back Larry's, 98 South 100 East, Kanab, 435-644-3636

Three Bears, 210 South 100 East, Kanab, 435-644-3300

Lodging and Camping

Parry Lodge, 89 East Center Street, Kanab, 435-644-2601, **parrylodge.com:**
Founded in 1931 by the three Parry brothers, Parry Lodge hosted some of the
biggest names during Hollywood's golden age.

Sun-n-Sands Motel, 347 South 100 East, Kanab, 435-644-5050: Inexpensive lodging
with free breakfast and Wi-Fi.

Outdoors Shops

Willow Canyon Outdoors, 263 South 100 East, Kanab, 435-644-8884,
willowcanyon.com: Full-service outdoors store and coffee bar.

Feed and Tack

Crosby Home & Farm Center, 723 East AZ 89, Kanab, 435-644-5116

Other Services

Laundry: Kanab Laundry & Car Wash, 260 East 300 South, Kanab, 435-644-5626

Massage: La Bella Salon, 30 East Center Street, Kanab, 435-644-3855

Area Attractions

Kanab is a popular hub for visits to **Zion, Bryce,** and **Grand Canyon National Parks;
Grand Staircase-Escalante National Monument;** and **Lake Powell National
Recreation Area.**

Geology Features of the AZT

By Rick Obermiller

THE ARIZONA NATIONAL SCENIC TRAIL (AZT) is unique among the long-distance trails of America—not because it's one of America's National Scenic Trails or because it's one of the most recently completed, but because of its geology, matched by few other places in the country. You can walk the storied Appalachian Trail from Georgia to Maine and see mostly forest, or hike along the Pacific Crest Trail and see the rugged ridges of the Sierra Nevada. But travel the AZT and you pass through almost 2 billion years of Earth's history. On the trail you'll see Arizona's geology at work. These structures and processes have shaped what's below your feet: from fiery volcanoes to uplifted plateaus, sedimentary mesas, river valleys, and a vast canyon, from hot spots to thrust faults, from limestone caverns to mineral porphyry. From the Proterozoic to the Pleistocene, take a step back through time, and then another and another.

THE KARST OF COLOSSAL CAVE
Passage 8: Rincon Valley

For an absorbing diversion from hiking, cycling, and horseback riding on the AZT, take a side trip to the karst topography of the underworld: Colossal Cave Mountain Park. On Old Spanish Trail, near Tucson, the park transports you to Mississippian times, 318–359 million years ago, when parts of Arizona were covered by shallow seas.

The natural sculpting visible at Colossal Cave started with ancient sea creatures. As their remains accumulated on the ocean bottom, the mass eventually transformed into limestone which, when subjected to mildly acidic rainwater, begins to dissolve. The result is sinkholes, depressions, and limestone caverns. Here, the block of what is known as Escabrosa limestone was uplifted, exposed, and folded under tortuous pressure during the formation of the Catalina–Rincon metamorphic complex. (See "The Mighty Santa Catalina and Rincon Mountains" discussion, next, and the "Rock Cycle" illustration, on page 42.)

Cracking and faulting, the limestone slowly fragmented into cave structures that filled, over a long period, with solution. As arid climates prevailed, the solution began to drain, and dripping material became *stalactites* (from above), *stalagmites* (growing upward), and *columns* (the meeting of stalactites and stalagmites). Thin sheets of water hardened into the ribboned walls, or *flowstones*, visible at Colossal Caves. Water no longer percolates into the complex, but the beautiful formations remain.

Also be sure to spend some time in the park's La Posta Quemada Ranch Museum to learn more about the 10th-century native Hohokam people, whose artifacts show that they used the cave's chambers for protection and shelter. They no doubt traveled all 3.5 miles of today's mapped cave system. For hours, fees, and more details about Colossal Cave Mountain Park, visit **colossalcave.com.**

THE MIGHTY SANTA CATALINA AND RINCON MOUNTAINS

Passages 9–13: Rincon Mountains, Redington Pass, Santa Catalina Mountains, Oracle Ridge, and Oracle

Nothing dominates the southern Arizona skyline like the Santa Catalina and Rincon Mountains, whose geology is complex. Crustal extension formed the mountains and basins in the Basin and Range Province, a process that sometimes also creates what is known as a *metamorphic core complex.* That serves as a modern explanation for ranges such as the Santa Catalinas in the Tucson area and the South Mountains in the Phoenix area that typically trend southwest to northeast (at right angles to Basin and Range mountains). There are a half-dozen other complexes in the state, but the Catalina–Rincon Complex is the largest.

What's known as the Catalina–Rincon Metamorphic Core Complex formed about 25 million years ago (and after the events that created the Basin and Range Mountains) when crustal extension caused deep crustal rocks (the lower plate) to be uplifted and forced overlaying crust (upper plate) to slide off in what's called a low-angle detachment fault. The detachment fault creates a domelike range on its lower plate (what we see as the current Catalina and Rincon Mountains) with a shell (carapace) of deformed rocks caused by the sliding. The upper plate, the Tucson Mountains, was displaced 20 miles to the east.

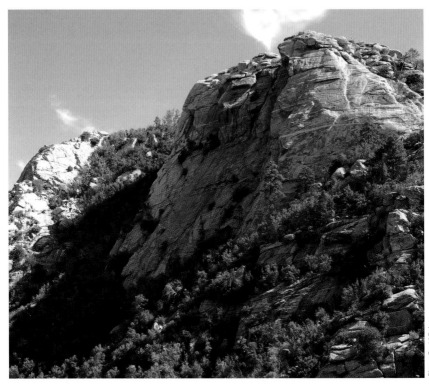

Photo: David Baker

The Santa Catalina Mountains are composed of beautiful granite and gneiss, evidence of crustal extension approximately 25 million years ago.

The uplifted, deep crustal rocks are the Catalina Granite (seen on the north part of the range) and the Catalina Gneiss (pronounced "nice"), which is a banded metamorphic rock seen on the south of the range. You can see further deformations of these rocks at the carapace because of the tremendous heat generated by the sliding of the upper plate off the lower plate. Of course, before the extension, the volcanic rocks of the Tucson Mountains sat on top of these older rocks.

Faulting between the upper and lower plates created the Tucson basin, which at one time was about 8,000 feet deep but has filled in about halfway (4,000 feet) with erosional elements from the surrounding mountains.

SUPERVOLCANOES OF THE SUPERSTITION MOUNTAINS

Passages 16-19: Gila River Canyons, Alamo Canyon, Reavis Canyon, and Superstition Wilderness

While there is much to appreciate along Passages 16, 17, 18 and 19, the Superstition Mountains are the dominant and most impressive landform. These mountains, known as the Superstition–Goldfield Volcanic Zone, represent the transition from the Basin and Range to the Central Highlands. If we could have observed what occurred in this area between 25 and 15 million years ago (the Middle Tertiary period), we would have been utterly astounded at the magnitude of the volcanic eruptions and the epic scale of the cataclysms that ensued.

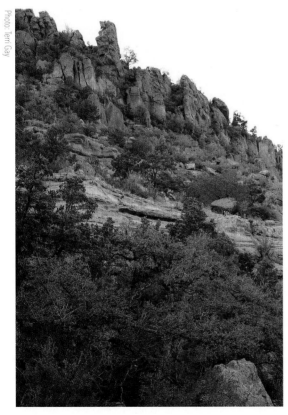

Photo: Terri Gay

Cliffs throughout the Superstition Mountains are evidence of cataclysmic volcanic eruptions during the Middle Tertiary period.

Just imagine this cycle, repeated many times in the Superstitions: plumes of ash and smoke that rose tens of thousands of feet and then collapsed into superheated volcano-rollers that destroyed everything in their path; ash so hot that it sometimes welded itself; volcanic bombs of lava the size of pickup trucks thrown like shotputs; heat lightning everywhere; toxic fumes of sulfur dioxide that asphyxiated any breathing animal; and the sheer heat of the cauldron. This place could have easily inspired Dante's descriptions in *Inferno*.

The most dangerous and powerful volcanoes are *supervolcanoes*—large, explosive events that eject more than 1,000 cubic kilometers of ash, gas, and molten rock. Such swift eruptions leave behind large a sunken depression called a caldera that represents a drained magma chamber. Currently the world's largest volcano (and supervolcano) is the 50-mile-diameter Yellowstone Caldera, which in its past eruptions literally blew a hole in the Rocky Mountain range.

While the Superstition Mountains' 8-mile-diameter caldera lacked the single eruptive strength of the Yellowstone eruptions, it still managed to pump out 2,500 cubic miles of ash and lava over the life of its explosions. The Superstition volcanoes were like Yellowstone's temperamental little brother, with eruptions so powerful because of the type of lava lying beneath the surface. It was high in silica and composed of a viscous type of magma that doesn't easily find its way to surface. When it does build up enough pressure to release, it does so explosively.

Once the Superstitions went through their most eruptive cycles, a large caldera formed. Because magma still bubbled beneath the surface, the caldera was pushed and arched up into what is called a resurgent dome. The current Superstitions are a resurgent dome that has eroded and faulted over time to give us the current dramatic range. Two of the most visible landmarks—Weaver's Needle and Picketpost Mountain—are resistant, erosional remnants of the cataclysm.

AMAZING MAZATZALS

Passages 20-24: Four Peaks, Pine Mountain, Saddle Mountain, Mazatzal Divide, and Red Hills

The Mazatzals are a very rugged mountain range divided into the Southern Mazatzals that end at Four Peaks to the south and the Northern Mazatzals that end at the town of Pine to the north. AZ 87 bisects the range just south of its juncture with AZ 188. This largest range in the Transition Zone Province is also known as the Central Highlands.

Passage 20 climbs right up to the Four Peaks Wilderness. The crest of Four Peaks is made up of 1.5 billion-year-old, very resistant metasediment called Mazatzal quartzite, a sandstone that has been changed by extreme heat and pressure. It was intruded with Precambrian Mazatzal granite in fingers at the peak level and also makes up the majority of the base. The less resistant granite eroded away, leaving the resistant quartzite that makes up the tops of the peaks. So it can be said that Four Peaks has quartzite teeth on granite gums. On the southernmost peak is the only commercial amethyst mine in North America—but it is private and cannot be accessed without permission. Four Peaks amethyst is renowned for its deep purple color with reddish tints.

The Mazatzals were formed in a mountain-building action (orogeny) caused by tectonic plate collisions 1.6 billion years ago when Arizona was at the continental margin of proto–North America. These collisions caused compression that uplifted mountains through folding and over thrust, where one block of rock is thrust over another. See this folding in detail for yourself in the Northern Mazatzals in Passage 23 (page 182) by taking the Barnhardt Trail junction and hiking about 3 miles down Barnhardt Canyon. On the northern side of the canyon, chevron folds are very striking and attest to the tectonic forces that are powerful enough to bend solid rock.

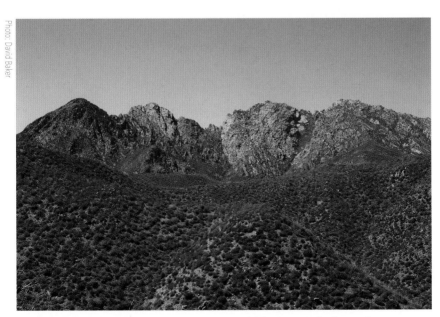

Photo: David Baker

Four Peaks feature quartzite and granite in chevron folds, showing the forces of a mountain-building episode strong enough to bend solid rock.

ELDEN MOUNTAIN: A VOLCANO UNLIKE THE OTHERS

Passage 32: Elden Mountain

Part of the San Francisco Volcanic Field, Elden Mountain is about 1 million years old. It flanks the impressive San Francisco Peaks but is a different kind of volcano. Unlike its stratovolcano neighbor, Elden is a volcanic dome formed by very silicic and viscous dacite and rhyolite lavas. Elden erupted quickly, but its lava was so thick that it piled on itself in steep, bulbous lobes forming a domelike structure. This is most apparent on its south face, which is most visible from Route 66 in Flagstaff. On its north face the eruption pushed up blocks of existing sedimentary rocks.

One interesting aspect of the Elden eruption is the columnar jointing visible on its south face. This is similar to the look of Devils Tower in Wyoming, made famous by the science-fiction movie *Close Encounters of the Third Kind*. The unique jointing is caused by rapidly cooling lava.

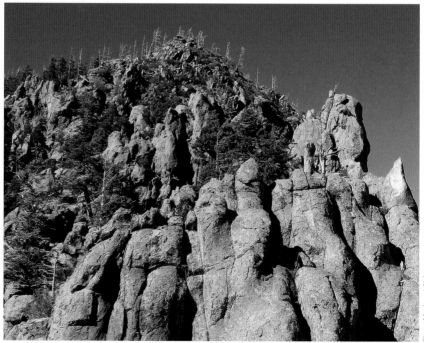

The distinctive columnar jointing on the south face of Elden Mountain is a result of rapidly cooling viscous lava.

THE SAN FRANCISCO PEAKS' VIOLENT PAST
Passage 34: San Francisco Peaks

Although Passage 34 crosses San Francisco Mountain (commonly referred to as the San Francisco Peaks, or Kachina Peaks), the mountain dominates the landscape from Passage 30 to 35. At 12,633 feet, San Francisco Mountain is the highest point in Arizona and, arguably, the most impressive massif in the Colorado Plateau Province. It is also the only stratovolcano in Arizona. A stratovolcano (also called a composite cone) fits the common conception of a cone-shaped volcano. Similar to Mounts Fuji and Rainier, such a volcano is composed of alternate layers of highly silicic and viscous volcanic rock, such as andesite or rhyolite and volcanic ash.

Andesitic San Francisco Mountain rises in the eastern portion of the San Francisco Volcanic Field. The field had its origins about 6 million years ago in the area of what is now the town of Williams. Some geologists believe that the volcanic field sits above a hot spot, where magma melts its way through the crust and as the North American

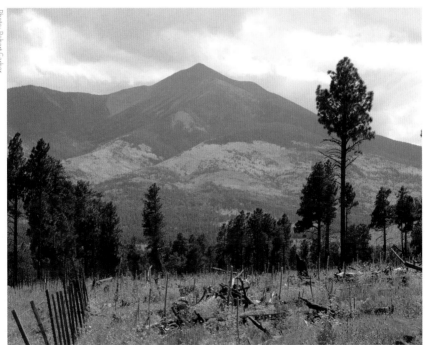

The San Francisco Peaks, the only stratovolcano in Arizona, mark the highest elevation in the state.

tectonic plate moves west, volcanoes erupt in a chain. Such a hot spot produced the Hawaiian Island chain. Currently, there are 600 volcanoes that trend northeast from Williams to the latest eruption at Sunset Crater, which is dated at AD 1064. It is highly possible that a new volcano could erupt in the future somewhere east of Flagstaff. The majority of volcanoes in the field are cinder cones.

San Francisco Mountain was built over a number of different eruptions between 1 million and 400,000 years ago. Geologists believe (by extrapolating the current peaks upward to a point) that the original volcano may have been as high as 15,000 feet. The eastern side of the mountain, called the inner basin, is a bowl-shaped depression that geologists believe was caused by landslides after an explosive eruption similar to that witnessed at Mount St. Helens, and by erosion and glaciation during the last 10,000 years.

THE GRAND CANYON: A GEOLOGICAL MASTERPIECE

Passages 37-39: Grand Canyon: South Rim, Grand Canyon: Inner Gorge, and Grand Canyon: North Rim

Nothing exemplifies the Colorado Plateau Province more than the passages through the Grand Canyon. And nothing is more iconic to the state than this spectacular system that formed through uplift of the plateau, downcut by the Colorado River, and massive erosion over a relatively short period of geological time. Most geologists believe that this process began about 6 million years ago.

Millions gaze from overlooks and scenic pullouts from the relative safety of the canyon rims, but from those vantage points, the scope of monumental vistas is almost too big to fathom. To truly experience Grand Canyon, hike or backpack your way into it. Hike down-canyon through a billion years of geological history, and you will begin to understand how little time our species has spent on this planet.

The Grand Canyon is 277 miles long, as wide as 18 miles across, and up to 6,000 feet thick. Almost 2 billion years of geological history are visible in its amazing vistas. The North and South Kaibab Trails are two of the most challenging sections of the AZT, specifically on the uphill, not because of the distances, but because of the relentless vertical climbs and the elevation changes. Even experienced backpackers will find

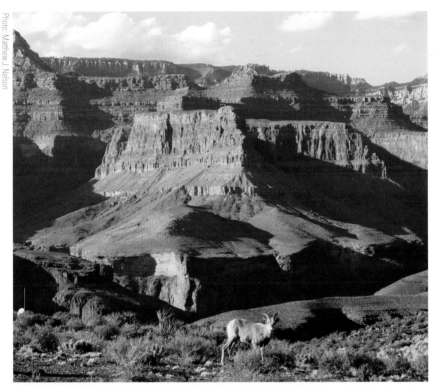

The Grand Canyon is one of the only places in the world where you can see nearly 2 billion years of geological history.

them arduous. One way to make the hikes more rewarding and less grueling is to set the geological layers as goals.

The sedimentary layers of the Grand Canyon are 4,000 feet thick and were formed during the Paleozoic Era. The resistant layers of sandstone and limestone form cliffs; the less-resistant layers of mudstone and shale form slopes. These layers were formed when Arizona was on the margin of the continent, when oceans advanced and retreated over time. The diagram on the following page shows the stratigraphy (layering) of the Grand Canyon.

A mnemonic for remembering the nine major geologic layers, or formations, is **K**now **T**he **C**anyon's **H**istory, **S**tudy **R**ocks **M**ade **B**y **T**ime. From the top of both rims going down-canyon, to the top of the Inner Gorge, the mnemonic reflects the layers

GRAND CANYON'S THREE SETS of ROCKS

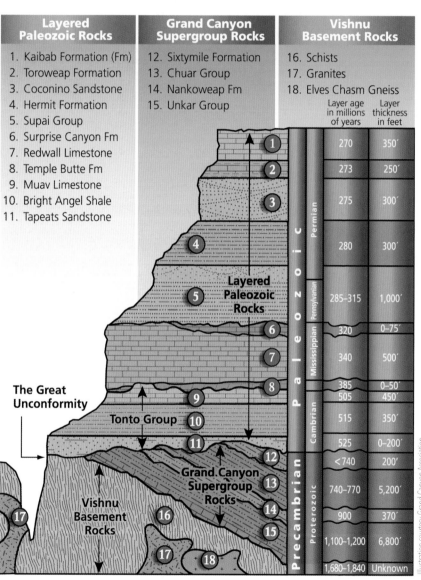

Layered Paleozoic Rocks	Grand Canyon Supergroup Rocks	Vishnu Basement Rocks
1. Kaibab Formation (Fm)	12. Sixtymile Formation	16. Schists
2. Toroweap Formation	13. Chuar Group	17. Granites
3. Coconino Sandstone	14. Nankoweap Fm	18. Elves Chasm Gneiss
4. Hermit Formation	15. Unkar Group	
5. Supai Group		
6. Surprise Canyon Fm		
7. Redwall Limestone		
8. Temple Butte Fm		
9. Muav Limestone		
10. Bright Angel Shale		
11. Tapeats Sandstone		

	Layer age in millions of years	Layer thickness in feet
1	270	350'
2	273	250'
3	275	300'
4	280	300'
5	285–315	1,000'
6	320	0–75'
7	340	500'
8	385	0–50'
9	505	450'
10	515	350'
11	525	0–200'
12	<740	200'
13	740–770	5,200'
14	900	370'
15	1,100–1,200	6,800'
16	1,680–1,840	Unknown

Layered Paleozoic Rocks

The Great Unconformity

Tonto Group

Grand Canyon Supergroup Rocks

Vishnu Basement Rocks

Paleozoic — Permian, Pennsylvanian, Mississippian, Cambrian

Precambrian — Proterozoic

Illustration courtesy Grand Canyon Association

listed below. (The mnemonic mirrors all but two minor formations that are not found throughout the canyon—Surprise Canyon and Temple Butte.)

K: Kaibab limestone made up of shallow ocean organic sediment, and fossils

T: Toroweap mudstone

C: Coconino sandstone cross-bedded due to the different position of Saharan-style sand dunes, with ancient critter tracks

H: Hermit shale and metamorphic mudstone

S: Supai Group made up of various layers of sandstone, limestone, and mudstone

R: Redwall limestone made up of shallow ocean organic sediment (In this section of Grand Canyon, the vertical walls of limestone are the major barrier to advancing down-canyon. Look for caves. The limestone is gray. The red color comes from the leaching of iron oxides from the Supai rocks above.)

M: Muav limestone

B: Bright Angel shale

T: Tapeats sandstone

Tapeats sandstone is the sloping formation that sits atop the Inner Gorge and creates the Tonto Platform. Trails on this platform connect many of the rim-to-river trails.

The Inner Gorge is composed of the Grand Canyon Supergroup, which is in turn composed of Proterozoic gneiss, schist, and other metamorphic rocks. Some younger volcanics have intruded these rocks or erupted over them. Some eruptions have even dammed the river in the past and created large lakes to the east until the river broke through the dams. The oldest exposed rocks in Arizona are found in the Inner Gorge upriver from the Kaibab Trails, the Elves Chasm granodiorite—dated at 1.82 billion years old.

For more information about the geological features that the Arizona National Scenic Trail passes, also see "Welcome to the Geology of Arizona" (page 36) in this book's introduction.

Appendix 1

WATER SOURCES ALONG THE ARIZONA NATIONAL SCENIC TRAIL

The table on the following pages provides information from both historical data and comprehensive on-the-ground reports from AZT users. Note that natural water sources in Arizona can rapidly change; water caches may be empty; and as temperatures continue their apparent rise, water will be among the resources most profoundly affected. Trail users should always verify water sources with local authorities, such as U.S. Forest Service ranger stations, the National Park Service, Bureau of Land Management offices, or Arizona Trail Association stewards. Water quality varies greatly by location, and you should always treat the water you find to reduce your risk of waterborne diseases.

Always remember that you are responsible for your own safety and hydration on the AZT, but review this chart and also check **aztrail.org** for regular updates.

Chart Notes

Passage miles: Indicates points along the AZT at which water is likely—though not always certain—to be found using mileage within each individual passage, measured from south to north.

S-N miles: Indicates points at which water may be found using cumulative trail miles from the Mexico–U.S. border (mile 0.0) to the Arizona–Utah border (mile 800.0).

Location: Indicates points at which water may be found. For example, the directional notation "16 m NW" indicates that a water source is 16 miles off-trail to the northwest of the S–N mileage point.

Type: Describes the source of the water or its container. Always be prepared to find a given source empty of water or unavailable.

Historical water reliability (scale):

0: not reliable

1: seasonal or "iffy"

2: probable

3: fairly reliable

4: definite source

Abbreviations:

m: mile(s)

N: North

E: East

S: South

W: West

~: approximately

Notes: Provides helpful commentary.

PASSAGE MILES	S–N MILES	LOCATION	TYPE	HISTORICAL WATER RELIABILITY	NOTES
Passage 1: Huachuca Mountains					
8.3	8.3	Bath Tub Spring	Spring	3	Usually good water
9.8	9.8	Bear Spring (0.5 m W)	Spring	3	Pool; steep trail; trees down
14.0	14.0	Sunnyside Canyon	Creek	1–2	Water in Sunnyside Canyon for next 2.5 miles
16.0	16.0	Cement water trough	Spring fed	1–2	
17.5	17.5	Scotia Canyon	Creek	1–2	Pools and intermittent flow
20.7	20.7	Parker Canyon Lake store (1.6 m NW)	Store	4	
Passage 2: Canelo Hills: East					
2.5	24.2	Parker Canyon Creek	Creek	2–3	Usually clear as it flows from lake
3.8	25.5	Trap Tank (0.1 m E)	Dirt tank	1	Little trap for holding livestock; good water if present
9.0	30.7	Pauline Canyon	Dirt tank	1	Water usually muddy if present
10.5	32.2	Middle Canyon	Intermittent pools	1	If low, can be nasty
Passage 3: Canelo Hills: West					
0.0	36.2	Flower Tank (1.5 m S)	Dirt tank	1	
3.5	39.7	Down Under Tank	Dirt tank	1	Often low or dry

PASSAGE MILES	S-N MILES	LOCATION	TYPE	HISTORICAL WATER RELIABILITY	NOTES
Passage 3: Canelo Hills West *(continued)*					
3.5	39.7	Down Under pipe at cement dam	Pipe	1–2	Pipe below dam or in streambed below dam
6.0	42.2	Cott Tank Enclosure (Red Rock Canyon)	Solar well and spigot	1–2	Solar pump on through May
6.9	43.1	Red Bank Well	Well	3	Solar pump; storage tank; water-leveler float in cattle trough; unpleasant taste
8.3	44.5	Gate Spring (0.08 m S)	Spring	2–3	Often flows in wash
16.6	52.8	Patagonia	Town	4	
Passage 4: Temporal Gulch					
4.9	57.7	Stock tank on FS 72	Dirt tank	1	Often muddy
7.0	59.8	Temporal Gulch	Intermittent pools	1	Often after trailhead sign
9.3	62.1	Anaconda Spring	Spring (seep)	1	Made into cow pool
13.1	65.9	Walker Basin Trailhead	Cement dam	1	If dry, there's a seasonal pool above dam
16.2	69.0	Bear Spring	Spring	2–3	Good, clear water
19.4	72.2	Tunnel Spring Trailhead	Creek	1–2	Gardner Canyon Creek along road
22.3	75.1	Cave Creek (just before Garden Canyon Trailhead)	Creek	0–1	Swampy; often has algae
Passage 5: Santa Rita Mountains					
3.7	78.8	Kentucky Camp	Spigot	3–4	Faucets usually on
7.0	82.1	Stock pond (0.1 m W)	Dirt tank	1	Hard to see until above pond
9.5	84.6	Bowman Spring– ***see below:***	Cement tank	3	Clear, good water

After passing through steel gate on FR 229 at m 9.5, trail turns N onto FR 7070; after ~0.1 m go through a wire gate to the west (off the road/trail); then follow a faint road paralleling the fence line N. Stay with this road as it jogs W then heads down into a secluded canyon. Where the road ends at the canyon bottom, continue up the wash to an old rusty trough, then walk up a small side canyon following a PVC pipe to a round cement tank with float valve.

13.0	88.1	Metal cattle trough with faucet (powered by pump when cattle present)	Faucet in corral	1–2	If cattle present, faucet usually on

PASSAGE MILES	S-N MILES	LOCATION	TYPE	HISTORICAL WATER RELIABILITY	NOTES
13.5	88.6	Tank ~0.6 m E down Oak Tree Canyon	Dirt tank	1	
Passage 6: Las Colinas					
13.3	101.9	The Lake (~1.25 m W)	Old dirt dam	2	An old dirt dam, now a murky stock pond
Passage 7: Las Cienegas					
0.2	102.1	Twin Tanks	Dirt tank	2	
7.6	109.5	Duck Tank (0.2 m NE of AZ 83)	Dirt tank	2	Even when low, has decent-quality water
Passage 8: Rincon Valley					
0.5	115.4	Cienega Creek	Creek	3	Usually water under the cool cottonwoods
4.7	119.6	La Posta Quemada Ranch (0.25 m W)	Store (faucets)	4	Sink outside restroom is on
7.3	122.2	La Selvilla Picnic Area	Faucet	3	Faucet at corner of stone ramada
13.9	128.8	Rincon Creek	Creek	1–2	
Passage 9: Rincon Mountains					
1.5	131.2	Drainage	Creek	1	Water after storms
8.3	138.0	Grass Shack	Chimenea Creek	1	Water after storms
12.8	142.5	Manning Camp	Creek	4	Big pool if spigots off
15.3	145.0	Italian Spring	Spring	3	Sometimes small, but clear
~16.2	~145.9	Unnamed canyon	Pools	1	
19.2	148.8	Tanque Verde Canyon	Creek (pools)	1	
21.6	151.3	Italian Trap Tank (~0.5 m W)	Tank	1	In a fenced pasture
Passage 10: Redington Pass					
6.8	158.1	The Lake	Large stock pond	2	If low, usually muddy
9.0	160.3	Agua Caliente Wash	Small creek	1	Flows after storms
10.8	162.1	West Spring	Big storage tank	1	If tank dry, a spring lies uphill about 0.1 mile

PASSAGE MILES	S-N MILES	LOCATION	TYPE	HISTORICAL WATER RELIABILITY	NOTES
Passage 10: Redington Pass *(continued)*					
13.2	164.5	Molina Basin Campground (see host)	Water trailer	0–2	No host in summer months
Passage 11: Santa Catalina Mountains					
2.5	169.5	Sycamore Reservoir	Reservoir	1	Water can be very nasty
3.5	170.5	Sycamore Canyon	Creek	1	
6.1	173.1	Sabino Canyon	Creek	1	
7.0	174.0	Hutch's Pool (0.25 m N)	Big pools	3–4	Large, reliable; camp by pool
11.7	178.7	Romero Pass and Canyon (~2 m NW)	Creek	2	
Passage 12: Oracle Ridge					
3.3	182.0	Lemmon Creek	Creek	1	Pools and creek for about 0.5 mile
8.0	186.7	Summerhaven	Town	4	
14.7	193.4	Rice Spring (SE of trail on FR 4475)	Spring	0–1	Hard to find; look in gulley to the left in ~100 feet
20.5	199.2	High Jinks Ranch	Faucet (troughs)	4	Hikers/riders welcome
22.1	200.8	American Flag Ranch Trailhead	Spigots	3	One on north side of ranch house; another near big tank behind house near RV
Passage 13: Oracle					
4.4	205.2	Kannally Wash	Windmill (tank)	0–1	Not in operation when park is closed
Passage 14: Black Hills					
0.0	209.1	Tiger Mine Trailhead (~170 feet N at switchback)	Resupply box	0–1	May be some water for public use
5.6	214.7	Section 31 windmill (~1 m SE)	Windmill	0–1	Windmill often not on
7.0	216.1	Dirt tank (cross-country ~0.1 m W)	Dirt tank	0–1	Usually dry
12.0	221.1	Mountain View Tank (0.3 m W)	Large tank	3	May have an aftertaste

PASSAGE MILES	S–N MILES	LOCATION	TYPE	HISTORICAL WATER RELIABILITY	NOTES
16.5	225.6	Cowhead Tank (0.2 m W) in Bloodsucker Wash	Large tank	3	Has had plenty of water
19.5	228.6	Beehive Well	Windmill	3	Often algae and bees are present in water
21.7	230.8	Antelope Tank (0.2 m N)	Dirt stock tank	0–1	Often dry
27.4	236.5	Freeman Road Trailhead (50 yards N)	Resupply box	0–1	May be some water for public use

Passage 15: Tortilla Mountains

PASSAGE MILES	S–N MILES	LOCATION	TYPE	HISTORICAL WATER RELIABILITY	NOTES
0.0	236.5	Freeman Road Trailhead (50 yards N)	Resupply box	0–1	May be some water for public use
17.2	253.7	New 100-gallon stock tank ~90 feet S; three fence posts in ground ~2 feet off-trail	Spring and tank	1–2	Fed by spring through plastic pipes
18.7	255.2	Ripsey Wash Spring (0.2 m S on road); water from a well-fed trough system closer to Florence-Kelvin Road	Spring and trough	0–1	Can be low and covered with algae
28.4	264.9	Gila River	River	2–3	Strong, muddy flow; low flow in November
28.4	264.9	Pinal County Maintenance Yard; 0.1 m N	Outside faucet	1–2	Available Monday–Thursday, 6:30 a.m.–3:30 p.m.
28.4	264.9	Wilson Trailer Court; 0.5 m N	Outside faucet	4	Phone also available if needed

Passage 16: Gila River Canyons

PASSAGE MILES	S–N MILES	LOCATION	TYPE	HISTORICAL WATER RELIABILITY	NOTES
0 to 15.9	264.9	Gila River (usually muddy)	River	3	Strong, muddy flow; low flow in November
0.2	265.1	Mineral Creek	Creek	1	Flows after storms
11.3	276.2	Walnut Canyon (~2.4 m N)	Creek	1	
11.3	276.2	Artesian well (3.4 m N)	Artesian well	4	Always warm
15.9	280.8	Rincon Road near the Gila (0.5 m SW)	Gila River	3	Strong, muddy flow; low flow in November
15.9	280.8	Red Mountain Seep (0.32 m N up wash to a small cairn)	Seep	2	Small pool

PASSAGE MILES	S–N MILES	LOCATION	TYPE	HISTORICAL WATER RELIABILITY	NOTES
Passage 17: Alamo Canyon					
1.0	291.1	NE corner of Section 8 (~25 yards NW)	Seep (wash)	1–2	If dry, check stock tank above and to the left
4.0	294.1	Trough Springs (~0.25 m N in wash)	Spring	0–1	If dry, follow pipe to spring
8.6	298.7	Small flow in wash		0–1	
11.5	301.6	Picket Post Trailhead (0.5 m SE)	Windmill (ponds)	0–1	Windmill working if cattle are present
11.5	301.6	Picket Post Trailhead (2.0 m E on US 60)	Faucets	4	Boyce Thompson Arboretum: 8 a.m.–5 p.m.; Superior about 5 m E
Passage 18: Reavis Canyon					
6.0	307.6	Whitford Canyon	Creek	1–2	If flowing for about 1 mile, or maybe big pools
12.0	313.6	Reavis Trail Canyon	Seeps (creek)	2	Few pools for about 1 mile
18.6	320.2	Rogers Trough Trailhead	Spring, creek, and pools	1	May be above and below trailhead
Passage 19: Superstition Wilderness					
3.6	323.8	Reavis Saddle Spring	Spring	0–1	Hard to find
6.0	326.2	Reavis Creek	Reavis Creek	2–3	Has not been seen dry in recent times
6.8	327.0	Reavis Ranch	Reavis Creek	3	Has not been seen dry in recent times
7.2	327.4	Reavis Gap Trail	Reavis Creek	3	Has not been seen dry in recent times
9.5	329.7	Pine Creek	Creek (pool)	1	Often dry
11.0	331.2	Walnut Spring	Spring	3	Usually clear and full
21.0	341.2	Cottonwood Spring and Creek (~0.5 m)	Spring (creek)	1–2	May flow in several places
25.1	345.3	Junction of Thompson Trail and Cottonwood Creek	Creek	1–2	Trough and creek
25.7	345.9	Cemetery Trail 0.25 m N to trailhead and then 0.4 m to info center and marina	Forest Service Information Center	4	After 5 p.m., water available from outside faucets

PASSAGE MILES	S-N MILES	LOCATION	TYPE	HISTORICAL WATER RELIABILITY	NOTES
Passage 20: Four Peaks					
7.7	356.6	Buckhorn Creek	Creek	1	If dry at trail, look downhill for pools
9.3	358.2	Granite Springs	Spring	0–1	Often dry
17.5	366.4	Shake Spring	Spring	0–1	
18.3	367.2	Bear Spring	Spring (pool)	1	Often OK
19.3	368.2	Pigeon Spring (~100 yards N)	Spring	1–2	Often OK
Passage 21: Pine Mountain					
4.0	372.4	Little Pine Flat along FR 422	Small flows (pools)	0–1	Water after rainstorms
11.3	379.7	Circle M Spring (0.5 m E)	Spring	0–1	Questionable source
12.5	380.9	Boulder Creek	Creek	1	May be pools above main crossing
15.6	384.0	Road crossing Boulder Creek; stock tank ~200 yards SE on road	Creek and pond	0–1	Ponds and potholes above road crossing
18.0	386.4	Sycamore Creek	Creek	3	Usually flowing
Passage 22: Saddle Mountain					
2.3	390.5	Spring ~80 yards E	Spring	1	
3.9	392.1	Stock pond	Dirt stock pond	0–1	
6.0	394.2	creek in Section 25	Creek (pools)	1	
13.0	401.2	wash	Creek	0–1	
12.2	400.4	McFarland Canyon (~0.5 m)	Creek	1	Pools may be downstream
14.9	403.1	Thicket Spring (30 yards S of junction)	Spring	1	Sometimes a big pool
Passage 23: Mazatzal Divide					
8.8	413.0	Bear Spring (400 yards E)	Spring box	3	
10.9	415.1	Windsor Seep (0.1 m S)	Seep (pools)	0–1	
15.2	419.4	Chilson Spring (150 feet uphill, to the right a little)	Spring box	2	Somewhat hard to find; look in ravine before Chilson

PASSAGE MILES	S-N MILES	LOCATION	TYPE	HISTORICAL WATER RELIABILITY	NOTES
Passage 23: Mazatzal Divide *(continued)*					
17.8	422.0	Horse Camp Seep	Seep (potholes)	2	Numerous potholes usually with some water if seep is dry
18.6	422.8	Hopi Spring (~75 yards E)	Spring	1	Flows across trail but hard to collect
Passage 24: Red Hills					
1.4	427.6	Wash	Pools and creek	1	
4.5	430.7	Red Hills Trail (~0.5 m)	Pools and creek	1	Pools in several places
7.7	433.9	Brush Spring (~50 yards up creek at crossing)	Spring	1	Creek is just beyond camping site
14.3	440.5	East Verde River and Rock Creek	River (creek)	3–4	Reliable; usually clear
Passage 25: White Rock Mesa					
0.6	441.1	Polk Spring (~30 yards E)	Spring	2	
3.8	444.3	Whiterock Spring ~50 yards E	Spring	2–3	Holding box can be seen downhill from trail
10.7	451.2	Saddle Ridge pasture tank	Dirt stock tank	1	If full, fairly clear
Passage 26: Hardscrabble Mesa					
3.3	455.2	Headwaters of Rock Creek	Creek	0–1	
6.1	458.0	East Tank	Dirt stock tank	0–1	If full, water turbid
7.5	459.4	Ridge Tank	Dirt stock tank	0–1	
8.3	460.2	Oak Spring (~20 yards E)	Spring	1–2	Generally good
10.9	462.9	Pine Creek	Creek	1	Usually dry
12.0	463.9	Pine (~0.7 m W)	Town	4	That Brewery & Pub, 3270 North AZ 87, milepost 267, is closest
Passage 27: Highline					
3.3	467.2	Red Rock Spring	Spring	1–2	If low, can be muddy
4.4	468.3	Pine Spring	Spring	1–2	Often OK

PASSAGE MILES	S-N MILES	LOCATION	TYPE	HISTORICAL WATER RELIABILITY	NOTES
7.5	471.4	Weber Creek	Creek	3	Usually flowing
9.4	473.3	Bear Spring (just below fence downhill)	Spring	1	
10.6	474.5	Bray Creek (usually spring water 0.1 m upstream or a tank or spigot 0.2 m downstream)	Creek	2-3	Often OK
11.9	475.8	North Sycamore Creek	Creek	2-3	Often OK
13.4	477.3	Chase Creek	Creek	2	
14.2	478.1	Tributary of Chase Creek	Creek	2	
16.9	480.8	East Verde River	River	2	Water from Blue Ridge Reservoir typically pumped only in October; usually has flow from Piper Hatchery Spring

Passage 28: Blue Ridge

1.5	484.1	General Springs Canyon	Creek	2-3	Generally good water along creek
8.0	490.6	Stock tank	Tank	1	
9.2	491.8	East Clear Creek	Creek	0-2	If dry, Blue Ridge Reservoir ~1-1.5 m E
10.9	493.5	Rock Crossing Campground	Spigot	1-3	Campground usually open mid-May–October
14.6	497.2	Blue Ridge Campground and Moqui Campground	Spigot	1-3	Campground usually open mid-May–October
15.2	497.8	Elk Tank	Dirt stock tank	1	
16.1	498.7	Blue Ridge Ranger Station (0.8 m E)	Outside faucets	4	On AZ 87

Passage 29: Happy Jack

6.8	505.5	Waldroup Tank	Dirt stock tank	0-1	Often dry
7.9	506.6	Sheepherders Tank	Dirt stock tank	1-2	
13.3	512.0	Gonzales Tank (~0.1 m N)	Dirt stock tank	1	Often scant and muddy

PASSAGE MILES	S-N MILES	LOCATION	TYPE	HISTORICAL WATER RELIABILITY	NOTES
Passage 29: Happy Jack *(continued)*					
18.8	517.5	Wild Horse Tank	Dirt tank	1–2	
21.0	519.7	Pine Spring (~0.1 m N)	Spring (tank)	2	Source of water for pioneers
22.3	521.0	Bargaman Park Tank	Dirt stock tank	1–2	
26.4	525.1	Shuffs Tank	Dirt stock tank	1	
28.0	526.7	Maxie Tank	Dirt stock tank	1–2	
Passage 30: Mormon Lake					
0.6	530.0	Allan Lake Tank W ~0.05 m	Tank	0–1	Often dry
1.3	530.7	Van Deren Spring (W of railbed)	Spring	0–1	
5.1	534.5	Spring 40 yards to the right of the trail	Spring (dirt tank)		
7.9	537.3	Navajo Spring (~0.1 m NE)	Seasonal spring	1–2	Pipe beyond cement building
7.9	537.3	Trail junction to Mormon Lake Lodge (0.5 m E)	Town	4	
12.5	541.9	Double Springs Campground	Springs and faucets	3	Faucet on mid-May–October; spring flows
14.3	543.7	Dairy Springs Campground	Springs and faucets	1–2	Faucet on mid-May–October; spring flows
15.5	544.9	Mayflower Spring (~0.25 m W)	Spring	1	Often dry
20.9	550.3	Railroad Tank (~0.25 m N)		0–1	Often dry
22.3	551.7	Pine Grove Camp on FR 651 (~0.2 m SW)	Faucets and showers	1–2	Water generally on mid-May–October
27.2	556.6	Horse Lake	Lake	0–1	Often scant and muddy
31.0	560.4	Vail Lake (~0.25 m N)	Lake	1	
32.5	561.9	Prime Lake (~0.1 m N)	Lake	1	Often scant and muddy
33.9	563.3	Marshall Lake Lower Tank (~0.7 m N)	Lake	1	Often scant and muddy

PASSAGE MILES	S-N MILES	LOCATION	TYPE	HISTORICAL WATER RELIABILITY	NOTES
Passage 31: Walnut Canyon					
1.6	564.9	Small tank (~0.2 m S)	Dirt tank	0–1	
4.1	567.4	Sandy's Canyon Trail Junction camp (~1 m S)	Creek and camp	0–3	Canyon Vista Camp faucets on May–October
4.1	567.4	Walnut Creek		0–1	Often dry
6.4	570.4	Flagstaff Urban Trail junction (~4.3 m W)	Flagstaff	4	
10.1	573.4	Wildlife tank (visible W of trail)	Wildlife tank	2–3	
12.8	576.1	Wildlife tank (visible W of trail)	Wildlife tank	3	
16.4	579.7	Walnut Canyon National Monument (~1.0 m SW)	Faucets	4	Open 9 a.m.–5 p.m. daily except Christmas
Passage 32: Elden Mountain					
7.0	588.8	Stores on AZ 89 (~0.25 m SW)	Flagstaff	4	
10.9	592.7	Little Elden Spring (by cliff and through fence)	Pool	1	6-foot pool about 200 feet left of old circular tank
10.9	592.7	Little Elden Spring Horse Camp (0.3 m N on road); ~0.5 m N a trail leads 0.3 m to trailhead and 0.9 m to camp	Faucets	3	Open May–mid-October
13.9	595.7	Schultz Pass Tank	Dirt tank	1	Sometimes dry
Passage 33: Flagstaff (Resupply Route)					
4.3	N/A*	Flagstaff: Route 66 and Switzer	Town	4	Multiple sources
7.2	N/A	Buffalo Park trailhead	Water fountain	3	Not on in winter
14.5	N/A	Schultz Creek for ~1.5 m	Creek	1	
Passage 34: San Francisco Peaks					
12.2	608.0	Aspen Corner trail junction; Alfa Fia Tank ~300 meters down a road (visible from trail)	Dirt tank	3	Usually clear and plentiful

*Mileages for Passage 33 are excluded from overall south–north AZT mileage.

PASSAGE MILES	S-N MILES	LOCATION	TYPE	HISTORICAL WATER RELIABILITY	NOTES
Passage 34: San Francisco Peaks (continued)					
12.9	608.7	Aspen Loop trail junction (~1.5 m E to Snowbowl)	Restaurant	2-3	
15.0	610.8	Lew Tank	Dirt tank	0	Always dry
15.5	611.3	Bismark Lake (~0.2 m W)		1	May have water sometimes
18.0	613.8	Little Spring (~0.6 m W to meadow, then left for ~25 yards)		2-3	
23.0	618.8	Kelly Tank	Dirt tank	0-1	Usually dry
27.6	623.4	Badger Tank (~0.1 m E)	Dirt tank	0-1	
28.1	623.9	Bonita Tank	Dirt tank	0-1	
35.1	630.9	East Cedar Tank (~0.25 m S)	Spring (tank)	0-1	If tank dry, water has been reported up pipeline
36.0	631.8	Trailhead: FR 9008A (~0.1 m left, S)		0-3	See below

The trailhead at Cedar Ranch may have water, but if it doesn't, take a left at the gate and follow the road for 0.1 mile. A water tank behind a fence has a black float that, when depressed, dispenses beautiful water.

PASSAGE MILES	S-N MILES	LOCATION	TYPE	HISTORICAL WATER RELIABILITY	NOTES
Passage 35: Babbitt Ranch					
6.4	638.2	Rabbit Tank (~0.5 m S)	Dirt stock tank	0-1	
10.1	641.9	Dirt tank at power line	Dirt stock tank	0-1	Visible from trail
16.7	648.5	Upper Lockwood Tank	Dirt stock tank	0-1	Often dry
18.5	650.3	Lockwood Tank (metal box)	Stock tank spring	1	Big tank but often low
Passage 36: Coconino Rim					
7.1	664.5	Russell Tank	Large dirt tank	2-3	Big tank but sometimes low and turbid
13.0	670.4	Wildlife tank (~0.2 m SW)	Fiberglass tank	1	Hard to find
18.3	675.7	Wildlife tank (~0.5 m toward Hull Tank and ~25 yards E of FR 307)		1	Visible from road
18.3	675.7	Hull Tank (1.5 m NE on FS 307)	Dirt tank	1-2	

PASSAGE MILES	S-N MILES	LOCATION	TYPE	HISTORICAL WATER RELIABILITY	NOTES
19.0	676.4	Grandview Lookout Tower	Water (when staffed in summer)	0–1	If not staffed, check large aboveground tank behind cabin, but treat water before using.
Passage 37: Grand Canyon: South Rim					
4.4	680.8	Watson Tank	Dirt tank	0–1	Often dry
7.3	683.7	Upper Tex X tank	Dirt tank	0–1	Often dry
14.5	690.9	Tusayan (~0.2 m W)	Town	4	Many places
20.8	697.2	Mather Campground (~0.2 m N)	Campground faucets	4	Restrooms; water spigots
22.0	698.4	Dirt tank	Dirt tank	0–1	
22.9	699.3	Mather Point Visitor Center (~1 m W)	Faucets	4	Faucets on year-round
23.5	699.9	South Kaibab Trail at Yaki Point	Spigot by corrals	3	At trailhead
Passage 38: Grand Canyon: Inner Gorge					
0.0	699.9	South Kaibab Trail at Yaki Point	Spigot by corrals	3	At trailhead
7.0	706.9	Footbridge	Bright Angel Creek	4	Campground with spigots
7.5	707.4	Phantom Ranch	Faucet	4	Faucets on year-round
10.8	710.7	Footbridges	Bright Angel Creek	4	Creek always flows
14.7	714.6	Cottonwood Camp	Spigot	4	Campground with spigots
16.2	716.1	Yard area at pumphouse residence	Spigot	4	Good water
19.8	719.7	Supai Tunnel	Spigot	1–2	Water on when North Rim is open
21.4	721.3	North Kaibab Trailhead (right of trail)	Water fountain	1–2	Water on when North Rim is open
21.4	721.3	North Rim Ranger Station; campground (~0.5 m W to ranger station and ~1 m W to camp)	Spigot	4	Faucets on year-round

PASSAGE MILES	S-N MILES	LOCATION	TYPE	HISTORICAL WATER RELIABILITY	NOTES
Passage 39: Grand Canyon: North Rim					
10.3	731.6	Log-cabin residence near park entrance	Two blue, 5-gallon jugs	1–2	On porch for AZT hikers– help yourself
Passage 40: Kaibab Plateau: South					
0.5	734.4	Upper North Canyon	Creek	0–1	Often dry
2.3	736.2	Sourdough Well (and pond 100 yards N)	Well	0	Cement cap on well, but seasonal pond is north of well
5.0	738.9	Crystal Spring	Spring	1	Usually clear
5.6	739.5	North Canyon Spring (~0.6 m E into canyon)	Spring	2	Good water, but down a steep trail
8.5	742.4	Dog Lake	Pond	1	Usually some water, often scummy
8.6	742.5	Wildlife drinker on left side of trail	Concrete drinker	0–1	
10.6	744.5	Kaibab Lodge (~5 m S)	Lodge	4	Kaibab Lodge on AZ 67 (about 4 m S to highway and then N about 1 m)
12.0	745.9	Kaibab Lodge (~5 m W)	Lodge	4	Kaibab Lodge on AZ 67 (about 1.5 m W to highway and then S about 3.5 m)
16.7	750.3	Little Pleasant Valley Tank	Two dirt tanks	1	
19.1	753.0	Crane Lake	Pond	2	Often scummy
Passage 41: Kaibab Plateau: Central					
7.0	762.9	Wildlife Tank	Cement tank	1	Usually good water
11.5	766.8	Ridge Tank (Buffalo Trick Tank)	Tank	1	
15.5	770.8	Big Ridge Tank	Dirt and metal tanks	1	
15.5	770.8	Jacob Lake Inn (~2.1 m W)	Store, café, motel, and gas	4	Spigot on in front of store
17.2	772.5	Jacob Lake Inn (2.4 m SW)	Store, café, motel, and gas	4	On US 89A

PASSAGE MILES	S-N MILES	LOCATION	TYPE	HISTORICAL WATER RELIABILITY	NOTES
Passage 42: Kaibab Plateau: North					
9.5	782.0	Government Reservoir	Dirt tank	0–1	Usually dry
Passage 43: Buckskin Mountain					
0.0	789.5	Wildlife tank W ~50 yards and then NW onto Honeymoon Trail for 0.2 m; north at campsite for another 0.2 m; at junction, take right fork; another 0.1 m	Metal trough	1	Hard to find
6.6	796.1	Wildlife tank	Cement tank	1	Off-trail about 50 feet to right; hard to see going north; easy to see going south
10.8	800.3	Arizona–Utah state line campground or ~1.2 m N at Wire Pass Trailhead	Campers and day-hikers	0–1	Campers or day-hikers usually present

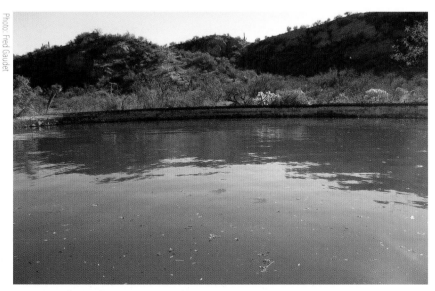

Photo: Fred Gaudet

All natural water sources along the AZT should be purified before use.

Appendix 2

LAND-MANAGEMENT AGENCIES

The following list (in alphabetical order) comprises the Land Managers that work with the Arizona Trail Association to maintain the Arizona National Scenic Trail.

ARIZONA STATE LAND DEPARTMENT
1616 West Adams Street
Phoenix, AZ 85007
602-542-4631
land.state.az.us

ARIZONA STATE PARKS
1300 West Washington Street
Phoenix, AZ 85007
602-542-4174
azstateparks.com

BABBITT RANCHES
P.O. Box 520
Flagstaff, AZ 86002
928-774-6199
babbittranches.com

**BUREAU OF LAND MANAGEMENT,
ARIZONA STRIP FIELD OFFICE**
345 East Riverside Drive
St. George, UT 84790
435-688-3200
blm.gov/az/st/en/fo/arizona
_strip_field.html

**BUREAU OF LAND MANAGEMENT,
TUCSON FIELD OFFICE**
3201 East Universal Way
Tucson, AZ 85756
520-258-7200
blm.gov/az/st/en/fo/tucson
_field_office.html

CITY OF FLAGSTAFF, PARKS DEPT.
100 West Birch Avenue
Flagstaff, AZ 86001

928-213-2192
flagstaff.az.gov

**COCONINO NATIONAL FOREST,
FLAGSTAFF RANGER DISTRICT**
5075 North Highway 89
Flagstaff, AZ 86004
928-526-0866
www.fs.usda.gov/coconino

**COCONINO NATIONAL FOREST,
MOGOLLON RIM RANGER DISTRICT**
8738 Ranger Road
Happy Jack, AZ 86024
928-477-2255
www.fs.usda.gov/coconino

COLOSSAL CAVE MOUNTAIN PARK
16721 East Old Spanish Trail
Vail, AZ 85641
520-647-7275
colossalcave.com

**CORONADO NATIONAL FOREST,
NOGALES RANGER DISTRICT**
303 Old Tucson Road
Nogales, AZ 85621
520-281-2296
www.fs.usda.gov/detail/coronado

**CORONADO NATIONAL FOREST,
SANTA CATALINA RANGER DISTRICT**
5700 North Sabino Canyon Road
Tucson, AZ 85750
520-749-8700
www.fs.usda.gov/coronado

**CORONADO NATIONAL FOREST,
SIERRA VISTA RANGER DISTRICT**
4070 South Avenida Saracino
Hereford, AZ 85615
520-378-0311
www.fs.usda.gov/land/coronado

CORONADO NATIONAL MEMORIAL
4101 East Montezuma Canyon Road
Hereford, AZ 85615
520-366-5515
nps.gov/coro

GRAND CANYON NATIONAL PARK
P.O. Box 129
Grand Canyon, AZ 86023
Backcountry Information Center:
928-638-7875
*Visitor Center (on the South Rim,
by Mather Point):* 928-638-7888
nps.gov/grca

**GRAND CANYON NATIONAL PARK,
PERMITS OFFICE**
1824 South Thompson Street, Ste. 201
Flagstaff, AZ 86001
nps.gov/grca

**KAIBAB NATIONAL FOREST,
NORTH KAIBAB RANGER DISTRICT**
430 South Main Street
P.O. Box 248
Fredonia, AZ 86022
928-643-7395
www.fs.usda.gov/kaibab

**KAIBAB NATIONAL FOREST,
TUSAYAN RANGER STATION**
176 Lincoln Log Loop
P.O. Box 3088
Tusayan, AZ 86023
928-638-2443
www.fs.usda.gov/kaibab

ORACLE STATE PARK
3820 Wildlife Drive
Oracle, AZ 85623
520-896-2425
azstateparks.com

**PIMA COUNTY
PARKS AND RECREATION**
3500 West River Road
Tucson, AZ 85741
520-877-6000
pima.gov/nrpr

**PINAL COUNTY
OPEN SPACE AND TRAILS
DEPARTMENT**
P.O. Box 2973
Florence, AZ 85123
520-866-6910
pinalcountyaz.gov/departments
/openspacetrails/pages/trails.aspx

SAGUARO NATIONAL PARK
3693 South Old Spanish Trail
Tucson, AZ 85730
520-733-5158
nps.gov/sagu

**TONTO NATIONAL FOREST,
GLOBE RANGER DISTRICT**
7680 South Six Shooter Canyon Road
Globe, AZ 85501
928-402-6200
www.fs.usda.gov/tonto

**TONTO NATIONAL FOREST,
MESA RANGER DISTRICT**
5140 East Ingram Street
Mesa, AZ 85205
480-610-3300
www.fs.usda.gov/tonto

**TONTO NATIONAL FOREST,
PAYSON RANGER DISTRICT**
1009 East Highway 260
Payson, AZ 85541
928-474-7936
www.fs.usda.gov/tonto

**TONTO NATIONAL FOREST,
TONTO BASIN RANGER DISTRICT**
28079 North Highway 188
Roosevelt, AZ 85545
928-402-3200
www.fs.usda.gov/tonto

Appendix 3

TRAIL RESOURCES

The guidebook you're holding is the most complete single resource compiled to date for the Arizona National Scenic Trail (AZT). Following are other collections to assist your planning for, navigation of, and enjoyment of this spectacular part of Arizona and the Southwestern United States.

Arizona Trail Databook

This document contains details on every turn, intersection, water source, and land-mark along all 800-plus miles of the AZT. It features mileage, elevation, reference to GPS waypoints, water sources, campsites, trailhead parking, and more. Arizona Trail Association (ATA) members may download the *Databook* as a PDF from **aztrail.org**. (Nonmembers may easily join the ATA on this same website.)

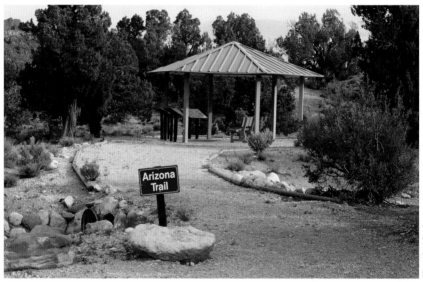

The Stateline Trailhead: the official end of the Arizona National Scenic Trail

Arizona Trail Mountain Bike Databook

Similar to the regular *Arizona Trail Databook,* this document contains details specific to mountain bikers, including preferred routes around wilderness areas. As with the *Databook,* ATA members may download the document from **aztrail.org.**

Arizona Trail Interactive Map

Using up-to-date GIS technology, the *Arizona Trail Interactive Map* allows you to view a variety of layers to get the most out of your pretrip research. Hosted by Esri online, this resource is available to the public at no charge at **aztrail.org;** ATA members are able to access additional layers for the most comprehensive resource available online.

Topo-Map Series

The ATA sells a complete set of AZT topo maps, compiled on one CD. Featuring 130 maps (1:24,000 scale) that you can easily print on letter-size paper from your home printer, the maps feature shaded relief, GPS grid marks, elevation profiles, and more. The map series is available for purchase at **aztrail.org.**

Garmin Trailhead Series

In collaboration with the ATA, Garmin International has developed a preprogrammed data card for handheld Garmin GPS devices, featuring the entire AZT route. The product provides highly detailed digital topographic maps comparable to 1:24,000-scale U.S. Geological Survey maps; a fully routable trail, plus basic road coverage for reference; searchable points of interests; 3-D terrain shading so you can estimate terrain difficulty; and township, range, and section. Look for it at **buy.garmin.com.**

Index

Profile

Executive Director
of the Arizona Trail Association

MATTHEW J. NELSON orchestrated *Your Complete Guide to the Arizona National Scenic Trail* and wrote many of its passages. His contributions to the Arizona National Scenic Trail (AZT) include volunteer trail-building on Passage 7, trail design for Passage 16, archaeological surveys along Passage 17, and explorations of the AZT on foot, mountain bike, and horseback. He also is a trail steward for Passage 16d. Matt has worked as an outdoor educator, Grand Canyon backpacking guide, archaeologist, editor, and freelance photojournalist. He has more than 500 published articles to his credit. A devotee of high mountains, deep canyons, vast deserts, and diverse cultures, he has a wanderlust that has led him to nearly every continent in search of adventure.

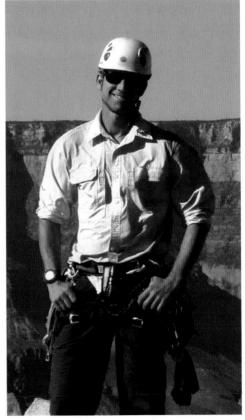

In 2012 Matt became executive director of the Arizona Trail Association. He lives off the grid in the Sierrita Mountains west of Tucson and spends summers in his hometown of Big Pine, California, volunteering for Inyo County Search and Rescue.

Photo: John R. Klein

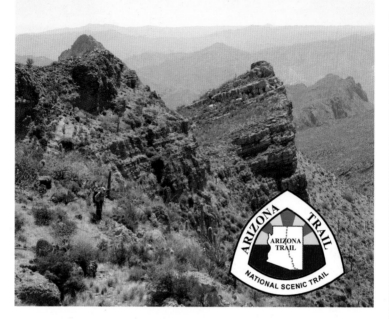

It took over three decades to make the dream

of a cross-state trail a reality. Thousands of volunteers contributed to the design and construction of the path that has quickly become one of the most popular destinations in the Southwest. In order for the Arizona Trail to be sustained into the future, your help is needed.

The **Arizona Trail Association (ATA)** is the nonprofit organization whose mission is to build, maintain, promote, protect, and sustain the Arizona National Scenic Trail as a unique encounter with the land. By becoming a member of the ATA, you support our mission and ensure the Trail will be here for future generations.

Over 100 trail stewards take responsibility for the care and mainte-nance of the Arizona Trail from border to border. Spending a few days each year caring for the trail is a great way to give back to a natural resource that positively affects so many people (and plants and animals). You are invited to join us for a trail work event, and to become a steward of the Arizona National Scenic Trail.

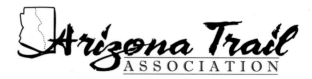

P.O. Box 36736 • Phoenix, AZ 85067 • (602) 252-4794
Please visit aztrail.org for more information.